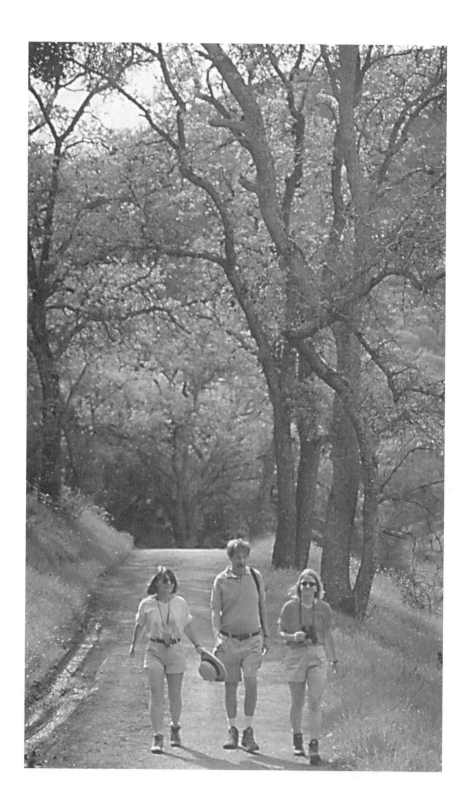

EAST BAY TRAILS

HIKING TRAILS IN ALAMEDA AND CONTRA COSTA COUNTIES

David Weintraub

 WILDERNESS PRESS · BERKELEY, CA

East Bay Trails: Hiking Trails in Alameda and Contra Costa Counties

1st EDITION May 1998
2nd EDITION June 2005

Front cover photo copyright © 2005 by David Weintraub
Interior photos, except where noted, by David Weintraub
Maps: Ben Pease, Pease Press
Cover design: Lisa Pletka
Book design: Margaret Copeland, Terragraphics
Book Editor: Jessica Benner

ISBN 0-89997-372-8
UPC 7-19609-97372-0

Manufactured in the United States of America

Published by: **Wilderness Press**
1200 5th Street
Berkeley, CA 94710
(800) 443-7227; FAX (510) 558-1696
info@wildernesspress.com
www.wildernesspress.com

Visit our website for a complete listing of our books and for ordering information.

Cover photo: Round Valley Regional Preserve: View northwest from high point, Hardy Canyon Trail
Frontispiece: Hikers in Mt. Diablo State Park

Acknowledgments

Many people contributed to the first edition of this book, some by sharing information and expertise, others by sharing miles on the trail. Thanks, then, to the fine folks at the East Bay Regional Park District, including Steve Fiala (who by now is enjoying retirement), Bert Johnson, Alan Kaplan, Juan Carlos Solis, Paul Ferreira, Anthony Fisher, and Maryanne Canaparo. Thanks as well to Bob Flasher and Pat Solo, East Bay Municipal Utility District; Cameron Morrison, Mt. Diablo State Park; John Steiner (staff) and Alvin Dockter (volunteer), Don Edwards San Francisco Bay National Wildlife Refuge; and Mike Koslosky, Hayward Area Recreation and Park District.

These friends also deserve my thanks: Laura Wood, Paul Ash, Silvia Fernandez, Elena Ash, Jed Manwaring, Brenda Tharp, Steve Gregory, Vickie Vann, Ken Kobre, Betsy Brill, Mary Thorsby, John Macchia, Angela Macchia, Susan Rouder, and George deTunq. Enjoying the trails vicariously, Denise Rehse transcribed countless hours of taped notes.

Two of the people involved with the first edition are, sadly, no longer with us—Dorothy L. Whitnah was a source of information and inspiration, and Galen Rowell graciously wrote the foreword.

Tom Winnett and his daughter Caroline at Wilderness Press took a chance on an untested author and helped me create what became my first book. Since then, I've worked on five more Wilderness Press books, and I thank all the wonderful people there who translated my words and photographs into printed form. Thanks to Ben Pease for the fine maps.

Finally I thank my wife, Maggi, for her love and support.

David Weintraub

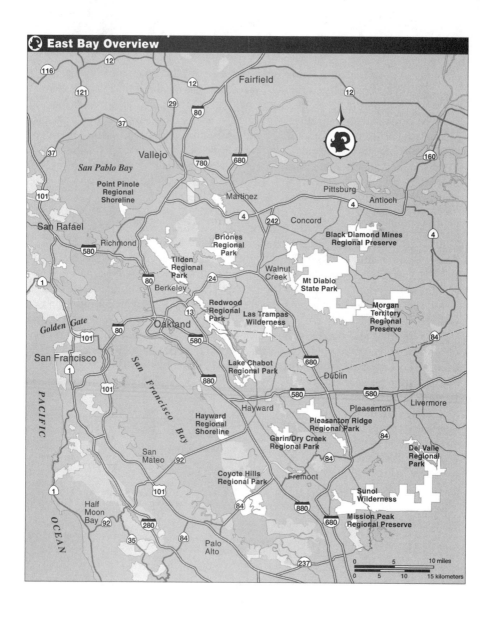

East Bay Overview

Table of Contents

Preface to the Second Edition

The task of checking and updating the information in this new edition of East Bay Trails fell primarily to three energetic and enthusiastic colleagues: Kate Hoffman, Hayden Foell, and Jed Manwaring. Because I no longer reside in the Bay Area, they were my eyes and ears on the trail, hiking each of the 53 original trips and providing corrections, comments, suggestions, additions, and annotated maps. The three new trips—Lime Ridge Open Space, Diablo Foothills Regional Park, and Round Valley Regional Preserve—were ones I completed before moving to South Carolina.

The purpose of this book is three-fold: first, to help you select an enjoyable trip; second, to guide you to the trailhead and along the trail; third, to provide information about some of the features you may see during the trip. My ultimate goal is to convey the excitement and wonder I felt as I explored the trails of the East Bay, and thereby encourage you to support efforts to preserve and expand the parklands.

I have tried to be as accurate and thorough as possible, but your experience of a trail will almost certainly be different from mine. Each day in nature is unique. I was on a particular trail for one or perhaps two days, and what I saw, heard, and felt will probably not be repeated, at least not exactly. I have indicated this in the text by using the word may instead of will, as in "you may see turkey vultures circling overhead," and by being specific about when things occur, such as the blooming of certain wildflowers.

As a matter of personal preference, most of the routes in this book are loops and semi-loops (a loop with a short out-and-back segment). I selected the direction of travel based on several factors, the most important being steepness of the downhill sections. As I get older, I find hiking steeply downhill more and more challenging. So if you follow the loop routes as described, you can expect to find the downhill sections less steep than the uphill ones whenever possible. If this is not to your liking, simply reverse the loop.

If you have comments, corrections, and/or suggestions, please send them to: mail@wildernesspress.com.

David Weintraub

✦ Introduction ✦

The East Bay

Imagine a landscape of oak-studded hills, grassy ridges, rocky peaks, forested valleys, and salt-marsh shoreline. Picture this landscape in a region blessed with a mild climate, where ocean breezes temper summer's heat and a winter freeze makes the evening news. Parts of this area have been protected from development and preserved for future generations, with more than 1000 miles of trails for hiking, bicycling, walking, jogging, and horseback riding. Often this kind of outdoor recreation paradise is only found tucked away in remote corners of national parks or set aside in wilderness areas, inaccessible to many of us. But all of these things can be found in the East Bay, within easy reach of millions of people.

The East Bay, which extends from San Francisco Bay to the edge of the Central Valley, and from Carquinez Strait and Suisun Bay to the foothills of Mt. Hamilton, is made up of two counties, Alameda and Contra Costa, a 1700-square-mile area that is home to some 2.5 million people. Most of the open space within the two-county area is administered by four public agencies which together control roughly 172,000 acres, or about 275 square miles: East Bay Regional Park District (EBRPD), East Bay Municipal Utility District (EBMUD), Mt. Diablo State Park, and the Don Edwards San Francisco Bay National Wildlife Refuge. (Appendix 3 contains a listing of the various federal, state, and local agencies that administer East Bay parklands.)

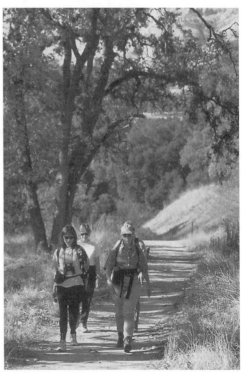

The East Bay contains one large city, Oakland, and a number of smaller ones, including Berkeley, Concord, Fremont, and Hayward. Interstate highways, along with Bay Area Rapid Transit (BART) and Alameda–Contra Costa Transit (AC Transit) link population centers in the two-county area. The region is a world-renowned center of learning, culture, and the arts, and is enriched by a diverse and growing population.

Hikers enjoy an autumn stroll on the Canyon View Trail in Sunol Wilderness.

Climate

The East Bay has one of the best climates in the United States for year-round outdoor recreation: it is rarely too hot or too cold to go hiking somewhere here. When summer's heat and humidity drive residents of other parts of the country to seek air conditioning or the beach, we can enjoy a stroll through cool, fog-shrouded groves of coast redwoods. And when the northern half of the United States is locked for months on end in winter's icy grip, we can often go outdoors with nothing more than a sweater and a windbreaker, taking advantage of clear skies to climb a peak and gaze at the snow-capped Sierra.

Instead of four seasons, the Bay Area has two: dry, lasting from May through October, and wet, generally from November through April. (Residents of San Francisco have a third season, fog, during the summer months, prompting Mark Twain's famous statement that the coldest winter he ever spent was the summer he spent in San Francisco.) Time of year can have a dramatic effect on trail conditions and the character of a particular hike. You can broil on some routes during the summer, and find others nearly impassable because of mud in the winter. Most of the trips in this book are enjoyable during spring and fall. Check Appendix 1 for the best summer and winter trips.

At the start of the dry season, the hills are green and decorated with blooming trees, shrubs, and wildflowers. But without rain, the hills gradually turn from green to brown, seasonal creeks dry up, and water levels in lakes and reservoirs fall. Skies are blue, but as spring gives way to summer, ocean breezes from the west and thermal low pressure over the Central Valley propel ocean fog over the western hills and through the Golden Gate into San Francisco Bay, where it often lingers for days on end, sometimes climbing up and spilling over the Berkeley Hills.

With the coming of fall, wind patterns shift and the fog is pushed out to sea. This is a time of extreme fire danger, with plenty of dry fuel and warm, dry winds. It is also a time of intense beauty in the East Bay, when the leaves of bigleaf maple, western sycamore, poison oak, and California wild grape take on autumnal hues, and the grasses that blanket the hills are golden brown. As high pressure over the Eastern Pacific weakens, the way is clear for storms to move in from the Gulf of Alaska or the sub-tropics. When the rains finally arrive, the East Bay undergoes a magical transformation, turning from brown to green almost overnight. Creeks fill and swell, often overflowing their banks and spilling onto the trail. Even as the calendar says winter, our early blooming manzanitas announce the coming of spring with clusters of white or pink flowers.

In addition to being influenced by time of year, conditions vary depending on where you are in relation to San Francisco Bay. The wind here generally blows from west to east, bringing cool, moist air inland from the Pacific Ocean. Starting with the Oakland and Berkeley hills and going east, each successive set of hills presents a further barrier to this marine air, making nearby valleys progressively hotter and drier in summer. So while Tilden Park in the Berkeley Hills might be comfortable in July, Mt. Diablo, farther east, would be unpleasantly hot. But the waters of the Bay also have a stabilizing effect on temperature, keeping areas near its shore cool in summer and relatively warm in winter. As you move east, away from the Bay, this effect lessens and temperature extremes increase. So in January, you might find it warmer in Berkeley than in, say, Concord.

Although our climate—average conditions over the course of a year—is mild, our weather—daily atmospheric conditions—can be exciting. Wind is perhaps the most unpredictable condition, sometimes blowing ferociously on an otherwise perfect day, at other times disappearing as you make a slight change in elevation or orientation. Strong winds can turn a pleasant hike into an ordeal, and can even be hazardous, knocking down trees and power lines. But wind can be a bonus too, bringing relief on a hot day or clearing the air after a winter storm. You can use a weather radio, available at Radio Shack, outdoor stores, and other outlets, to receive broadcasts from the National Weather Service. You can also find up-to-the minute weather information on the Weather Channel or on the Internet at www.weather.com.

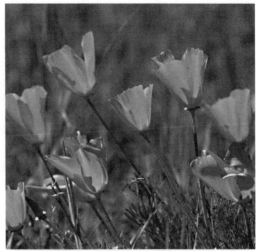

California poppies, among the East Bays most common wildflowers, bloom from February through November.

Geology

The geology of the Bay Area is a complex story, written in stone, with a plot line constantly changing and an ending yet to be determined. The principal actors in this drama are the major fault lines, fractures in the earth's crust, that run along the east and west sides of San Francisco Bay. It is the release of tension along these fault lines that we feel as an earthquake, a natural phenomenon both awe-inspiring and terrifying. Anyone who experienced the 1989 Loma Prieta quake felt in a mere 15 seconds some of the power of the geological forces that have been at work in the Bay Area for millions of years.

California's most famous fault, the San Andreas, runs from the Gulf of California, near the Salton Sea, northwest to Cape Mendocino and the Pacific Ocean. In the Bay Area, the fault goes through San Mateo and Marin counties, passing San Francisco just outside the Golden Gate. Two major faults associated with the San Andreas—the Hayward and Calaveras faults—cross the East Bay from southeast to northwest. The Hayward fault starts in the southern Santa Clara Valley and passes through the hills of Oakland and Berkeley. The Calaveras fault, farther east, follows a stretch of Interstate 680, passing near Pleasanton and San Ramon.

San Francisco Bay, actually the flooded mouth of the Sacramento–San Joaquin river system, lies in a basin between the San Andreas and Hayward faults. Over the past several hundred thousand years, changes in sea level caused by waxing and waning ice ages filled and drained this basin many times, the most recent being about 5000 years ago, when water trapped in great sheets of ice that covered parts

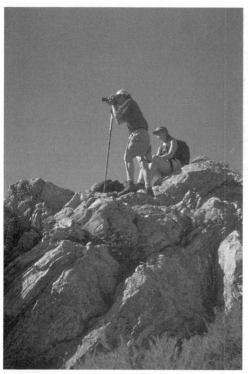

Lizard Rock, Coyote Hills Regional Park, makes a fine photo vantage point.

of North America was released into the oceans, raising sea level by hundreds of feet.

Rising astride the Hayward and Calaveras faults, and a network of smaller faults which crisscross our area, are the hills of the East Bay, part of the Coast Ranges of northern California. The Coast Ranges—a complex system of ridges and valleys that stretches from Arcata to near Santa Barbara, and inland to the edge of the Central Valley—were formed millions of years ago, as the floor of the Pacific Ocean was dragged under the western edge of North American continent. This process scraped material from the ocean floor and piled it higher and higher on the continent's edge, in what is now California. The East Bay hills, built mostly from sedimentary rock and some basalt lava, were uplifted, folded, and eroded into their present shape by geological activity that began three to five million years ago and continues today.

Two parks of interest to geology buffs are Sibley Volcanic Regional Preserve, in the Oakland Hills, and Mt. Diablo State Park. Sibley Preserve contains an extinct volcano, Round Top (1763'), which, along with three others nearby on private property, erupted around 10 million years ago, spewing lava, rock fragments, and ash. There is a self-guiding tour into the volcanic area, and an excellent brochure available at a small visitor center. (See the route description for "Round Top Loop.") Mt. Diablo (3849'), the highest point in the East Bay, resembles a volcano but was actually formed when a large, rocky mass pushed up through layers of sedimentary rock and soil, sometime between one and two million years ago, twisting the layers and in places turning them upside down. You can see interesting rock formations at Rock City, on South Gate Road about 1 mile past the entrance kiosk.

Plant Communities

California has a rich diversity of plant life. Some species, like coast redwoods, date back to the dinosaurs, whereas others have evolved within the past several thousand years. Roughly 30 percent of the state's native plants grow nowhere else. These endemics, as they are called, include many types of manzanita (*Arctostaphylos*) and monkeyflower (*Mimulus*). Botanists divide the plant kingdom into several major groups: flowering plants, conifers, ferns and their allies, mosses, and algae. A plant community consists of species growing together in a distinct habitat. Here are the principal plant communities you will encounter along the trail. (The common names for plants in this book are mostly from *Plants of the San Francisco Bay Region,* by Eugene N. Kozloff and Linda H. Beidleman.)

Oak Woodland

No tree symbolizes the East Bay better than the oak, a sturdy, long-lived tree whose leaf makes a fitting symbol for the East Bay Regional Park District, and whose name echoes in cities throughout California. Oak woodlands are found generally at low elevations on gentle slopes; foothill woodlands, where trees such as California buckeye and gray pine accompany oaks, occupy steeper or higher ground. If the trees have considerable room between them, making the terrain seem park-like, the area is called a savanna. Park visitors with an interest in plant identification will soon learn to recognize the six common East Bay oaks—three deciduous and three evergreen or "live": valley, blue, and black, and coast live, canyon live, and interior live. Oaks are islands of life: they produce acorns that are eaten by animals and birds (and until recently, by Native Americans), and provide both shade and shelter in a sea of grass. More than 100 species of birds are associated with oak woodlands in California.

Mixed Evergreen Forest

Mixed-evergreen forests contain oaks and other species, usually California bay and madrone, and perhaps California buckeye and bigleaf maple as well, in a habitat that is cooler and wetter than the one occupied by oak and foothill woodlands. The understory often contains shrubs such as toyon, blue elderberry, hazelnut, buckbrush, snowberry, thimbleberry, oceanspray, and poison oak. Carpeting the forest floor may be an assortment of wildflowers, including milk maids, fairy bells, hound's tongue, and western heart's-ease.

Riparian Woodland

Riparian, or streamside, woodlands often contain large, deciduous trees such as western sycamore, bigleaf maple, Fremont cottonwood, and white alder. Growing with them will be willows and perhaps California bay, California buckeye, hazelnut, and blue elderberry. Other streamside plants

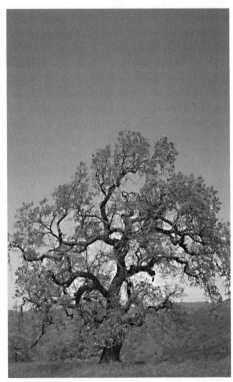

Oaks, such as this one in Black Diamond Mines Regional Preserve, symbolize the East Bay.

include snowberry, creek dogwood, vine honeysuckle, and California wild grape. This type of habitat provides the best display of fall colors in the East Bay.

Redwood Forest

At one time coast redwoods blanketed the Pacific coast from central California to southern Oregon. These giants are the world's tallest trees and are among the fastest growing. Commercially valuable, they were heavily logged, especially in the Santa Cruz Mountains. All of the East Bay's virgin redwoods are gone, most having been logged between 1840 and 1860. A few pockets of second-growth redwoods still exist in Redwood and Anthony Chabot regional parks, and in the City of Oakland's Joaquin Miller Park. Tall redwoods, with their extensive system of needle-covered branches, shade out most other species. Often western sword ferns are the only plants able to grow beneath these towering giants. Near streams in a redwood forest, where some light penetrates from above, look for evergreen huckleberry, thimbleberry, and hazelnut.

Chaparral

This community is made up of hardy plants that thrive in poor soils under hot, dry conditions. Chaparral is very susceptible to fire, but some of its members, such as various species of manzanita, survive devastating blazes by sprouting new growth from ground-level burls. Although chaparral foliage is mostly drab, the flowers of many species are beautiful, with some blooming as early as December. The word chaparral comes from a Spanish term for dwarf or scrub oak, but in the East Bay it is chamise, various manzanitas, and various species of ceanothus that dominate the community. Other chaparral plants include mountain mahogany, bush poppy, toyon, and chaparral pea.

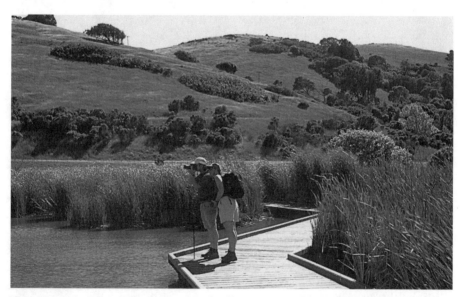

Main Marsh, in Coyote Hills Regional Park, offers opportunities for photography and nature study.

Grasslands

Where we see green, rolling hills in East Bay parklands, the botanist sees "disturbed" areas of nonnative plants and weeds which show the effects of civilization—farming, grazing, road building, and burning. Before humans intervened to alter the landscape, the grassland community in the East Bay contained mostly native bunchgrasses and a wide variety of wildflowers, and supported large grazing animals such as tule elk and pronghorn. Today those grazers are gone, replaced by cattle, and most of the grasses we see here, including wild oats, Italian rye, and fescue, are aliens from Europe and the Middle East. Also noticeable are invasive nonnative thistles that often border the trail or dominate an entire hillside. In spring the East Bay's grasslands are beautifully decorated with bright wildflowers, some of the most common being California buttercup, California poppy, red maids, and shooting stars.

Coastal Scrub

Among the plants that make up coastal scrub, also called soft chaparral, are coyote brush and poison oak, found almost everywhere, along with California sagebrush, coffee berry, bush monkeyflower, black sage, and yerba santa.

Salt Marshes

Around the edge of San Francisco Bay you will find salt marshes—wetlands exposed to tidal flooding but protected from the high winds and waves found along ocean beaches. Three of the most characteristic salt marsh plants are cord grass, which grows in the lowest marsh zone and gets a twice-daily soaking from the tide; pickleweed, a middle zone plant which can tolerate some salt water; and salt grass, an upper zone resident, out of reach of all but the year's highest tides.

When the first Europeans arrived here in 1769, San Francisco Bay contained more than 300 square miles of marsh; today only about 20% of the original marshland remains, the rest having been diked, drained, or filled for salt production, agriculture, housing, or industrial development. Efforts are underway by governmental and conservation organizations to protect the Bay's marshlands by controlling industrial and residential development in sensitive areas. Some former marshlands along the East Bay shoreline previously lost to diking have been restored by breaching dikes and allowing Bay waters to flow unhindered once more.

Animals

Mammals

Other than squirrels, rabbits, and the occasional deer, you probably will not see many mammals on your hikes in the East Bay. Most of the mammals here, such as skunk, raccoon, gray fox, bobcat, coyote, and mountain lion, are shy and active mostly at night, after the parks close. Cottontail rabbits are present in the grasslands, where they sit tight to avoid the notice of predators, bounding away at the last minute. California ground squirrels live in large colonies, and you will often see them standing by their burrows or running furtively through the grass. Black-tailed deer inhabit chaparral, as do gray fox, coyote, and bobcat. If mountain lions are present, deer are their prey of choice. Oak woodlands support deer, rabbits, and western gray squirrels, along with foxes, bobcats, and mountain lions.

Birds

More than 350 species have been recorded in the East Bay, making it one of the best places in California to look for birds. The region is doubly blessed: first, it lies on the Pacific Flyway, a major migratory route; and second, it contains a wide variety of habitats. In a single day, traveling west to east, a dedicated birder could scan a salt marsh for shorebirds in the morning, search a redwood forest for songbirds at lunch time, and spend the afternoon looking for hummingbirds and hawks on the oak-and-pine covered flanks of a mountain. (Bird names in this book follow the American Ornithologists' Union's (AOU) checklist: www.aou.org/checklist/index.php3.

Your success in finding birds depends on looking in the right place at the right time. Some birds are present year-round, while others are seasonal visitors. Avid birders often revisit the same spot throughout the year, turning up an impressive list of species. Summer brings dense vegetation that offers birds plenty of places to hide from predators and from you; instead, try your luck in late winter or early spring, when many of the tree and shrub limbs are still bare. Time of day is important—many birds sit tight during the hotter part of the day. The tide determines when shorebirds will be active and within viewing range: rising or falling is best.

Reptiles and Amphibians

Lizards and snakes are the most common reptiles in the East Bay parklands, and it is sometimes starling to have your hiking reverie interrupted by a scurrying sound from right beside the trail. The only harmful snake in our area is the western rattlesnake (see page 16), and it is rarely encountered. The warning sound of a rattlesnake shaking its rattles is instantly recognizable, even if you have never heard it before. A harmless snake that resembles a rattlesnake is the gopher snake, California's largest snake. Whereas a rattlesnake has a triangular head, thick body, and rattles at the end of its tail, a gopher snake has a slender head, a slender, shiny body, and a pointed tail. Other common snakes in the East Bay include California kingsnake, yellow-bellied racer, and garter snake. One species, Alameda whipsnake, is federally listed as a threatened species.

Common lizards of the East Bay parks include western fence lizard, alligator lizard, and western skink. Lizards often sit motionless on a tree trunk or rock, then dart quickly away as you approach. An animal resembling a lizard but that is actually an amphibian is the California newt, which spends the summer buried under the forest floor, then emerges with the first rains and migrates to breed in ponds and streams. Briones Regional Park is the site of one of the largest of these migrations, and in Tilden Regional Park, South Park Dr. is actually closed during migration to protect the newts. Other amphibians you might see or hear include western toad and Pacific tree frog.

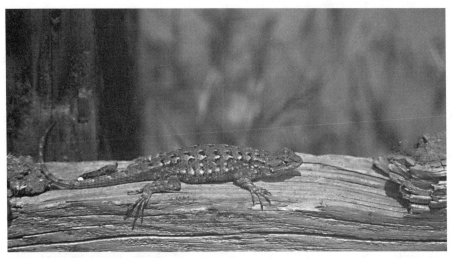

The western fence lizard is the East Bays most commonly seen reptile.

Human History

The East Bay today is an exciting and vibrant place, where many cultures and communities contribute their history and heritage, where industry and commerce thrive, and where open space has been preserved and protected for all to enjoy. Agriculture still dominates land use in the East Bay, as it did 100 years ago, but land for crops and cattle grazing is steadily being lost to residential and industrial development, much of it densely packed along freeway and highway corridors. The area is an important transportation hub, with major air, rail, and port facilities. It is a world-renowned mecca for learning and research, a lively center of culture and the arts, and a place where the latest trends in politics, lifestyles, and fashion are conceived and then, sometimes, carried to extremes.

Since the mid-19th century, the East Bay has been a place of farms, orchards, dairies, and cattle ranches, supporting a diverse population of laborers from around the globe, including China, Japan, the Philippines, India, Mexico, Hawaii, and Portugal. During the Gold Rush and the years that followed, the East Bay helped feed the rest of California with produce from large farms centered in Alameda County. (One of these, which belonged to George Washington Patterson and his family, can be visited at EBRPD's Ardenwood Regional Preserve in Fremont.) Alameda County also became known for its wines, and in 1889 one of its winery owners, Charles Wetmore of Cresta Blanca, won a gold medal at the Paris Exposition. Hops and hay grown in the Livermore Valley gained world-wide reputations for quality.

Cattle ranching in the East Bay, which continues today on public lands under a multi-use policy, began in the 1820's after Mexico overthrew Spanish rule and made California, then called Alta (Upper) California, part of its republic. The Spanish mission system, in place in California since the 1760s, was dismantled in the 1830s, and former mission lands in the East Bay became large Mexican ranchos, supplying cowhides for leather goods and tallow for candles to manufacturing plants in the northeastern United States. The ranchos and the rich lifestyle they supported lasted only until 1846, when war broke out between Mexico and the United States. At the war's conclusion in 1848, Mexico signed the treaty of Guadalupe Hidalgo and ceded California, which became a state two years later, to its increasingly powerful northern neighbor.

The first Europeans to explore California extensively by land were the Spanish, and in 1769 Gaspar de Portola led an expedition from Baja California to the San Francisco Peninsula. Members of a scouting party from this expedition, under Jose Ortega, were the first Europeans to gaze on San Francisco Bay, whose opening at the Golden Gate had eluded such 16th and 17th century maritime explorers as Juan Rodrigues Cabrillo, Francis Drake, Sebastian Rodrigues Cermeno, and Sebastian Vizcaino. Residents of the Bay's east shore, the Ohlone Indians, met the Spanish with a combination of hostility and fear, but contact continued over the next few years, as more of the East Bay was explored. Native Americans, who had been here for thousands of years, lived in thatched houses framed with willow wood, depended on hunting and gathering for survival, and organized themselves into various towns and nations. It is estimated that 10,000 native people lived in the Bay Area when the Spanish arrived.

In 1776 the Spanish established their first mission in the Bay Area, Mission San Francisco de Assis (now called Mission Dolores) and built the Presidio of San Francisco. More missions and settlements soon followed, including Mission Santa Clara and Mission San Jose, and the Spanish began converting the Indians to Christianity and moving them onto the missions, where their freedom was curtailed. Resistance to the mission system came from some groups of native people who refused to give up their centuries-old way of life, but their efforts were overcome by Spanish military action, along with European diseases such as measles and small pox. (A cemetery near Mission San Jose holds 4000 Indian dead, the

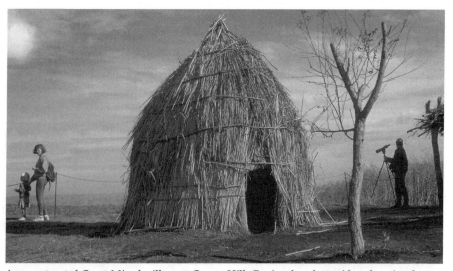

A reconstructed Coast Miwok village at Coyote Hills Regional park provides educational opportunities for visitors of all ages.

result of a 10-year epidemic. In 1971, descendants of the Ohlone people incorporated as the Ohlone Indian Tribe and received title to the cemetery.)

The dismantling of the Spanish mission system in the 1830s did nothing to improve conditions for the remaining native people; instead many of them became serfs and slaves on the new Mexican ranchos. When the cry of "Gold!" echoed from the Sierra foothills in 1848, what had been a trickle of immigration to California from the United States and other countries turned into a flood. During the Gold Rush, newcomers used dubious means to seize many of the ranchos, and then relied on Indians serfs and slaves to work the land. When California entered the Union in 1850, the California legislature initially denied its native people citizenship.

Despite hardship, disease, and efforts to exterminate them, the East Bay's Indians clung to their cultural and spiritual values, and today Ohlone descendants work to keep alive their history, culture, religion, and language. You can learn more about this fascinating aspect of the East Bay by visiting Coyote Hills Regional Park, where there are displays, information, and interpretive programs about the Ohlone people, some presented by Ohlone descendants themselves.

East Bay Regional Park District

The agency responsible for overseeing most of the open space in the East Bay is the East Bay Regional Park District (EBRPD), governed by a publicly elected board of directors and headquartered in Oakland. With more than 95,000 acres of land under its jurisdiction, EBRPD administers 65 regional parklands and about 1150 miles of trails, including 29 regional inter-park trails. This extensive network of parks and trails, which has put regional park areas within 15 to 30 minutes of each and every resident of Alameda and Contra Costa County, had its genesis in 1928, when the East Bay Municipal Utility District (EBMUD) completed its consolidation of local water systems and declared surplus approximately 10,000 acres of former watershed land.

But the true beginning of the regional park system goes back another 60 years or so, to a suggestion by Frederick Law Olmsted, famed designer of New York's Central Park, that "scenic lanes" be constructed in the Oakland and Berkeley Hills. In the years following the Civil War, however, the Bay Area was experiencing rapid growth, and Olmsted's was an idea whose time had not yet come. After the turn of the century, two prominent city planners, Charles Mulford Robinson and Werner Hegemann, each called for the creation of East Bay parklands, but they too were ignored.

It took the threat of development—EBMUD's 10,000 acres were up for grabs—to get the ball rolling. Prominent citizens like Robert Sibley, executive manager of the University of California Alumni Association, joined with outdoor groups like the Sierra Club to petition EBMUD to preserve its surplus land and open it to the public for recreation, but the District refused. In 1930, the landscape architecture firm Olmsted Brothers—run by the sons of Frederick Law Olmsted—and Ansel F. Hall of the National Park Service were hired to produce a survey of possible East Bay parks. Their 41-page report was far-sighted: It emphasized preserving easily accessible land for a variety of uses.

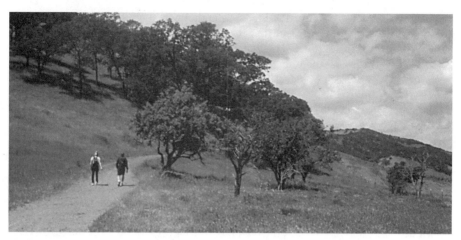

The Miwok Trail at Round Valley Regional Preserve traverses oak-studded hillsides where wildflowers bloom.

Supporters of parklands, now banded together in the East Bay Regional Park Association, used the Olmsted-Hall report to again petition EBMUD to open its surplus lands. When the District declined, the East Bay Regional Park Association called for the formation of a regional park district, unprecedented at the time, to include parklands in Alameda and Contra Costa counties. State Assemblyman Frank K. Mott, a former mayor of Oakland, drafted AB 1114, which was passed and signed into law in 1933, to authorizing the establishment in California of regional park districts, a new concept.

The next step, under California law, was to get approval from the voters in nine East Bay cities—Alameda, Albany, Berkeley, El Cerrito, Emeryville, Oakland, Piedmont, Richmond, and San Leandro—who would have to pay for the new parks. In response, some 14,000 people signed an initiative petition placing a measure on the November 1934 ballot to approve an East Bay Regional Park District, elect its board, and assess property owners five cents per $100, not an inconsiderable sum during the Depression, to pay for it all.

Now the plan hit a roadblock: the Contra Costa County Board of Supervisors decided against sanctioning the initiative, causing the cities of El Cerrito and Richmond to withdraw from the proposed district. The Supervisors were responding to concerns of farmers in the mostly rural county who did not see the need for additional taxes to acquire parklands when there was plenty of remaining open space at their doorsteps. The Supervisors were also concerned about taking too much land off the tax rolls, and there was sentiment in the county against creating a new tax-and-spend agency with broad powers. So voters in the remaining seven cities—all in Alameda County—would have to support the initiative on their own. (It was not until 1964 that most of Contra Costa County was annexed to the East Bay Regional Park District, and it was in 1981 that the remaining part of the county joined.)

Although it was approved by a more than two-to-one majority, the East Bay Regional Park District still had no land, and it took more than a year and a half of negotiating with EBMUD to make the first purchase. But on October 18, 1936, opening ceremonies were held to dedicate three new regional parks: Wildcat Canyon (now Tilden Regional Park), Roundtop (now Sibley Volcanic Regional Preserve), and Lake Temescal. New Deal agencies—the Civilian Conservation Corps (CCC), the Works Progress Administration (WPA), and the Public Works Administration (PWA)—contributed money and workers to the District for projects that included the construction of parts of Skyline Blvd. and the administration building at Lake Temescal.

Next came the acquisition of Redwood Regional Park in 1939, and after World War II, Grass Valley (now Anthony Chabot Regional Park) in 1952. The 1960s brought a tremendous increase in EBRPD land acquisition under the leadership of William Penn Mott, Jr., including Briones and Coyote Hills regional parks, and Las Trampas and Sunol wildernesses. Mott, a former Oakland Superintendent of Parks, was the District's general manager from 1962 to 1967, and later went on to become director of California's Department of Parks and Recreation and then head of the National Park Service. Mott Peak in Briones Regional Park is named in his honor.

Attention turned in the 1970s to the shores of San Francisco Bay, which were losing open space and salt-marsh habitat at an alarming rate. The District responded by acquiring land for Point Pinole, Miller/Knox, Hayward, San Leandro Bay (now Martin Luther King, Jr.), and other regional shorelines. At the same time, inland parks such as Mission Peak, Morgan Territory, and Black Diamond Mines regional preserves were being developed. A system of regional inter-park trails, including the East Bay Skyline National Recreation Trail, was conceived at this time; many of the trails are in place now, with more to be developed in the years to come.

The twenty-first century will undoubtedly see a steady increase in the East Bay's population, along with an increased demand for accessible outdoor recreation. Future District plans call for continued parkland acquisition and the improvement of existing park facilities. Other priorities include working to complete the planning of Eastshore State Park, creation of an environmental education camp for students at Arroyo Del Valle, and the continued development of programs to increase public awareness of the regional parks system.

Comfort, Safety, and Etiquette

Most of the trips in this book can be enjoyed with a minimum of preparation and equipment, calling for nothing more than sturdy footwear and plenty of water. Probably the biggest safety concern is driving around the Bay Area. And trail etiquette means simply being considerate of others and picking up after yourself (and your pet). However, the more detailed information that follows may enhance your outdoor experience.

Preparation and Equipment

A little common sense goes a long way when preparing for the outdoors. Be realistic about your level of physical conditioning—there are trips in this book to suit all abilities. None of the routes require anything more complicated than putting one foot in front of the other. Some, however, require you to do this for several hours or more, uphill and down. In addition to terrain, weather conditions such as heat, cold, and wind, can affect individual performance.

Although hiking is a "low-tech" sport, requiring little in the way of equipment, a pair of sturdy, well-fitting boots will increase your enjoyment and help prevent sore feet and mishaps like a fall or a twisted ankle. Today's boots, many of them made of a combination of leather and synthetic materials, are designed more like running shoes—lightweight, flexible, yet supportive. Some models are lined with Gore-Tex, making them waterproof and breathable. Second only to boots in importance, socks are your next line of defense against sore feet and blisters. Use socks made only of synthetics or wool. Cotton socks retain moisture and will almost certainly give you blisters.

The East Bay climate is, for the most part, benign, so hiking here requires little in the way of specialized clothing. Whatever you wear should be comfortable and offer protection from the sun and hazards such as ticks and poison oak. Lightweight long pants and a long-sleeved shirt, combined with a hat, give the best protection. Avoid cotton: it retains moisture next to your skin and is slow to dry. The biggest challenge is coping with changing conditions. By carrying several layers—a lightweight pile vest and a waterproof/breathable jacket, for example—you can be prepared for sudden changes in the weather, such as wind, fog, and rain. Stashing a pair of lightweight gloves and an insulating headband in your pack is a good idea too.

Other items to take along include plenty of water, snacks, sunglasses, sunscreen, insect repellent, map and compass, flashlight, knife, and basic first-aid supplies. Many hikers use a walking stick, or trekking pole, for stability and comfort. Binoculars, a hand-lens for plant study, and a pad and pencil are also useful. Try leaving your heavy field guides at home and instead make notes and sketches of birds or flowers you wish to identify. Please do not collect plant or flower specimens.

Maps

The East Bay Regional Park District has maps available at its trailheads, by mail, and from its website. A trail map of Mt. Diablo State Park is available at the park's visitor centers and from the Mt. Diablo Interpretive Association. EBMUD has downloadable maps on its website. A map of the Don Edwards San Francisco Bay National Wildlife Refuge is available at the refuge visitor center. Walnut Creek Open Space & Trails Division has a downloadable map of Lime Ridge Open Space on its website.

There are two Olmsted maps for the East Bay, available at REI stores. The Northern Section map covers Tilden, Wildcat Canyon, and Briones regional parks, and EBMUD lands around San Pablo, Briones, and Lafayette reservoirs. The Central Section map covers Redwood and Anthony Chabot regional parks, Las Trampas Wilderness, Sibley and Huckleberry regional preserves, and EBMUD lands in the Upper San Leandro reservoir watershed.

Getting to the trailhead requires some navigation too. The California State Automobile Association (CSAA) gives its members free road maps. Most useful for the routes in this book is *San Francisco Bay* in the California Regional Series. The Thomas Guide's *Metropolitan Bay Area Street Guide and Directory* is helpful for driving around the East Bay.

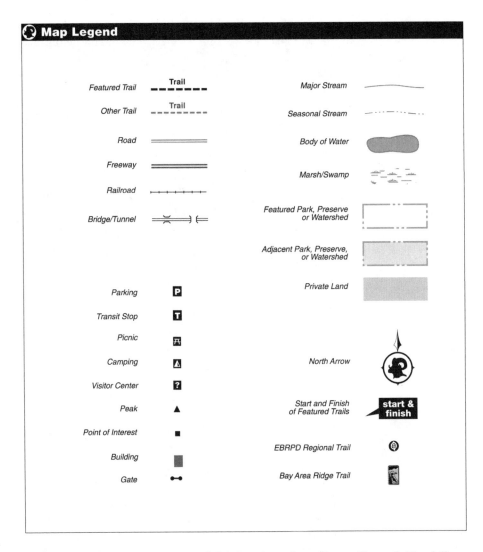

Transit Outdoors is a project of the Bay Area Open Space Council. The following address takes you to a web page devoted to accessing Bay Area parklands by public transit: http://maps.openspacecouncil.org/Outdoors.

Special Hazards

Most of the trails in the East Bay are clearly marked, and anyone with a map and basic map-reading skills will probably not get lost. Still, there are times when you get confused, make a wrong turn, or head off the beaten track to explore and lose your way. If this happens, don't panic. Backtrack to the last point where you are sure of your position. Use map and compass, if you have them, to establish your position by sighting on identifiable landmarks. Altimeters are very useful if you have a map with elevation lines. A GPS (Global Positioning System) device may also be useful, but only if you have programmed the route in advance. Also, GPS devices vary in their ability to record an accurate position if the view skyward is obstructed.

Poison oak is a common Bay Area plant that comes in three forms—herb, shrub, and vine. Contact with any part of the plant produces an itchy rash in allergic individuals. "Leaflets three, let it be," is the rule. In fall the shrub's leaves turn yellow and red, adding color to the woods. In winter, upward-reaching

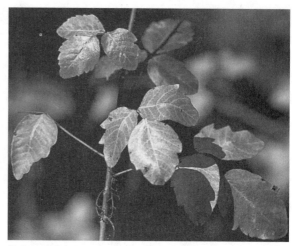

Poison oak is a common trailside plant: Leaflets three, let it be!

clusters of bare branches identify the plant. Avoid contact with poison oak by staying on the trail and wearing protective clothing. Wash anything that touches poison oak—clothing, pets—in soap and water.

Ticks cause a variety of illnesses, but in recent years most attention has been focused on Lyme disease, which is produced by bacteria carried in our area by western black-legged ticks. These tiny insects are almost invisible, and often the victim doesn't know he or she has been bitten. Sometimes a "bull's-eye" rash appears, and the victim has flu-like symptoms. The best prevention against tick bites is to wear protective clothing, with pant legs tucked into socks and shirt tucked into pants, and stay on the trail. You can also treat clothing with a spray containing Permethrin, available at outdoor stores. When you return from your trip, shake out and brush all clothing, boots, packs, etc., before bringing them indoors. Shower immediately after hiking and check your body for ticks.

If you find an attached tick, remove it at once with small tweezers by grasping the tick's head as close to your skin as possible and using a gentle, rotational motion to pull it out. Be careful not to squeeze the tick's body, as that might cause it to inject bacteria into you. Wash the bite area and apply antiseptic; call your doctor. Latest research indicates that a single dose of doxycycline 200 mg, given within 72 hours of a tick bite, is effective in preventing Lyme disease.

Another animal of concern in the East Bay is the western rattlesnake. Despite their fearsome reputation, rattlesnakes are shy creatures, preferring flight over fight, and they attack only when provoked, either intentionally or accidentally. If you do hear a rattling sound, stand still until you have located the snake, and then back slowly away. Protective clothing and boot material may absorb venom if the snake succeeds in biting. Prevention includes staying on the trail, wearing high-top boots and long pants, and not putting hands or feet anywhere beyond your vision. If you are bitten, seek medical attention as quickly and effortlessly as possible, to avoid spreading the venom.

Mountain lions, though present in the East Bay, are rarely seen. However, sightings have been reported even from parks close to urban areas. These nocturnal hunters feed mostly on deer. If you do encounter a mountain lion, experts advise standing your ground, making loud noises, waving your arms to appear larger, and fighting back if attacked. Above all, never run. Report all mountain lion sightings to park personnel.

Trail Etiquette

The trails of the East Bay are shared by hikers, bicyclists, equestrians, joggers, dog-walkers, parents pushing strollers, and, where paved, in-line skaters. In many parks, cows use them too. Bicyclists can generally ride on all dirt roads that are open for hiking, but are not allowed on single-track trails, with a few exceptions. (Bicycles are not allowed on EBMUD lands.) Most trails open to hiking, including single-track trails, are also open to horses, although some are for hiking only. Hikers who see or hear horseback riders approaching should give them the right of way by stepping off the trail, remaining quiet, and waiting for them to pass. Bicyclists should slow down and call out when approaching people, and dismount when near horses. Whenever possible, if a route described in this guide has a segment closed to bicycles, alternate trails are suggested.

The common injunction to "leave only foot prints, take only photographs" is a good one to follow. Nothing you leave behind improves the environment, and it is easy to pack out your trash (and other people's too, if you see some on the trail and have room in your pack). Similarly, everything you take, such as plants or wildflowers, detracts from nature's beauty and other people's enjoyment of the parks. The practice of cutting switchbacks causes erosion and damage to the trails, and gains you little in terms of time or effort saved.

East Bay parklands are at high risk for fire, especially in the fall when grasses that carpet the hills have dried out and summer's cooling blanket of fog has retreated off shore. Although lightning-caused wild fires are part of the natural cycle and play an important role in maintaining the health of certain ecosystems, fires caused by human

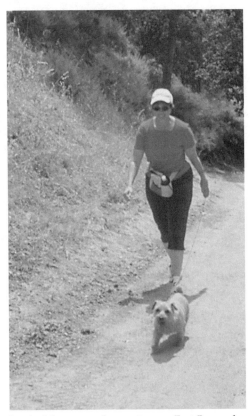

Leashed dogs are welcome at many East Bay parks. See Appendix 1 for trips that dont allow dogs.

carelessness should be prevented. Each jurisdiction has its own rules about when and where fires are permitted; if you plan to have a barbecue or camp fire, obey the rules and use extreme caution. If you must smoke, do so only when stopped and never while walking. Pack out your butts. Smoking is prohibited in Mt. Diablo State Park and on EBMUD lands.

Each jurisdiction has its own rules about dogs. Where permitted at all, dogs must be leashed when in developed areas such as parking lots and picnic sites, and under voice command at all other times. Dogs frighten and chase wildlife; they may also frighten people who do not want to be approached by an unfamiliar animal. Carry plastic bags to clean up after your dog, and dispose of the waste in a garbage can. For a list of trails on which dogs are prohibited, see Appendix 1.

Cattle graze in many of the East Bay parklands. As you hike in parks where cattle graze, you will pass through many gates designed to keep them in or out of certain areas. Close all gates as instructed by signs; leave others in the position you found them.

Using This Book

The trips in this book are organized in eight chapters, with each chapter covering a specific area of the East Bay. Chapter 1, Bayside, includes trips along the shores of San Francisco and San Pablo bays. From there, the chapters (and trips) proceed roughly west to east and north to south, ending with the Livermore area. Thus the book reflects geography, and parklands that are neighbors will be found on neighboring pages. (Appendix 1 is a selection of highly recommended trips.)

Information about length, time, and difficulty, along with a summary of the trip and its highlights, is presented at the start of each route description. Also here is information about fees, trail use, and the facilities available. Driving directions are given from the closest major roadway or roadways, and include the location of the trailhead in relation to where you park your car. Car-shuttle trips have travel directions to both trailheads. Remember to check park hours, usually posted at the entrance, and make sure you can return before the parking-area gates close.

The following is an explanation of the terms used at the start of each route description.

Length: An estimate of the total mileage of the trip, exactly as described. Mileages for out-and-back trips include both the outbound and return legs.

Time: An estimate of the time it takes an average hiker to complete the trip, including stops along the way.

Rating: A subjective evaluation based on distance, total elevation gain/loss, and terrain. Here is an explanation of the four categories:

Easy. Short trips with little or no elevation gain.

Moderate. Trips of several hours or more, with some ups and downs but no significant elevation changes.

Difficult. Extended trips with significant elevation changes.

Very Difficult. The longest, most rigorous trips in this book.

Regulations: The agency or agencies having jurisdiction over the route as described, along with information about fees and trail use. A listing of agencies, along with the abbreviations used in this book, is in Appendix 3.

Within each route description, the steepness, or grade, of various sections is indicated by the terms gentle, moderate, and steep. For uphill travel, a gentle grade is one that can be walked without much effort by someone who is reasonably fit. A moderate grade may cause you to slow your pace somewhat, but should not interrupt the flow of the hike. A steep grade involves a slow, steady pace, much huffing and puffing, and perhaps rest stops. For downhill travel, a gentle grade means easy walking, while moderate and steep descents require an increasing amount of caution, especially over rough terrain such as loose dirt or gravel.

Most of the trips in this book are loops or semi-loops (a loop with a significant out-and-back section.) The rest of the trips fall into two categories: out-and-back and point-to-point. Trips which are point-to-point, such as the Ohlone Wilderness Regional Trail, segments of the East Bay Skyline National Recreation Trail, and the Ramage Peak hike, involve a car shuttle; this is noted and explained in the Directions section of the route description. The few out-and-back routes either have no loop possibility, or none that is worth pursuing.

Alameda-Contra Costa Transit (AC Transit) runs buses to some of the parklands in the East Bay; these buses often connect to Bay Area Rapid Transit (BART) stations. If you plan to use public transit, it is best to check current AC Transit (www.actransit.org) and BART (www.bart.gov) schedules for routes, days of operation, and frequency of trains and buses. The Bay Area Travelers Information System phone number is (510) 817-1717.

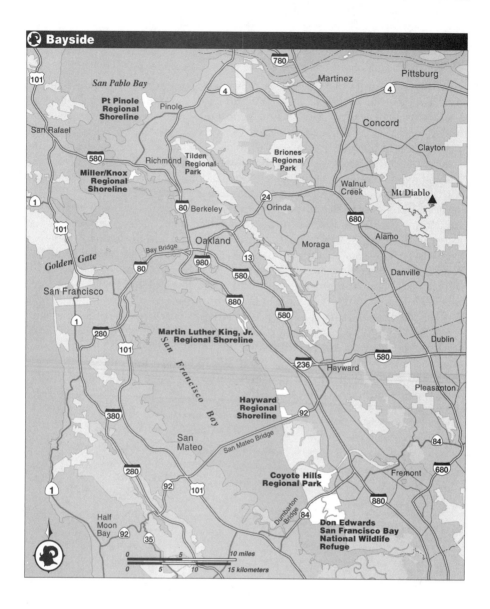

Bayside

◆ Bayside ◆

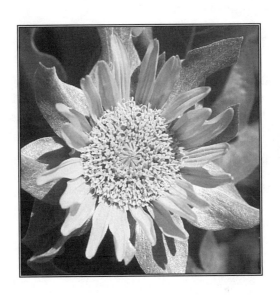

◆ Point Pinole Regional Shoreline ◆

BAY VIEW TRAIL

Length: 5.2 miles

Time: 2 to 3 hours

Rating: Moderate

Regulations: EBRPD; fees for parking and dogs; dogs not allowed on fishing pier and must be leashed at all times.

Facilities: Picnic tables, water, toilet, phone, children's play area. A shuttle van from the parking area to a fishing pier at the end of Point Pinole runs daily except Tuesdays and Wednesdays; there is a small fee, but seniors, the disabled, and children under age 6 ride free. Dogs are not allowed on the shuttle. The shuttle leaves the parking area at half past every hour beginning at 7:30 A.M. Return trips leave the pier turnaround area at a quarter past every hour. The last trip back to the parking area is at 3 P.M.

Directions: From Interstate 80 in Pinole, take the Richmond Parkway/Fitzgerald Dr. exit and follow Richmond Pkwy. west 1.9 miles to the Giant Highway exit. After exiting, go 0.3 mile to a stop sign, turn right, and go another 0.2 mile to Giant Highway. Turn right and follow Giant Highway as it jogs left, crosses railroad tracks, and jogs right for a total of 0.7 mile to the park entrance, left. Go 0.1 mile to the entrance kiosk, then turn left into the parking area. The trailhead is at the northwest corner of parking area.

Point Pinole juts north like a thumb into San Pablo Bay, and the more than 10 miles of easy trails through its marshlands, grassy fields, and groves of eucalyptus offer a sanctuary from the almost continuous industrial and residential development stretching along the East Bay shoreline from San Leandro to the Carquinez Bridge. This loop trip follows The Bay View Trail to the tip of the point, then returns via the Marsh and Cook's Point trails.

History buffs will especially enjoy this hike, because Point Pinole was the location of a large explosives manufacturing industry, which, from 1880 to 1960, turned out 2 billion pounds of dynamite. A few remnants, in the form of sunken bunkers and half-buried railroad ties, of this dangerous yet prosperous enterprise are still visible. Before starting out, you might take a moment to visit a commemorative plaque, just west of the entrance kiosk and beyond the parking-area fence, which designates Point Pinole a California Historical Landmark and tells more about the area's unique history.

Leave the parking area and walk north along the left of two paved roads that soon join (the right one is used by a shuttle van ferrying people to the fishing pier). Turn left to cross a bridge over railroad tracks. Just past the bridge, turn left again and follow the Bay View Trail, here a dirt path, leading downhill through a grove of eucalyptus, Point Pinole's dominant tree, to Parchester Marsh, a large expanse of pickleweed and other marsh plants at the edge of San Pablo Bay. The Bay View

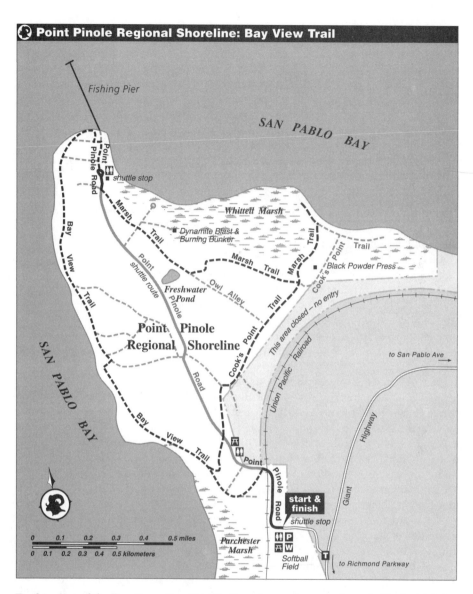

Point Pinole Regional Shoreline: Bay View Trail

Trail is part of the San Francisco Bay Trail, a planned route, about half of which has been completed, which someday will encircle the Bay. As you come out into the open, past large toyon bushes, you can see Mt. Tamalpais and the Marin County shoreline across the bay, and, closer at hand, the industrial areas of Richmond.

San Francisco and San Pablo bays combined are one of the largest wintering grounds in the United States for migratory shorebirds, with an estimated one million visiting here each year. It is also the most important stop on the Pacific Flyway, a migration route between northern breeding grounds and wintering areas in Southern California, Mexico, and Central and South America. The bays are visited by a number of threatened and endangered species, such as brown pelican, least tern, and snowy plover, and its salt marshes are home to two endangered ones, clapper rail and salt marsh harvest mouse.

Upon reaching the upper edge of the marsh, you come to a T-junction with a broad dirt path; here you turn right and walk past a small sandy beach, then through another fragrant eucalyptus grove. As you pass the Cook's Point Trail (COOKES on the trail post), right, be on the lookout for hummingbirds and, especially in winter, beautiful orange-and-black monarch butterflies. If the tide has exposed the mud flats to your left, look with binoculars or a spotting scope for feeding shorebirds. Once in a while, a northern harrier will cruise by, causing panic and putting up the birds. Farther out in the bay, you may see rafts of ducks floating on the water.

The route, parallel to the shoreline, is open here, with no shade and no protection from the wind. Just past the 0.5-mile point, a rest bench, left, invites you to sit for a moment and look out over San Pablo Bay. In the East Bay, access by foot to the shoreline is prevented in many places by levees, highways, and industrial development, so it is a pleasure to be able to walk down to the water's edge, which you can do at several points on this loop. Partially exposed railroad ties indicate that this section of the route was probably used to transport explosives. According to the EBRPD brochure, Point Pinole was crisscrossed with "a system of two broad-gauge and extensive narrow-gauge rail lines." Electric and gas-operated locomotives were used to transport dynamite over these rail lines between manufacturing plants, storage areas, and a shipping pier, which was east of the present-day fishing pier.

Just past a beach-access point, you turn right and follow the Bay View Trail as it climbs gently through a grove of eucalyptus, while the path you've been on goes straight, through a fence guarding a restricted area. At a T-junction, your route, now a dirt road, turns left and continues in the shade, soon passing two unsigned roads, less than 0.1 mile apart, on the right. After a brief descent, you reach a four-way junction. The path that went into the restricted area now rejoins your route from the left, and another road goes right. As you continue straight, you pass through an area where EBRPD has used fire to maintain the health of the eucalyptus growing here and remove forest floor debris.

At about the 1.3-mile point, you reach a fork and a cement bunker, another reminder of the area's dynamite days. Take the left-hand fork and soon reach a bluff. Here a rest bench overlooks the bay, and an access path winds down to a gravel beach, perhaps inhabited by a snowy egret. Old wood pilings, more reminders of Point Pinole's past, jut out of the water close to shore. A lone California buckeye and a hillside of California sagebrush, coyote brush, poison oak, and lupine add variety to the plant life.

Just past the bluff, near a clearing planted with pines, your road is joined by another coming from the right. Now you pass several more rest benches, and soon you can see across Point Pinole—an expanse of meadows and eucalyptus—to the east edge of San Pablo Bay. With the fishing pier in sight, you leave the Bay View Trail as it turns right, and continue straight on a narrow trail along the edge of cliffs overlooking the water. Near the present pier are the remains of a much older shipping wharf used by dynamite manufacturers.

Following the trail around the tip of Point Pinole, you soon join a paved path coming from the fishing pier, and turn south through a picnic area, where water and toilets are available. Just past the shuttle bus turn-around, you leave pavement and bear left on the Marsh Trail, a gravel road; Whittell Marsh, habitat for herons, egrets, and shorebirds, is left. After passing through a four-way junction, you can see another historical remnant, the Dynamite Blast and Burning Bunker, in the marsh. A fresh-water pond bordered by cattails marks an upcoming junction, where the gravel road, now called Owl Alley, continues straight, and your route, the Marsh Trail, a wide dirt path, turns left. (Both lead to the Cook's Point Trail, your return route.)

Turn left and follow the Marsh Trail as it winds past a rest bench along the upland edge of Whittell Marsh, with eucalyptus and acacia bordering your route. In the fall portions of this pickleweed marsh turn brilliant ruby red. Just past the 3-mile point, you come to a rest bench and a junction with the Cook's Point Trail, a dirt road. Just east of the junction is a machine used in making explosives—a black-powder press. From this junction, go sharply left to stay on the Marsh Trail. Near the edge of San Pablo Bay is a T-junction. Turn left again and follow the Marsh Trail to its dead end overlooking Whittell Marsh, where a beautiful view extends northwest past the tip of Point Pinole to the hills of Marin County.

Now return to the previous junction, turn right, and retrace your route to the junction of the Marsh and Cook's Point trails, near the black-powder press. (To explore more of the shoreline, go straight from the junction mentioned at the start of this paragraph on a short connector that leads to the Cook's Point Trail, which traces the shoreline east for a short distance. After these wanderings, retrace your route to the junction of the Marsh and Cook's Point trails.)

Now follow the Cook's Point Trail southwest, through a corridor of eucalyptus. At the junction with Owl Alley, you pass the ranger's residence and continue straight, now on broken pavement, until you reach a fork in the route. Take the right-hand fork and climb slightly on solid pavement, passing a junction, left, with a gravel road. A few feet beyond, you reach another junction; here a paved road goes right and uphill, but your route, now a gravel path, bends left. Ahead you can see a picnic area and children's play equipment. Just past the 4.5-mile point, you cross paved Point Pinole Road, which goes from the parking area to the fishing pier. Continue straight, now on a dirt path in a ravine, and walk downhill toward the water, enjoying a view of Mt. Tamalpais rising in the distance. About 0.3 mile past Point Pinole Road, you come to a trail post which points you left to the parking area. Ignore this, and continue toward the water, soon joining the Bay View Trail. From here, turn left and retrace your route to the parking area.

◆ Miller/Knox Regional Shoreline ◆

SCENIC LOOP

Length: 1.8 miles

Time: 1 to 2 hours

Rating: Moderate

Regulations: EBRPD; hiking only.

Facilities: Picnic tables, toilet, water (just past the north end of the parking area), phone.

Directions: From Interstate 580 eastbound in Richmond, take the Canal Blvd./Garrard Blvd. exit, turn right and go 0.1 mile to Cutting Blvd. Turn right, go 0.3 mile to S. Garrard and turn left. Follow S. Garrard, which becomes Dornan Dr. on the south side of a tunnel, 0.7 mile to the first of two park entrances, right. The trailhead is at the south end of the north parking area, at the entrance from Dornan Dr.

From Interstate 580 westbound in Richmond, take the Canal Blvd./Garrard Blvd. exit, turn left and go 0.2 mile to Cutting Blvd., then follow the directions above.

One of the East Bay's more urban regional parks, Miller/Knox demonstrates the value of setting aside land for recreation and preservation. Less than a mile from the parking area, and barely hidden from a heavily industrialized site, is one of the region's most scenic spots, a 322-foot vantage point straddling San Francisco and San Pablo bays, with views extending in all directions. This loop, using the West Ridge, Crest, and Marine View trails and Old Country Road, also lets you

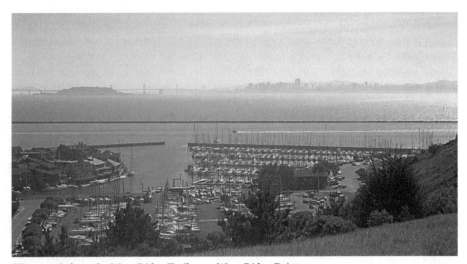

View south from the West Ridge Trail near West Ridge Point

enjoy a lovely assortment of trees, shrubs, and wildflowers. This 306-acre regional shoreline was named for two EBRPD supporters in the state legislature, the late Senator George Miller, Jr. and former Assemblyman John T. Knox.

Cross carefully to the east side of busy Dornan Dr. and find a dirt turnout just left of EBRPD's Golden State Model Railroad Museum. From here a dirt path heads southeast to a boardwalk that zigzags across an open marshy area and then enters a stand of willow and coast live oak. After the boardwalk ends, the trail, now a single track lined with bush monkeyflower, toyon, and coyote brush, angles steeply uphill via two sets of wooden steps. Just past the first set of steps, you pass a path heading right and uphill, then continue climbing via switchbacks and a second set of steps.

At a T-junction marked by a trail post, you turn right on Old Country Road, a single track, and follow it south and then southwest toward West Ridge Point. As you make the turn, you have a beautiful view of the Richmond–San Rafael Bridge and Mt. Tamalpais, which dominates the western skyline. The route continues climbing, now on a moderate grade, past overgrown thickets of blackberry and manroot. In spring, the grassy hillsides here are splattered yellow with California buttercup. A short steep pitch brings another scenic reward, as you get a sweeping view of San Francisco and San Pablo bays, Angel Island, and the hills of Marin County.

Passing a trail post and an unsigned path, left, you continue straight and begin descending to a clearing where California poppies bloom from late winter through fall on an eroded hillside. Tall Monterey pines stand guard on a ridgetop, and the slopes below are graced with toyon, willow, and bush monkeyflower. A cool breeze off the water is welcome here on a warm day. The trail crosses a ditch on two wood planks, continues through the clearing, and then negotiates a steep hillside that drops to your right. Passing a path going right and downhill, and another heading left and uphill, you continue straight to a T-junction, marked by a trail post, with the West Ridge Trail.

Here you turn left, enjoying a fine view of Brooks Island, Richmond Inner Harbor, and, in the distance, the huge cargo cranes at the Port of Oakland. The route, a rocky dirt path, climbs in the open on a moderate grade, and as you gain elevation, landmarks such as Emeryville, UC Berkeley, and the Berkeley Hills come into view. If you turn around, you are treated to a grand vista: San Francisco, Alcatraz, Angel Island, and the Bay Bridge. As you climb higher you can look southwest into Raccoon Strait—the body of water between Angel Island and Tiburon—and beyond to the just-visible north tower of the Golden Gate Bridge.

A steep climb brings you, at about the 0.8-mile point, to an exposed hilltop. This vantage point, one of the most impressive in the East Bay, gives you a 360-degree panorama of the Bay Area, making this a must-visit spot for people who enjoy learning the geography of the region in which they live. After descending briefly, you begin to climb again, soon reaching a paved summit with a rest bench and a trail junction. From this lofty perch you can see east to Wildcat Canyon and Tilden regional parks, and southeast toward Sibley Volcanic Regional Preserve, Round Top, and Redwood Regional Park. Here the West Ridge Trail ends, the Crest Trail goes straight, and an unnamed trail goes left over False Gun Vista Point.

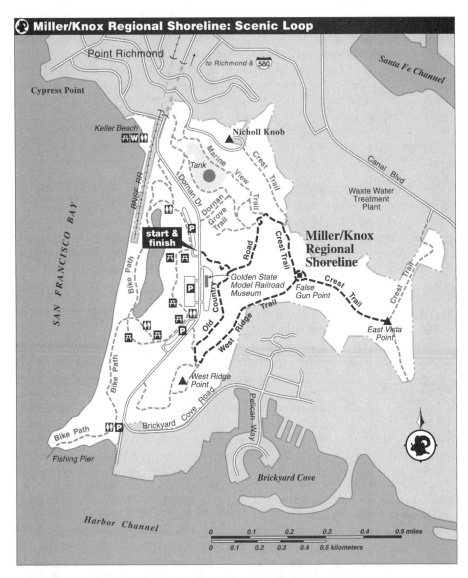

Continuing straight and descending gently on the Crest Trail, a paved path, you approach East Vista Point, ahead, with a refinery left and downhill. Here you may see an American kestrel, a small falcon well-adapted to a variety of habitats, gliding on the wind or hovering aloft, searching for prey. At about the 1-mile point you reach East Vista Point, where a dirt path leads to a viewpoint, right. When you have finished enjoying the view, retrace your route to the previous junction.

From here, turn right, traverse False Gun Point, and soon reach a notch with a four-way junction. From here, the Crest Trail angles right and climbs steeply via steps to Nicholl Knob, and an unsigned trail veers sharply left. You angle slightly left on the Marine View Trail.

Soon, as you begin to cross a steep hillside where poppies cling to rock outcrops, you can see down to Dornan Dr., the parking area, and the trailhead. Once across a plank bridge, you turn left at a junction and descend moderately on a single track, eventually coming to a set of wooden steps. At the bottom of the steps you come to an unsigned fork in the route. Here you bear left and follow Old Country Road, a dirt path, across a wooden bridge, and soon close the loop at the trail coming up from the boardwalk. Now turn right and retrace your route to the parking area.

✦ Martin Luther King, Jr. Regional Shoreline ✦

ARROWHEAD MARSH

Length: 3.7 miles

Time: 2 to 3 hours

Rating: Easy

Regulations: EBRPD; dogs on leash.
Facilities: Picnic tables, water, toilet, phone.
Directions: From Interstate 880 in Oakland, take the 66th Ave./Coliseum exit and go briefly west on Zhone Way to Oakport St. Turn left and go 0.6 mile to Hassler Way. Turn right and go 0.2 mile to Edgewater Dr. Turn right again and go 0.2 mile to the end of Edgewater Dr. Continue straight 0.1 mile on the entrance road to the Garretson Point parking area. The trailhead is at the southwest edge of parking area.

The San Leandro shoreline, in one of the East Bay's busiest industrial corridors, hosts a wonderful array of waterbirds, from long-legged waders such as the great blue heron, to small shorebirds like the least sandpiper. This out-and-back trip follows a level, paved pathway that runs from Garretson Point to Swan Way, passing San Leandro Bay, Elmhurst Creek, San Leandro Creek, Arrowhead Marsh, and Airport Channel, all productive birding areas. Birds will be most numerous in fall through spring, because the San Francisco Bay, on the Pacific Flyway, attracts large numbers of migrating and wintering species, many of which are on northern breeding grounds during the late spring and early summer. Plan your visit for a rising or falling tide when the birds are active but not too far away to identify. Benches and picnic tables along the way provide plenty of opportunities to sit, watch birds, and enjoy the view.

With binoculars and a bird guide or note pad handy, walk toward the water from the parking area and turn left on the Garretson Point Trail, a paved pathway along the shoreline. In front of you is San Leandro Bay, nestled between Oakland International Airport and Alameda. To your left, jutting northwest into the bay, is Arrowhead Marsh, a wildlife sanctuary that attracts large numbers of coots, ducks, grebes, herons, egrets, gulls, terns, and shorebirds. Arrowhead Marsh is part of the Western Hemisphere Shorebird Reserve Network, a collection of sites identified as

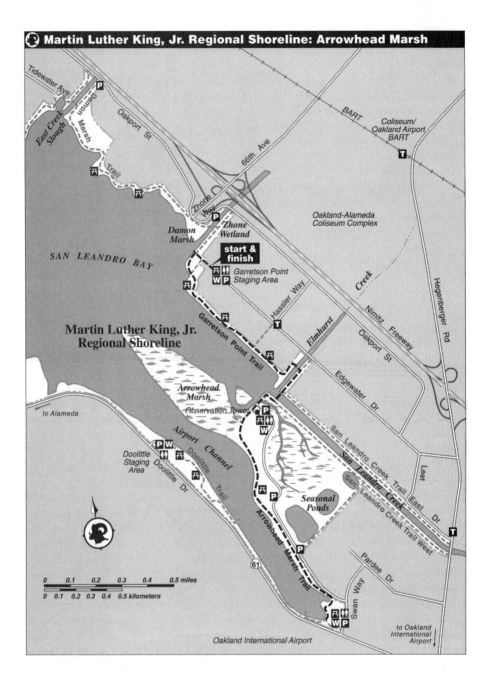

Martin Luther King, Jr. Regional Shoreline: Arrowhead Marsh

Tidewater Ave

East Creek Slough

Marsh Trail

Oakport St

BART

Coliseum/ Oakland Airport BART

66th Ave

Zhone Way

Damon Marsh

Zhone Wetland

Oakland-Alameda Coliseum Complex

SAN LEANDRO BAY

start & finish

Garretson Point Staging Area

Creek

Martin Luther King, Jr. Regional Shoreline

Hassler Way

Elmhurst

Nimitz Freeway

Oakport St

Hegenberger Rd

Garretson Point Trail

Edgewater Dr

Arrowhead Marsh

Observation Tower

to Alameda

Airport Channel

Doolittle Staging Area

Doolittle Dr

Doolittle Trail

San Leandro Creek Trail East

San Leandro Creek

San Leandro Creek Trail West

Seasonal Ponds

Leet Dr

Arrowhead Marsh Trail

61

Pardee Dr

Swan Way

0   0.1   0.2   0.3   0.4   0.5 miles
0   0.1 0.2 0.3 0.4   0.5 kilometers

to Oakland International Airport

Oakland International Airport

critical to shorebird survival. To your right is the much smaller Damon Marsh, also a wildlife sanctuary. In 1998, tidal flow was restored to 71 acres of previously filled tidal and seasonal wetlands, thanks to the efforts of EBRPD, the Port of Oakland, the Golden Gate Audubon Society, and numerous other groups.

Soon you reach Fred (Skip) Garretson Memorial Point, named for an Oakland Tribune reporter whose stories inspired shoreline conservation efforts. Here is a picnic area surrounded by white alder, western sycamore, eucalyptus, and acacia trees.

Although this park is situated in a heavily industrial area, it is one of the best places to observe birds in the East Bay. Looking south across the bay with binoculars or a spotting scope, you should be able, depending on the tide and time of year, to pick out a wide variety of birds, including common ducks such as American widgeons, mallards, northern pintails, ruddy ducks, scoters, and scaups, and shorebirds such as American avocets, dowitchers, and willets. Perhaps a great blue heron will pay you a visit, landing silently on a nearby rock.

Where there are ducks and shorebirds, especially in the fall, there may be falcons—merlin and peregrine—hunting them. Be alert for something "putting up" the birds: when panicked, great clouds of waterbirds will lift from the mud flats or water in a noisy attempt to evade and confuse their predators. Nothing sets a birder's heart pounding like the glimpse of a dark shape, wings swept back, streaking seemingly out of nowhere in hot pursuit of a meal.

At about 0.7 mile, the paved path bends left, away from the water. Here a set of railroad tracks dead-end at an exercise station, and a small spit of land juts southwest into the water beside Elmhurst Creek. At high tide, look for large numbers of shorebirds roosting at the end of this spit. Species here may include American avocet, black-necked stilt, willet, marbled godwit, dowitcher, and small sandpipers. Roosting is a crucial part of a shorebird's daily activity, when the rising tide covers feeding areas and forces the birds to seek out protected high ground. Disturbing roosting or feeding birds threatens their delicate, life-and-death struggle to balance energy, rest, and food requirements. It may be fun for kids or dogs to chase birds, but it is cruel sport.

After crossing Elmhurst Creek on a bridge and scanning its banks for more birds—perhaps a greater yellowlegs—you reach a T-junction with the Elmhurst Creek Trail. Turn right and follow it back toward the marsh. Soon you reach another bridge, this one across the mouth of San Leandro Creek, here a wide channel. Just before the bridge, you pass a junction on your left with San Leandro Creek Trail East; just after the bridge is a junction with San Leandro Creek West. Once across the bridge, bear right on the Arrowhead Marsh Trail as it passes a large parking area, fishing pier, and picnic area. (Toilets and water are available here.)

Although your attention may be focused on birds, you may also notice large numbers of California ground squirrels, standing at attention by their burrows or scurrying through the grass in the open field, left. A squirrel hole is sometimes taken over by a pair of burrowing owls, so it is worth scanning with binoculars all squirrel colonies you come across. Ahead, past the fishing pier, is a boardwalk jutting a few hundred yards into the marsh. This is a great spot to scope the mud flats and pickleweed for ducks and shorebirds, but also look under the boardwalk for Virginia rails—dark brown, robin-sized waders that prowl the overgrown areas of the marsh. In addition to pickleweed, other common salt-marsh plants found here

include cord grass and salt grass. Each of these plants is tolerant of salt water to a
different degree, and this accounts for its distribution, relative to the high-tide line,
in the marsh.

Arrowhead Marsh and the nearby mud flats that are exposed at low tide occupy a large part of San Leandro Bay. With the sun at your back, the boardwalk is a
fine vantage point for viewing shorebirds. Because the tide dictates shorebird
behavior, you should plan your viewing for a few hours before or after high tide.
This will allow you to observe birds as they feed, while they are still close enough
to identify. Once the tide goes all the way out, the birds disperse and are hard to
see clearly. You may notice broken mussel shells near the end of the boardwalk;
these are deposited by gulls, which drop them from the air in an attempt to crack
them open.

You may see a white, heron-like bird feeding on fish in the shallows near the
walkway, and then do a double-take when you notice one just like it, but almost
twice as big. The smaller is called a snowy egret, and the larger is the great egret.
Careful study reveals other differences besides size. The snowy has a black bill and
golden feet, while the great has a yellow bill and black feet. Both are graceful fliers,
and, with their cousin the great blue heron, add an exotic touch to marshes and
wetlands of North America.

Southwest of Arrowhead Marsh are Airport Channel, Doolittle Dr., and the
hangars of Oakland International Airport. Being in the midst of urban hustle and
bustle gives you an appreciation for this 739-acre wildlife sanctuary, opened to the
public in 1979 as the San Leandro Bay Regional Shoreline, and renamed in 1992 to
honor the slain civil-rights leader. Along the southwest edge of Arrowhead Marsh
is another good place to look for shorebirds, but you will probably need a spotting
scope to identify individual species. Closer in, birds may be feeding along the near
shoreline of Airport Channel.

Besides pickleweed and marsh grasses, you may notice tall, thick-leaved plants
with bright yellow flowers, growing along the upper edge of the marsh. This is
gumplant, which is named for the sticky resin that oozes from the daisy-like flower
buds. These attractive plants bring color to marshes around San Francisco, San
Pablo, and Suisun bays from late summer through fall. A dirt road, left, parallels
your route from the Arrowhead Marsh parking area to another just off Swan Way,
your turn-around point. A grassy field, home for ground squirrels and perhaps a
pair of burrowing owls, lies between you and this road.

As you continue southeast on the Arrowhead Marsh Trail, other shorebirds to
look for include dunlin, a chunky sandpiper with a long bill curved down at the
tip; and black-necked stilt, a black-and-white wader with shocking pink legs. A bit
farther along, as you near Swan Way, look for a large black pipe that runs under
your path and into Airport Channel. On the mud flats, right, you may find least
sandpipers, small brown and white birds with pale legs; on the pipe itself there
may be black turnstones, pecking at barnacles. When you reach the parking area at
Swan Way, which has water, a toilet, a picnic table, and a grove of trees planted to
honor Dr. King, turn and retrace your route to the Garretson Point parking area.

✦ Hayward Regional Shoreline ✦

COGSWELL MARSH

Length: Approximately 3.3 miles

Time: 2 to 3 hours

Rating: Easy

Regulations: EBRPD; no dogs.

Facilities: A small visitor center, open only on weekends, 10 A.M. to 5 P.M., with toilets, water, books, maps, exhibits, and information.

Directions: From Highway 92 eastbound at the east end of the San Mateo Bridge in Hayward, take the Clawiter Road/Eden Landing Road exit. At a four-way stop, turn left onto Clawiter Road, cross over the highway, and at the next four-way stop turn left onto Breakwater Ave. Almost immediately, Breakwater Ave. turns left, then veers right and heads west, parallel to Highway 92. Follow Breakwater Ave. to the Hayward Shoreline Interpretive Center, about 1 mile from Clawiter Road. Park on the right side of the road. The trailhead is behind the visitor center.

From Highway 92 westbound at the east end of the San Mateo Bridge in Hayward, take the Clawiter Road/Eden Landing Road exit, and from the four-way stop at the end of the exit ramp go directly across Clawiter Road onto Breakwater Ave., then follow the directions above.

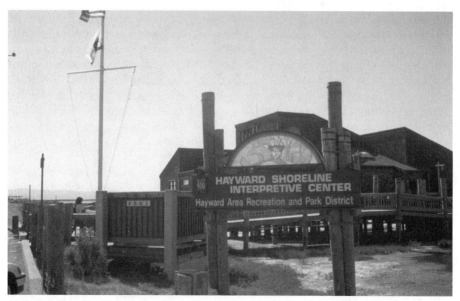

Hayward Shoreline Interpretive Center, located on Breakwater Ave., just north of Highway 92. The Hayward shoreline is a good place to see shorebirds, ducks, geese, gulls, herons, and egrets. It is also home to the endangered salt marsh harvest mouse.

The Hayward Regional Shoreline is one of the best places in the East Bay to view shorebirds. The trails are easy and bring you close to the water. The birds are used to people and will generally stay put. This semi-loop route goes through a restored marsh—a great example of how nature, with a little help, can reclaim areas previously altered by human intervention. The area gets windy in the afternoon, especially during spring and summer.

From just behind the visitor center, operated by the Hayward Area Recreation and Park District, take a moment to look out over the system of marshes around you. To your left are the Oliver Ponds, remnants of a vast salt-harvesting industry that began during the mid-19th century in San Francisco Bay and still exists today in limited areas of the Bay. Four generations of the Oliver family farmed salt on the Hayward shoreline, and the Hayward Area Recreation and Park District (HARD) purchased the ponds from the Oliver estate in the mid-1990s. The area directly in front of you is the HARD Marsh, former salt ponds restored to tidal action in 1986. Beyond lies the fresh and brackish water Hayward Marsh, an EBRPD project created in 1988 to naturally cleanse and release into the Bay some one million gallons per day of secondary treated sewage discharge water. To your right is habitat managed for the endangered salt marsh harvest mouse.

Turn left and begin walking west on a wide, hard-packed dirt path; your route will be along the levees that crisscross this area. The 1-mile trail from the visitor center to the Bay honors Arthur Emmes, a prominent Castro Valley optometrist and member of the Hayward Area Shoreline Planning Agency's citizen advisory committee, who championed acquisition and development of trails along the shoreline. After reaching the Bay, this trail joins EBRPD's trail system, which continues north about 7 miles to the San Leandro Marina.

As you walk toward San Francisco Bay, following a slough on your left, scan the marsh to your right for shorebirds, a tribe that includes oystercatchers, avocets, stilts, plovers, willets, curlews, godwits, small sandpipers, dowitchers, and phalaropes. In just a few minutes you may see a fine assortment, including black-necked stilts, American avocets, long-billed curlews, marbled godwits, dowitchers, and sandpipers, along with other water-loving birds such as egrets, ducks, and gulls. In the grassland areas, watch for resident savannah sparrows and blacktail jackrabbits.

Once you reach the shoreline, in about 0.8 mile, the route turns north and runs along the water. From here you have terrific views, on a clear day, of San Francisco, Oakland, the Bay and San Mateo bridges, the Oakland and Berkeley hills, Mt. Diablo, and Mt. Tamalpais. If the tide is out, you will see shorebirds during most of the year, feeding on the mud flats at the edge of the Bay. Some species, such as American avocets and black-necked stilts, breed in the Bay Area, but many others fly north in May and June to breed in Canada, Alaska, and the Arctic, which accounts for their absence from our area during those months. But during the rest of the year, and especially in winter, San Francisco Bay hosts one of the largest concentrations of shorebirds in North America, sometimes more than one million strong. The Bay is also the most important stop on the Pacific Flyway, the aerial route between northern breeding grounds and wintering areas in southern California, Mexico, and Central and South America.

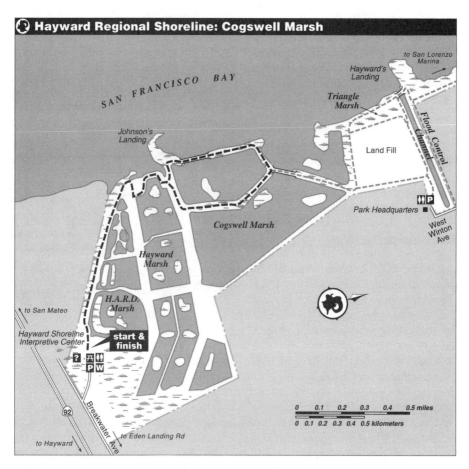

Hayward Regional Shoreline: Cogswell Marsh

to San Lorenzo Marina
Hayward's Landing
Triangle Marsh
SAN FRANCISCO BAY
Johnson's Landing
Land Fill
Flood Control Channel
Park Headquarters
West Winton Ave
Cogswell Marsh
Hayward Marsh
H.A.R.D. Marsh
to San Mateo
Hayward Shoreline Interpretive Center
start & finish
92
Breakwater Ave
to Hayward
to Eden Landing Rd

0   0.1   0.2   0.3   0.4   0.5 miles
0 0.1 0.2 0.3 0.4 0.5 kilometers

As you turn north, the route crosses another slough, whose water passes under a short bridge and makes several jogs on its way around the west edge of Hayward Marsh. Two of the most common marsh plants, pickleweed and cord grass, are evident here. Pickleweed, a low-growing plant with many stubby branches, thrives in the middle marsh, where it is moistened only briefly by the tide's salty flow. Light green in spring and summer, pickleweed brightens marshes in the fall as it turns red and purple, but winter finds it dull brown. Cord grass, 1 to 4 feet tall and dark green, lives low in the marsh and is well adapted to twice-daily flooding by the tide. Cord grass, like other plants, is an air purifier, consuming carbon dioxide and carbon monoxide, and releasing oxygen into the atmosphere. The orange threads that you may see wound in the pickleweed is salt-marsh dodder, a parasitic plant.

After walking about a mile, you reach a junction with a path going right, which you will use later on your return. But for now, turn left and return to the shoreline at Johnson's Landing, a cove with a small beach and breakwater. John Johnson began harvesting salt from San Francisco Bay by putting levees around natural pools in the marsh. This landing, like others along the shoreline, was built in the 1850s for boats that carried salt, waterfowl, agricultural products, and passengers to San Francisco.

As you turn north and continue walking along the water's edge, a sweeping view of the Alameda County shoreline stretches before you all the way to Oakland. This part of the route is also a segment of the San Francisco Bay Trail, which uses existing trails and roadways owned and maintained by various public agencies and will some day encircle the Bay. More than half of the Bay Trail's proposed 400-mile route has been completed. On your right is Cogswell Marsh, named in honor of Dr. Howard L. Cogswell, a well-known Bay Area shorebird biologist, educator, and member of EBRPD's board of directors from 1971 to 1982. This large marsh consists of several former ponds restored to tidal action by an EBRPD levee-breaching project completed in 1980.

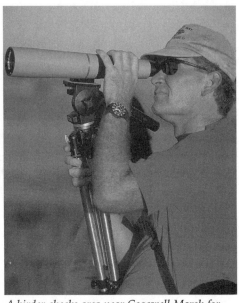

A birder checks area near Cogswell Marsh for shorebirds.

Soon you reach the first of two bridges that span breached levees in this section of the shoreline. Here is an excellent vantage point from which to study shorebirds feeding on the mud flats below. Time your arrival just after high tide, when the water begins to recede and more and more of the flats are being continuously exposed. Different shorebirds have evolved different strategies for feeding, from the avocet's side-to-side swiping motion, to the dowitcher's rapid, machine-like drilling. The largest North American shorebird, the long-billed curlew, probes deep in the mud for small clams using its long, down-curved bill. The bird will then rinse off its muddy prize before swallowing it whole.

After crossing the first bridge, continue north, with the Bay on your left and the salt marsh spreading out to your right. Soon the route turns right, away from the bay, and heads east. On your left is a large inlet, with the second bridge ahead. On a rising tide, shorebirds feeding in the shallows of this inlet are pushed toward shore, so this is another great vantage point for observing their antics. And because you are facing north as you look out across the inlet, the sun is behind you for most of the day, another plus when viewing birds. Across the Bay to the northwest, the light-colored buildings of San Francisco are thrown into relief by the dark background of Mt. Tamalpais.

At the second bridge, after you've had your fill of birding, turn right and begin your return trip along a dike with a slough and salt marsh to the left. (If you want a longer hike, cross the bridge and follow the route northeast, then west to Triangle Marsh and Hayward's Landing.) Check the slough for ducks; especially pretty are ruddy ducks in bright plumage. After walking south for about 0.5 mile, turn right on a dike leading back to the bay. If the tide is coming in, especially just before sunset, you may see large flights of shorebirds coming to roost in Hayward Marsh, left. Soon you rejoin the original route near Johnson's Landing; turn left here and retrace your route to the visitor center.

◆ Coyote Hills Regional Park ◆

This is one of the most user-friendly of the East Bay parks. It has a visitor center with informative displays and helpful staff; a lovely, shaded picnic area; rewarding but not-too-taxing trails; ample opportunity for nature study; and a rich history dating back thousands of years. Children will enjoy the Muskrat Trail, a self-guiding nature walk through the park's Main Marsh, as well as special cultural programs presented by descendants of Native Americans who lived in this area for more than two thousand years. There is a paved pathway, the Bayview Trail, which circles the Coyote Hills on a mostly level course, and connects at its north end with the paved Alameda Creek Trail.

The Coyote Hills themselves are the tips of an ancient mountain range, composed of iron-rich Franciscan chert, which lies between the Hayward Hills, east, and the Coast Range on the west side of San Francisco Bay. Mud, gravel, and silt washed down from the Hayward Hills created the flat plain at the Bay's southern end. One of the best views of this area is from the summit of Red Hill, just a few minutes from the visitor center. At the end of the last ice age, when sea levels rose and the Bay filled, the Coyote Hills became islands. Gradually, sedimentation deposited by Alameda Creek created marshlands around the islands—on the west side, a salt marsh; and on the east, a marsh flooded with freshwater from the creek.

Wetland areas in the park today consist mostly of brackish marshes, dominated by cattails and bulrushes. These areas provide important habitat for many species of birds and aquatic animals. The Coyote Hills bird check list, revised in 1990, contains 210 species in more than 40 categories, including grebes, pelicans, cormorants, herons, egrets, geese, ducks, raptors, shorebirds, gulls, terns, and songbirds. One wetland area, called the DUST (Demonstration Urban Stormwater Treatment) Marsh is a research project, begun in the early 1980s, to study the effectiveness of using marshes to remove pollutants from urban runoff.

Coyote Hills Regional Park was opened to the public in 1968, and the area has a colorful history. The building that today houses the visitor center served in the 1960s and early 1970s as a lab where Stanford Research Institute scientists studied seals and other marine animals. (After the park opened, tours of the lab for the public were arranged.) In the 1950s the building served as an Army barracks for Nike missile crews; the missiles themselves were atop the hills.

Like other regional parks, Coyote Hills has a long ranching history, going back to an 1844 land grant establishing Rancho Potrero de los Cerritos ("Pasture of the Little Hills"). This 10,000-acre parcel, owned by Augustin Alviso and Tomas Pacheco, included land that became today's 978-acre park. After California became a state in 1850, the U.S. Congress allowed challenges to the land-grant system, and many owners were forced to sell their land to pay legal fees; this fate befell the rancho. One of those who purchased a part of the rancho was George Washington

Patterson, who eventually came to own nearly 6000 acres of farm land, including the current park. The Patterson family, whose farm can be visited at nearby Ardenwood Regional Preserve, and whose name is on the park entrance road, held the land until 1968.

The original occupants of the Coyote Hills area were the Ohlone Indians, whose village sites can be visited on naturalist-led tours. The sites, raised areas that were created by the debris of everyday life, are called "shell mounds," or "kitchen middens," because they contain mostly shells, animal bones, and ashes. But archaeological excavations of village sites have also uncovered jewelry, pieces of mortars and pestles, and remnants of hearths and house floors, along with human remains. Native people lived in willow-framed huts thatched with tule, and navigated the Bay's waterways in kayak-like crafts made of bundled tules. Park naturalists and volunteers have built replicas of Indian buildings at the shell-mound site, and in 1979 they constructed a tule boat, which they paddled across San Francisco Bay. The Spanish referred to all Indians west of the Diablo Range from the Bay Area to Big Sur as Costanoans, or coast people, but today's East Bay descendants prefer the term Ohlone.

Park gates open: 8 A.M. to 8 P.M., April–October; 8 A.M. to 6 P.M. November–March

Visitor center: (510) 795-9385; open 9:30 A.M. to 5 P.M.; closed Mondays, Thanksgiving, and Christmas.

LIZARD ROCK

Length: 0.8 mile

Time: 1 hour or less

Rating: Easy

Regulations: EBRPD; fees for parking and dogs; the single-track Lizard Rock Trail is for hiking only.

Facilities: Visitor center, picnic tables, water, toilet.

Directions: From Highway 84 at the east end of the Dumbarton Bridge in Fremont, take the Thornton Ave./Paseo Padre Pkwy. exit, and go north 1.1 miles on Paseo Padre Pkwy. to Patterson Ranch Road. Turn left, and go 0.5 mile to the entrance kiosk. Another 1.0 mile brings you to the parking area for the visitor center. The trailhead is at the west end of parking area, at its entrance.

Short and easy, this loop uses the Bayview, Lizard Rock, and Chochenyo trails to give you a quick sample of what this park has to offer, including an overview of the Main Marsh. If you have more time to spend here, consider also doing the "Red Hill" trip.

From the west end of the parking area, where the entrance road makes a 180-degree bend, head northwest on the paved Bayview Trail, passing the Quail Trail, a dirt road, left. The Bayview Trail is gated just beyond the parking area. After passing the gate, you have the Main Marsh on your right and beautiful grassy hills rising on your left. The Main Marsh, a brackish body of water bordered in places with cattails and bulrushes, is a haven for birds. There are several vantage points along the Bayview Trail to look for herons, egrets, ducks, and shorebirds. Black-necked stilts, which nest in marshes around San Francisco Bay, are sometimes here in flocks of 20 to 30—look for a black-and-white shorebird with shocking pink legs. Besides a few willows and London planetrees (introduced hybrids related to sycamores), the vegetation is mostly scrub—coyote brush, fennel, and poison hemlock.

When you reach a junction with the Nike Trail, about 0.1 mile from the trailhead, continue straight on the Bayview Trail. Across the Main Marsh is Lizard Rock, a large pinnacle of light-colored chert, reached by the single-track trail that bears its name. Chert was used by local Native Americans for arrowheads and spear points when they could not obtain obsidian. After about 0.25 mile you reach a junction with the Lizard Rock Trail, where you turn right and climb on a gentle grade to the rock, passing it on the left. This is a wonderful vantage point from which to look out over the marsh.

You might also take a moment here to scan the eastern skyline, picking out such landmarks as Mission Peak and, to its right and beyond, Mt. Hamilton. Once past Lizard Rock, the trail descends gently across an open hillside of grass mixed with clumps of California sagebrush. After an unsigned single track joins from the left, you reach a T-junction with the Chochenyo Trail. Turn right and follow the dirt-and-gravel road back toward the visitor center, passing deeper water where white pelicans sometimes float lazily about. The marsh wren, a chickadee-sized bird mostly heard but not seen, is likely to keep track of your progress with its raspy, buzzing call.

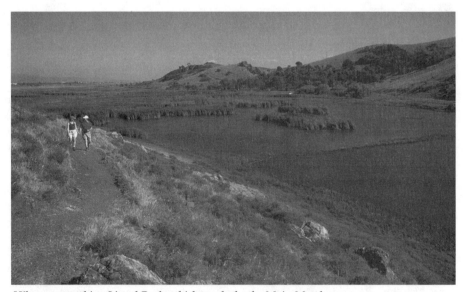

Hikers approaching Lizard Rock, which overlooks the Main Marsh.

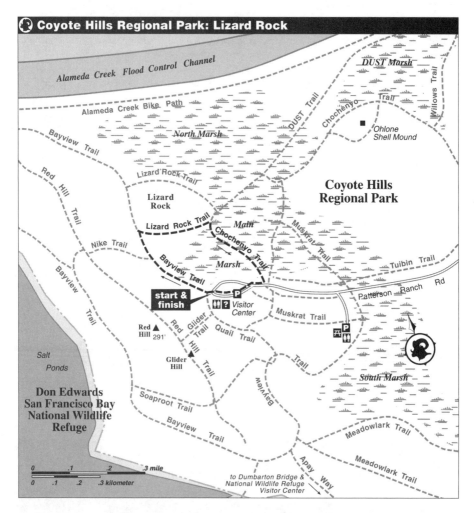

Coyote Hills Regional Park: Lizard Rock

Here is a good opportunity to learn the difference between cattails and bulrushes, both of which are found along this stretch of the route. Cattail (genus *Typha*) is a familiar perennial marsh plant, found where there is at least some fresh water, best identified by its brown, cigar-like flower clusters held aloft on tall stems. Bulrush, also called tule, refers to plants of the genus *Scirpus*, which has 9 species in coastal California and 17 throughout the state. The ones found here have tall, round stems tapering to a sharp point, and tipped during late spring and summer with brown flower clusters. Red-winged blackbirds share the cattails and bulrushes with the marsh wrens. Blackbirds are vocal wizards, keeping up a constant refrain of odd gurgles, chortles, whistles, and other sounds.

A gate marks the south end of the Chochenyo Trail. Beyond the gate, you come to a T-junction with a paved path that parallels the park entrance road. To the left is a short paved path leading to a boardwalk that goes into the marsh, a route followed by the self-guiding Muskrat Trail. To return to the parking area, turn right and follow the paved path.

RED HILL

Length: 1.5 miles

Time: 1 hour or less

Rating: Moderate

Regulations: EBRPD; fees for parking and dogs; the Quail Trail is for hiking only.

Facilities: Visitor center, picnic tables, water, toilet.

Directions: From Highway 84 at the east end of the Dumbarton Bridge in Fremont, take the Thornton Ave./Paseo Padre Pkwy. exit, and go north 1.1 miles on Paseo Padre Pkwy. to Patterson Ranch Road. Turn left, and go 0.5 mile to the entrance kiosk. Another 1.0 mile brings you to the parking area for the visitor center. The trailhead is at the west end of parking area, at its entrance.

Combining portions of the Bayview, Nike, Red Hill, Soaproot, and Quail trails, this short loop over the summits of Red and Glider hills offers more scenery per calorie expended than any other hike in the East Bay. Besides open summits, which provide 360-degree views that extend from San Francisco to the Santa Cruz Mountains, this park contains an extensive brackish marsh, habitat for waterfowl and shorebirds. If you have more time to spend here, consider also doing the "Lizard Rock" trip.

From the west end of the parking area, where the entrance road makes a 180-degree bend, head northwest on the paved Bayview Trail, passing the Quail Trail, a dirt road, left. The Bayview Trail is gated just beyond the parking area. After passing the gate, you have the Main Marsh on your right and beautiful grassy hills rising on your left.

When you reach the Nike Trail, about 0.1 mile from the trailhead, you climb left, leaving the Bayview Trail to its straight and level course. (The Nike Trail is named for the missiles perched atop these hills during the cold war, not the running shoe.) As you gain elevation on a moderate grade, take a moment to look back and admire the view, which takes in Mt. Diablo, the hills of Garin and Dry Creek Pioneer regional parks, Sunol Ridge, Mission Peak, and Mt. Hamilton. In late spring, the grasses of the Coyote Hills turn a rich, golden brown, especially pleasing an hour or two before sunset; after the autumn rains arrive they become lush green.

Soon you reach a flat spot—a saddle between Red Hill and an unnamed hill to the north—and a four-way junction. The view from here stretches across San Francisco Bay, with its system of levees and salt ponds, to the hills of San Mateo County. Turning left here onto the Red Hill Trail, a dirt road, you continue your ascent over open terrain, with views of the marshes that compose much of this regional park. To the northeast lies Alameda Creek, which gets its start high on the flanks of Mt. Hamilton, flows through the Sunol Wilderness, and empties into San Francisco Bay northwest of here. The Alameda County flood-control channel, which diverts water from the creek, borders the north side of Coyote Hills Regional Park, where the 12-mile Alameda Creek Regional Trail—actually two trails, one on each side of the channel—connects to the Coyote Hills trail system.

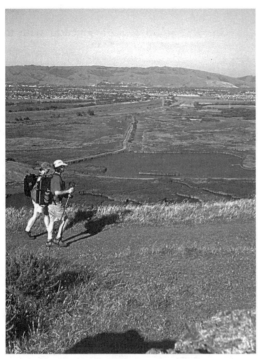

Red Hill is an easy destination for hikers and run-ners, and offers spectacular views

As you reach a short, steep pitch just below the summit of Red Hill, you may see California poppy, blue bush lupine, wild radish, and wild mustard in bloom, their bright colors contrasting with the red dirt underfoot. The only trees up here are acacias, imports from Australia. The summit itself is studded with rock outcrops of Franciscan chert, giving you a pleasant perch from which to take in the 360-degree view. To the northwest is the faint outline of San Francisco, with the dark hulk of Mt. Tamalpais looming behind. Oakland is also in view, beyond Hayward, San Leandro, and Alameda, and just north of this park vast tracts of new housing push almost to the shoreline. To the south, the vista extends past the Dumbarton Bridge and the Don Edwards San Francisco Bay National Wildlife Refuge, all the way to the Santa Cruz Mountains.

While on Red Hill, you may find yourself distracted from the view by the flutter of large yellow and black butterflies. These are swallowtails; there are several species, including one associated exclusively with fennel. Only hardy plants take root on this windy site, where California sagebrush and poison oak sprout from the red, rocky soil. After crossing the level summit, you descend steeply to a saddle between Red Hill and Glider Hill, the next rise south. Just as the route begins to climb once more, you arrive at a four-way junction. From here, single-track trails go left and right (but only the left-hand one, the Glider Hill Trail, is shown on the EBRPD map). Continuing your climb over moderate and then steep ground, you soon reach the top of Glider Hill, where the views equal those from Red Hill. The open, grassy summit even has a convenient picnic table; from here another unsigned single-track trail heads left.

Now a short, steep descent brings you to another saddle and a four-way junction. At this point, the Red Hill Trail, which continues straight, is crossed by the Soaproot Trail, a dirt road. Turn left and begin a gentle descent. From here, the paved Bayview Trail, Dairy Glen picnic area, and South Marsh are all in view. Heading southeast, the Bayview Trail becomes Apay Way, which climbs over South Red Hill and continues to the San Francisco Bay National Wildlife Refuge.

Your route zigzags moderately downhill. At a bend are several unofficial trails heading north. Pass these by and continue descending to a junction with the Bayview and Quail trails. Turn left onto the Quail Trail, a wide dirt-and-gravel road that climbs north. Just after the road crosses a rise, a single-track trail, right, offers you an easy side trip to Castle Rock, a jumble of pinnacles made from the same red chert as Red Hill.

Following the Quail Trail downhill, you may see and hear its namesake, the California quail. On your way, you pass the Hoot Hollow Trail, left, and the Hoot Hollow picnic area, with its beautiful assortment of trees and shrubs, including acacia, coast live oak, madrone, toyon, and California buckeye. Late spring bloomers, buckeyes in flower resemble fireworks, with exploding white blossoms tinged pink and beige against bright green leaves.

Beyond the picnic area, you pass an unsigned path heading left up some wooden steps, and a paved path, right, that leads to the visitor center. About 200 feet downhill from these paths you reach a gate and the entrance to the parking area.

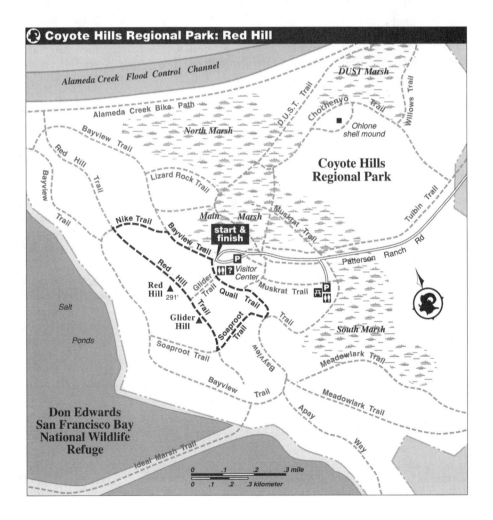

•Don Edwards San Francisco Bay •
National Wildlife Refuge

TIDELANDS TRAIL

Length: 1.3 miles

Time: 1 to 2 hours

Rating: Easy

Regulations: Pets are permitted only on the Tidelands Trail and must be leashed at all times. Pets are prohibited inside the visitor center and elsewhere on the refuge.

Facilities: Visitor center with helpful staff, interpretive displays, books, maps, and information about guided nature walks and other programs; picnic tables, water, toilet, phone.

Directions: From Highway 84 at the east end of the Dumbarton Bridge in Fremont, take the Thornton Ave./Paseo Padre Parkway exit, and go south 0.5 mile to Marshlands Road, the refuge entrance. Turn right and go 0.5 mile to a stop sign, then left into the parking area. The trailhead is at the west side of parking area, just below the large flagpole.

This easy loop, with habitat ranging from upland to salt marsh, is a perfect introduction to the amazing variety of plants and animals, especially birds, found in the refuge. Fall, winter, and spring, when bird populations are highest, are the best times to visit; avoid afternoons, when wind and glaring sunlight may make viewing difficult. Binoculars and/or a spotting scope, along with bird and plant guides, are recommended. Consider also taking one of the guided walks, offered by refuge personnel and volunteers, which concentrate on either birds or plants. (Coyote Hills Regional Park is just north of the refuge, across Highway 84; it would be easy to explore both areas on the same day.)

As you walk up the stairs from the west side of the parking area toward the visitor center, you pass a native plant garden containing coyote brush, black sage, toyon, and bush monkeyflower. When you reach a T-junction with a paved path, turn left and continue uphill to the visitor-center entrance, passing eucalyptus, coast live oak, and coast silk tassel on the way. After exploring the visitor center, with its many exhibits, books, and other publications, walk back outside to an observation area overlooking San Francisco Bay.

Looking southwest, the section of the refuge in front of you extends roughly to the middle of the Bay, and includes salt ponds enclosed by levees, as well as Newark Slough, a river of tidewater flowing through the salt marsh just below the visitor center. Salt ponds, remnants of an extensive salt industry that flourished here in the mid-1800s, still exist on the Bay today. Water moves from pond to pond via channels, the salinity concentrates through evaporation, and the highly saline water is eventually processed into salt.

This is our nation's largest urban wildlife refuge, with more than 20,000 acres of open space set aside to protect wildlife. Three hundred species of birds and other wildlife, including a number of threatened and endangered species, live here year-round or pass through on migration. The refuge extends from Newark to Alviso and contains a variety of habitat, including open water, salt ponds, mudflats, salt marshes, and upland areas. The refuge was renamed to honor Don Edwards, a congressman from San Jose, now retired,

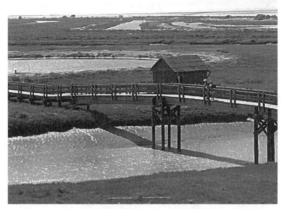

Tidelands Trail, bridge over Newark Slough.

who was instrumental in creating and then expanding the refuge through Congressional acts.

Walking uphill from the visitor center, you follow the self-guiding Tidelands Trail, a loop that will take you through an upland area, beside a salt marsh, across Newark Slough, and along the shore of a salt pond. Gaining elevation on a gentle grade, you can see east to a large salt marsh bordering Marshlands Road, a good area to search for shorebirds on a rising or falling tide. As you climb to a high point, you pass some of the plants growing on the refuge, including toyon, California sagebrush, curly dock, pearly everlasting, and California buckwheat.

A few hundred yards from the visitor center you reach a fork. Going left takes you uphill to an observation deck perched on a bluff overlooking Newark Slough; staying right bypasses the bluff. Bear left, and when you reach the observation deck via steps on your right, take a moment to enjoy a 360-degree view that encompasses much of San Francisco Bay, one of the world's great wildlife areas. Approximately 250 species of birds can be found here, including more than one million shorebirds and waterfowl that use the Bay as a wintering area. Descending from the observation deck on a gentle grade that soon steepens, you pass some picnic tables and then the bypass trail, merging from the right.

As you descend, the route bends left and heads toward the marsh. Shorebirds, terns, ducks, and grebes are the main avian attractions of this refuge, but there are other birds to watch for, including raptors, hummingbirds, and songbirds. A dried fennel stalk may offer a perch for the tiny Anna's hummingbird, while the tall spike of a century plant may hold a white-tailed kite. Descending past beautiful acacia trees, which bloom in mid-winter, and a grassy area brightened by yellow Bermuda buttercups, you reach the edge of the marsh, flooded at high tide, where a trail joins from the left.

As the route turns right and heads toward the Bay, you pass a trail heading left into the marsh. Tide and time of year will determine the level of bird activity here,

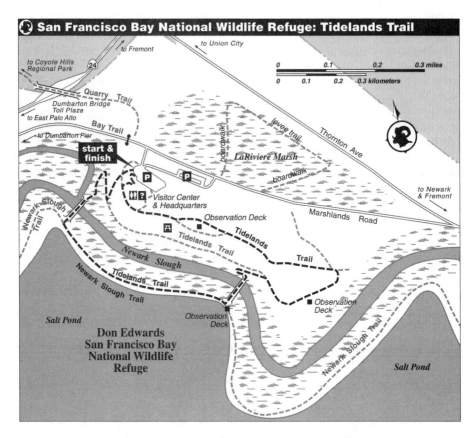

especially for shorebirds, a tribe that includes oystercatchers, avocets, stilts, plovers, willets, curlews, godwits, small sandpipers, dowitchers, and phalaropes. Most of these birds breed elsewhere, usually during May and June, and arrive here as either migratory visitors or winter residents. Some shorebirds, however, including American avocets, black-necked stilts, and snowy plovers, a threatened species, nest in the marshes around San Francisco Bay.

At low tide, shorebirds will be dispersed along the many miles of mudflats around the Bay that provide fertile feeding grounds, and at high tide, rising water will force them to congregate in elevated roosting areas, just above the flood. Thus a rising or falling tide is best for viewing shorebirds. If shorebirds are present, you are almost certain to see one of their tribe called a willet. With its long legs and long bill, this large, drab gray sandpiper transforms itself in flight into a thing of beauty, flashing a bold black-and-white wing pattern as it skims low over the marsh.

As you begin to climb through a rocky area with outcrops of serpentine, California's state rock, you pass some large century plants, residents of southern California, whose tall stalks offer perches for winged hunters in this treeless part of the refuge. At a rest bench, the route levels and bends right, leading you to another observation deck.

Here the route forks, the right-hand path staying level and the left-hand path dropping past a tangle of blackberry vines to a bridge over Newark Slough. Descend to the bridge, which makes a great vantage point for observing birds as they fly over the marsh and swim in the slough. You can also study the marsh plants—pickleweed, cord grass, salt grass, alkali heath—spread out below and adapted in varying degrees to their salty surroundings. In the late summer and early fall, marsh gum-plant sports bright yellow flowers, pickleweed adds touches of red and magenta, and dodder, a parasitic plant, paints everything it touches a garish orange.

After crossing the bridge, you reach a T-junction with a dirt path running along the top of a levee next to a salt pond. If the pond is flooded, you may see shorebirds such as western and least sandpipers, dunlin, and black-necked stilts scampering along its edge, probing for invertebrates or picking brine flies off the water's surface. Turning right, you come to a picnic table and another observation deck, a good vantage point from which to observe the Bay's salt ponds.

Although definitely a drastic alteration of the natural habitat, salt ponds have created a unique environment, similar to saline Mono Lake in the eastern Sierra, that supports a breeding population of American avocets, black-necked stilts, phalaropes, and snow plovers, along with California gulls and Forster's terns. (Because of the snowy plover's threatened status, Marshlands Road beyond the visitor-center parking area is closed from April through approximately the end of August).

Endangered species, such as brown pelicans, peregrine falcons, least terns, clapper rails, and salt marsh harvest mice, call the refuge home or pass through on migration; despite habitat loss, they have survived thanks to efforts by conservationists, scientists, and government agencies. Other animals that used to roam the Bay Area, such as grizzly bear and tule elk, are no longer found here.

Stories of the Bay's huge supply of waterfowl attracted sportsmen and market hunters to these marshes beginning in the late 1800s. A low red hunting shack, right, was built in the 1930s by Joe Pine of Niles, California, and was occupied by him until the 1960s. A nearby sunken blind, left, offers a hidden site for bird observation and photography. Just past the blind, the route turns right to cross Newark Slough on a long wooden bridge. (The Newark Slough Trail, a 5-mile circuit, starts here and follows the slough west into the marsh.)

Partway across the bridge, another shack, left, has a picnic table and information about the creatures—brine flies and brine shrimp—that live in salt ponds. Once across the bridge, you switchback right, passing a trail leading left to a small amphitheater used for outdoor meetings and programs, and climb to an observation deck flanked by picnic tables in the shade of a eucalyptus. At a T-junction you turn left, joining the path coming from above the first bridge. As you come over a low rise, you reach the paved path leading right and uphill to the visitor center. With the large flagpole directly ahead, follow a dirt-and-gravel path straight to the parking area.

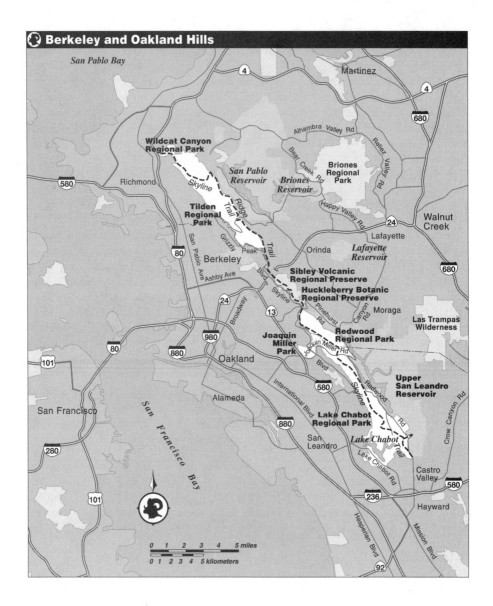

Berkeley and Oakland Hills

◆ Berkeley and Oakland Hills ◆

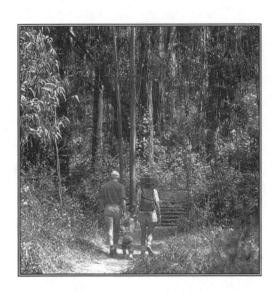

◆East Bay Skyline National Recreation Trail ◆

The East Bay Skyline National Recreation Trail was the nation's first nonfederal national recreation trail, a designation granted by the U.S. Department of the Interior to publicly owned or controlled routes that are close to an urban or metropolitan area; have scenic value; are wide enough to provide for hiking, horseback riding, nature study, and, in some cases, bicycling; and do not allow motor vehicles. The Skyline Trail certainly fulfills all of these requirements and more: it is one of the gems of our East Bay parklands.

When the Skyline Trail opened in 1970, it ran through only Anthony Chabot and Redwood regional parks. Today the 31-mile route stretches from the Wildcat staging area in Wildcat Canyon Regional Park to Proctor Gate in Anthony Chabot Regional Park, meaning it is possible to walk or ride a horse on an unbroken path from Richmond to Castro Valley. (Bicycles are not permitted on a 6.3-mile section from Lomas Cantadas in Tilden Regional Park to Skyline Gate in Redwood Regional Park.) The Skyline Trail passes through six EBRPD regional parks and preserves: Wildcat Canyon, Tilden, Redwood, Anthony Chabot, Sibley Volcanic, and Huckleberry Botanic. The route also briefly crosses EBMUD land between Tilden Regional Park and Sibley Volcanic Regional Preserve.

While it is possible to hike or jog the entire trail in one day, most people do it in stages. In this book, the trail is divided into four segments, each of which is easily completed in a day, with a not-too-difficult car shuttle. Be sure to take plenty of water and snacks; there is only limited water along the way. Food, drinks, and cold beer are available at the Willow Park Golf Course, near Proctor Gate, the trail's southern end. There is currently only one overnight camp for individuals and groups, at Anthony Chabot Campground near the southern end of the route. For campground information call (510) 636-1684.

WILDCAT CANYON
TO LOMAS CANTADAS

Length: 10.2 miles

Time: 4 to 6 hours

Rating: Difficult

Regulations: EBRPD

Facilities: Water and picnic tables are available in the Alvarado Area picnic grounds, northwest of the parking area in Wildcat Canyon, and at Lomas Cantadas near Tilden Regional Park's Steam Trains parking area. Toilets are available at the Wildcat staging area, Inspiration Point, and Lomas Cantadas.

Directions: This is a car shuttle trip, starting at the **Wildcat Canyon staging area** in Wildcat Canyon Regional Park, and ending at **Lomas Cantadas**, near the Steam Trains in Tilden Regional Park. Drive first to Lomas Cantadas, leave a car there, and proceed to the Wildcat Canyon staging area.

To reach **Lomas Cantadas:** From Highway 24 just east of the Caldecott Tunnel, take the Fish Ranch Road exit and go uphill 1 mile to a four-way intersection with Claremont Ave. and Grizzly Peak Blvd. Turn right on Grizzly Peak Blvd. and go 1.1 miles to Lomas Cantadas Dr. Turn right and then immediately left onto a road signed for Tilden Regional Park's Steam Trains, Fire Station, and Corporation Yard. Pass the entrance to the Steam Trains, left, and at a fork bear right and slightly uphill to a large gravel parking area.

To reach the **Wildcat Canyon staging area:** From Lomas Cantadas, return to Highway 24 and follow it west to Interstate 580 westbound, then get on Interstate 80 eastbound. From Interstate 80 in Richmond, take the Solano Ave. exit, which puts you on Amador St. Turn left and go 0.4 mile to McBryde Ave. Turn right and follow McBryde Ave. 0.2 mile, staying in the left lane as you approach a stop sign. (Use caution at this intersection; traffic from the right does not stop.) Continue straight, now on Park Ave., for 0.1 mile to the parking area, left. The trailhead is at the east end of the parking area.

This northernmost segment of the 31-mile East Bay Skyline National Recreation Trail uses the Wildcat Creek, Belgum, San Pablo Ridge, Curran, Sea View, Lupine, and Vollmer Peak trails, along with Nimitz Way, to traverse Wildcat Canyon and Tilden regional parks. Although there is steep climbing at the outset, much of the point-to-point route is along the top of San Pablo Ridge, a generally level course, and views are among the best in the East Bay.

From the east end of the parking area, head uphill past stands of coast live oak, eucalyptus, acacia, and Monterey pine on paved Wildcat Creek Trail, a remnant of Wildcat Canyon Road, which was closed in the early 1980s by landslides. After about 0.3 mile the pavement ends, and you continue on a rocky and eroded dirt road, past an unsigned path, left. Willows signal the presence of Wildcat Creek, downhill and right, which gets its start high on Vollmer Peak and empties into San Pablo Bay north of the Richmond–San Rafael Bridge.

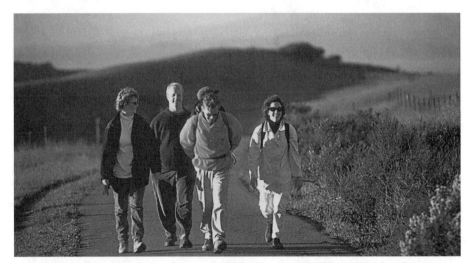

Nimitz Way offers a paved route between Wildcat Canyon and Tilden regional parks.

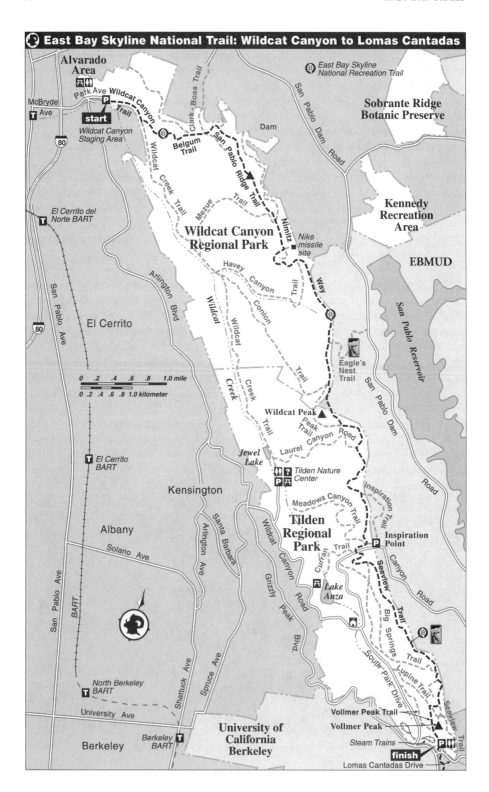

East Bay Skyline National Trail: Wildcat Canyon to Lomas Cantadas

At about the 0.5-mile point, you come to a junction with the Belgum Trail, here a paved road, where you turn left and begin to climb. There is a trail post at the junction with an emblem for the East Bay Skyline National Recreation Trail. As you walk uphill, you pass an area, left, that has been invaded by cardoon, an artichoke relative in the thistle family. A program by EBRPD to control this nonnative pest is underway. Passing through a gate, you stay on pavement for about 100 feet and then the Belgum Trail continues as a dirt road. There is a large eucalyptus grove ahead, and if you turn and look west, you have a beautiful view of Mt. Tamalpais.

The route alternates between wooded and open areas, and at one point passes several large palm trees, the site of Belgum's Grand Vista Sanitarium, which has since burned down. As you gain elevation on a moderate grade, the view gets even better, taking in Angel Island and the Golden Gate Bridge. Open areas here, mostly grassland, will be decorated in spring with blue bush lupine and California poppy. Beyond another large stand of eucalyptus, the route stays in the open, passing occasional groves of California bay. With every step, more of the Bay Area is revealed, including the San Francisco skyline, which on a clear day appears etched on a background of hills and blue sky.

After reaching a shoulder, the route passes a rest bench, bends left and continues its climb, aiming for the high ground of San Pablo Ridge, just east across an open valley. As the route levels and then drops slightly, the vista extends north across San Pablo Bay to the hills of Napa and Sonoma counties and Mt. St. Helena. At the next flat spot, several junctions sprout trails in different directions. The first junction is a fork; here an unsigned road heads straight but you veer left, reaching a trail post in about 50 feet. At the post, the Clark–Boas Trail heads left and downhill, a faint trail climbs right, and your route, the Belgum Trail to San Pablo Ridge Trail, continues straight. A field of California buttercup brightens the scene here, and nearby is an active California ground squirrel colony. You may see an American kestrel hovering overhead, on the lookout for small reptiles and rodents.

Soon you reach the next junction, a fork marked by a trail post, where you veer right and steeply uphill on the San Pablo Ridge Trail, a rough dirt road. As you crest San Pablo Ridge, you have your first view today of Mt. Diablo, dead ahead. The route now climbs over several high summits, each one affording 360-degree views of almost the entire Bay Area; this park provides some of the best vantage points in the East Bay hills. As you head southeast along the ridgetop, the side of San Pablo Ridge drops steeply left to the narrow valley filled by San Pablo Reservoir. Ahead in the distance lies Tilden Regional Park, crowned by Vollmer Peak (1913'), a forested summit with communication towers; a parking area just south of the peak is your goal for today.

Descending in open terrain, the San Pablo Ridge Trail ends at a junction, at about the 2.8-mile point, with the Mezue Trail, which goes left and right. You turn right and walk past a large cattle pen. Whatever trees and shrubs grow here, mostly bay and coyote brush, are kept low and flat-topped by the wind, which usually blows from the west. About 100 yards beyond the previous junction, you pass a dirt road, left. Some 50 feet farther, you pass Old Nimitz Way, another dirt road merging from the left. Now on Nimitz Way, you continue southeast on a mostly level course, go through a cattle gate, and soon reach a T-junction at the base of a hill used during the Cold War as a Nike missile site.

Here a gravel road heads left to the concrete base of the Nike site, and your route, Nimitz Way, now a paved road, goes right. As you curve around the hill, Oakland's skyline appears, and you begin to get views toward the south end of San Francisco Bay. In spring, poppies, red maids, and other wildflowers color the grassy hills beside Nimitz Way. A short distance beyond the Nike site you pass a junction, right, with the Havey Canyon Trail. Soon a rest bench beckons, and you can enjoy a glorious view of Mt. Diablo and, to its right, Las Trampas and Rocky ridges, the high walls that form Bollinger Canyon. A bit farther, the Eagle's Nest Trail, a segment of the Bay Area Ridge Trail, joins from the left. From here to near the south end of Anthony Chabot Regional Park, the Bay Area Ridge and East Bay Skyline National Recreation trails follow the same route.

Continuing on Nimitz Way, a poplar route for hikers, bicyclists, in-line skaters, equestrians, and joggers, you next pass the Conlon Trail, which goes straight and uphill to the edge of Tilden Regional Park, then switches back and descends to the Wildcat Creek Trail. Stay left to continue on Nimitz Way. At about the 5-mile point, you cross into Tilden Regional Park and enter the shade of a large eucalyptus grove. Soon a connector to the Peak Trail, signed WILDCAT PEAK TRAIL, joins Nimitz Way from the right, and if you look up the trail you can see a planted stand of cone-shaped trees, giant sequoias, called the Rotary Peace Grove. (These trees achieve their giant status only on the western slope of the Sierra Nevada, their natural habitat.)

Now you are walking in filtered sunlight and shade, thanks to the eucalyptus and bay trees that line the route. Beside the road you may find snowberry, blackberry, vine honeysuckle, and much poison oak. At the next junction, Laurel Canyon Road leads right and downhill through the Tilden Nature Area. As you continue on Nimitz Way, you pass several large stands of mostly Monterey pine, right, and a seasonal wetland bordered with willows, left. Another collection of giant sequoias, right, called the Redwood Grove, was planted by the Berkeley Hiking Club.

The route soon swings left and follows a set of power lines, and now, rounding a bend, you can see Inspiration Point and its parking area ahead. Rest benches on this part of Nimitz Way are strategically placed to take advantage of the best views, especially of Mt. Diablo and Mt. Tamalpais. Just before reaching Inspiration Point, a little past the 7-mile point, Nimitz Way bends left and comes to a gate. Before the gate, just past some toilets, look for a trail post, right, with the Bay Area Ridge Trail and East Bay Skyline National Recreation Trail emblems. Here you turn right, descend a dirt-and-gravel path, and in about 30 feet turn right again on the Curran Trail, a dirt road.

Continuing to descend over rough ground, you enter an area shaded by bay, coast live oak, and pine. A few hundred yards down the road you pass the Meadows Canyon Trail, right, and in about 50 feet come to a junction with a single-track trail going left and uphill. Climbing up it on a moderate grade across a brushy hillside, you soon reach Wildcat Canyon Road, a paved thoroughfare that runs through the heart of Tilden Regional Park. Cross the road carefully and find the Sea View Trail, a dirt road, taking off left and uphill. This rocky road makes a sweeping S-bend to gain altitude on a moderate grade. Eucalyptus trees, which here shade the route, look and smell lovely, but besides being a fire hazard they can fall during wind storms.

As the route bends left you pass a trail, right, to the Quarry picnic area, then continue on a moderate uphill grade, with views extending from Mt. St. Helena to the San Francisco skyline. If you look carefully, you can even pick out your earlier route along San Pablo Ridge in Wildcat Canyon Regional Park. Soon you pass the Big Springs Trail, right; afterwards the uphill grade eases somewhat as you enter a stand of Monterey and Coulter pines. The view now extends west past the Golden Gate Bridge to the Pacific Ocean, and east to Briones Reservoir and the hills of Briones Regional Park. On this stretch you will pass several paths that head left to viewpoints, but your route continues straight and soon begins to climb steeply over rocky, eroded ground.

Reaching a high point, you are rewarded by a 360-degree panorama and a conveniently placed picnic table. In spring, large sunflower-like blossoms of mule's ear appear, giving a festive appearance to the grassy slopes, which are also decorated with lupine and fiddleneck, sporting yellow-orange flowers along a coiled stem. Now the route descends, in preparation for the final push up Vollmer Peak. Reaching a flat spot at about the 9-mile point, you pass the Big Springs Trail, heading right and downhill. Beginning to climb again on a moderate grade, you pass a west-facing hillside covered with clumps of California sagebrush and black sage, chaparral plants that seem out of place in the fog belt. The road now makes a series of S-bends to gain elevation, and soon reaches a junction marked by a trail post.

Here the Lupine Trail, a single track, goes right, bending away from Vollmer Peak, and the Sea View Trail continues over the peak, then descends to the Lomas Cantadas parking area. (Bicyclists must use the Sea View Trail.) Turning right, you pass in about 20 feet a junction with the Arroyo Trail, right, but you continue straight on the Lupine Trail. After several hundred feet, you pass an unsigned trail, right, and then climb through a brushy area to a clearing and a T-junction marked with a trail post. Here the Lupine Trail turns right, but you turn left onto an unsigned trail and continue to climb, now on a rocky path. In about 150 feet you meet the Vollmer Peak Trail, which goes straight (uphill) and also right. You veer right and contour around the west side of the peak. Crossing a steep hillside brightened by buttercups, lupine, mule's ear, and poppies, you soon reach a junction. Here the Vollmer Peak Trail turns right, but you angle left and enter a dense bay forest. After about 200 feet you emerge at the Lomas Cantadas parking area.

Lomas Cantadas to Skyline Gate

Length: 6.3 miles

Time: 3 to 4 hours

Rating: Moderate

Regulations: EBMUD, EBRPD; no bicycles, no dogs; horses in Huckleberry Regional Preserve are allowed only on the East Bay Skyline National Recreation Trail.

Facilities: Water and toilets are available at Lomas Cantadas in the Steam Trains parking area; at Sibley Volcanic Regional Preserve visitor center (about half way); and at Skyline Gate. There are picnic tables across the road from the Steam Trains entrance. A phone is available at Skyline Gate.

Directions: This is a car shuttle trip, starting at **Lomas Cantadas,** near the Steam Trains in Tilden Regional Park, and ending at **Skyline Gate** in Redwood Regional Park. Drive first to Skyline Gate, leave a car there, and proceed to Lomas Cantadas.

To reach **Skyline Gate:** From Highway 24 just east of the Caldecott Tunnel, take the Fish Ranch Road exit and go uphill 1.0 mile to a four-way intersection with Claremont Ave. and Grizzly Peak Blvd. Turn left on Grizzly Peak Blvd. and go 2.5 miles to Skyline Blvd. Turn left and follow Skyline Blvd. for 2 miles, staying left at an intersection with Snake Road, to Skyline Gate, on the left, 0.1 mile beyond Shepherd Canyon Road.

To reach **Lomas Cantadas:** From Skyline Gate, return on Skyline Blvd. 2 miles to Grizzly Peak Blvd., which is just beyond the entrance to Sibley Volcanic Regional Park. Turn right onto Grizzly Peak Blvd. and go 3.6 miles, passing the four-way intersection with Claremont Ave. and Fish Ranch Road, to Lomas Cantadas Dr. Turn right and then immediately left onto a road signed for Tilden Regional Park's Steam Trains, Fire Station, and Corporation Yard. Pass the entrance to the Steam Trains, left, and at a fork bear right and slightly uphill to a large gravel parking area. The trailhead is at the southeast end of the Lomas Cantadas parking area.

From Highway 24 just east of the Caldecott Tunnel, take the Fish Ranch Road exit and go uphill 1 mile to a four-way intersection with Claremont Ave. Grizzly Peak Blvd. Turn right on Grizzly Peak Blvd. and go 1.1 miles to Lomas Cantadas Dr. Turn right and then immediately left onto a road signed for Tilden Regional Park's Steam Trains, Fire Station, and Corporation Yard. Pass the entrance to the Steam Trains, left, and at a fork bear right and slightly uphill to a large gravel parking area. The trailhead is at the southeast end of the Lomas Cantadas parking area.

This segment of the East Bay Skyline National Recreation Trail, here also part of the Bay Area Ridge Trail, heads southeast from the edge of Tilden Regional Park, crosses EBMUD land and the Caldecott Tunnel, and then traverses Sibley Volcanic and Huckleberry Botanic regional preserves on its way to the northwest corner of Redwood Regional Park. A point-to-point trip of many ups and downs, and terrains ranging from open grasslands to deep wooded canyons, its rewards include dramatic views of Mt. Diablo and a wonderful assortment of trees, shrubs, and wildflowers. (Much of this trail follows the ridgeline, where tall trees collect water from the fog and drop it onto the paths below, making for possibly muddy trails even in summer.)

From the southeast end of the parking area, walk along the entrance road—passing a paved road that climbs Vollmer Peak, left, and a road to the Steam Trains, right—until you reach a crosswalk at Lomas Cantadas Dr. Cross carefully and look left for a trail post with emblems for the East Bay Skyline National Recreation Trail and the Bay Area Ridge Trail. Here you get on a single-track trail and follow it downhill, passing through several gates into a weedy area overgrown with coyote brush, cow parsnip, vine honeysuckle, and poison oak. You are now on EBMUD lands, and the view, when you reach a clearing, extends east toward Orinda and Mt. Diablo. The trail is rough and eroded in places, lined with California sagebrush, bush monkeyflower, toyon, and thimbleberry, and shaded by California bay and California buckeye.

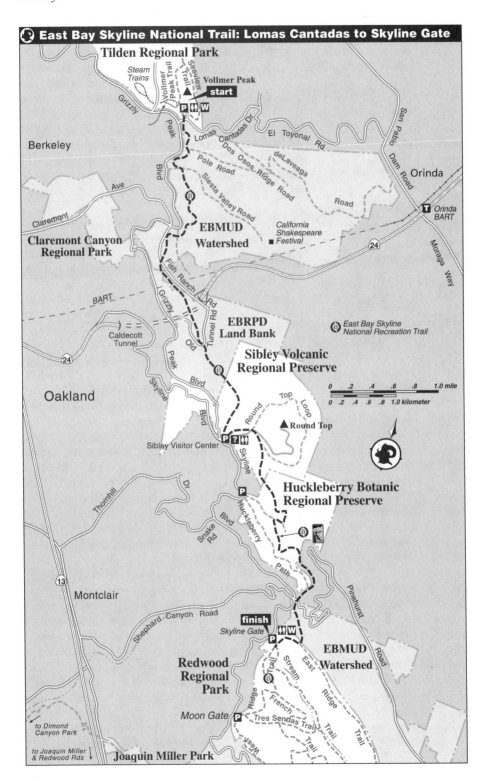

East Bay Skyline National Trail: Lomas Cantadas to Skyline Gate

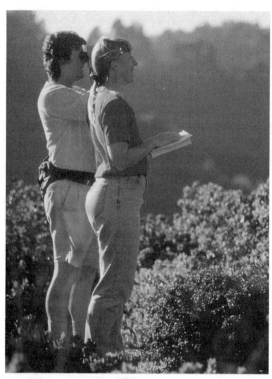

Huckleberry Botanic Regional Preserve is within easy access of Berkeley and Oakland.

The route levels, then climbs, and soon reaches a T-junction with the deLaveaga Trail, a dirt road. Here you turn right, climb a short steep section, and then enjoy a level walk with a beautiful view, left, of Mt. Diablo. (Another beautiful, if startling, sight when I hiked here was a large male peacock, perhaps someone's pet.)

The road bends sharply left, descends slightly, then levels and comes to a four-way junction, poorly signed, with a dirt fire road, closed to the public. Here you proceed straight, finding a single-track trail that leads through a brushy area decorated with Chinesehouses, mule's ear, and woodland star.

The trail crosses a steep hillside, reinforced to help prevent landslides, that drops left, and then alternates between open and wooded areas, where blackberry, coffeeberry, and hillside gooseberry grow in the shade of bay and coast live oak. Passing the Berkeley Hills Reservoir, a large EBMUD water tank, you soon you reach an open grassy area where the trail turns sharply west toward the Golden Gate Bridge. Below you is Fish Ranch Road, which you will soon cross. Entering a stand of eucalyptus, you pass a faint trail heading right and uphill, but here your route bends sharply left and goes downhill over rough ground. Then, at about the 1.5-mile point, you reach two gates and a paved path leading, in approximately 200 feet, to Fish Ranch Road.

Fish Ranch Road is a busy, high-speed thoroughfare, so take care when crossing. Once on the other side, you will see signs for the East Bay Skyline and Bay Area Ridge trails. Now on a wide dirt trail, you wind on mostly level ground through a wooded area of coast live oak, bay, and blue elderberry. Soon the route begins a moderate descent, then rises slightly to a four-way junction with an overgrown dirt road. The Caldecott Tunnel, built in 1937, runs through the Berkeley Hills near this spot. Here you continue straight, descending past bigleaf maple, hazelnut, and madrone, on a trail lined with French broom, coyote brush, and poison oak. Several tight S-bends take you downhill quickly, but then a short climb wins back some of the lost elevation.

Where Old Tunnel Road merges from the right, you join it briefly, then continue straight as the road makes a sharp left-hand bend. You are now on a dirt road, heading southeast and climbing on a gentle grade. Willows beside the road indicate water is near; in fact it may be flowing across your path. Soon the road narrows, crosses several eroded gullies that may have water in them, and then begins a gradual climb beside a creek nestled in a shallow ravine, right. This is a beautiful area, deep in a shady forest. A wooden bridge takes you across the creek, and now the route climbs on a moderate grade below a high ridge, right, topped with eucalyptus.

After a long, steady climb, you arrive at the Sibley Volcanic Regional Preserve visitor center, just a few paces north of a small parking area off Skyline Blvd. Here are water, toilets, and an interpretive display with information about the preserve's geology, plants, and animals. You have come about 3.4 miles, and have approximately 2.9 miles more to reach Skyline Gate at Redwood Regional Park. When you are ready to continue, follow a paved road around the west side of the visitor center. Just before reaching a gate, angle right and uphill on a single-track trail, signed for the East Bay Skyline/Bay Area Ridge Trail and the Round Top Loop Trail.

Follow the trail northeast through a wooded area, parallel to and just above a paved road that climbs Round Top (1763'), an extinct volcano and one of the highest peaks in the Oakland and Berkeley hills. As you emerge into a clearing, you pass a trail, left, and in about 100 feet come to a confusing four-way junction. Left, the dirt-and-gravel Round Top Loop Trail, described elsewhere in this book, leads to the volcanic area. Right, a paved path leads downhill, and, in about 50 feet, joins a paved road that goes uphill to a well-hidden EBMUD water tank. Your route continues straight, crosses the water-tank road, and now as a single track heads southeast through a corridor of tall Monterey pines. Your trail soon crosses the paved road to Round Top's summit and in about 125 feet reaches a junction where you leave the Round Top Loop Trail. Here you bear right and follow the East Bay Skyline/Bay Area Ridge Trail.

On a gentle descent through eucalyptus and pine, the route makes a sharp bend right and passes tangled thickets of blackberry, coyote brush, and evergreen huckleberry, then switchbacks on a steeper grade into a dense forest of bay and coast live oak. Soon a clearing brings dramatic views of Mt. Diablo and the high ground around Bollinger Canyon, including Las Trampas and Rocky ridges. More switchbacks over rocky and eroded terrain lead you down a ridge with steep drop-offs on either side, and eventually you reach the bottom of heavily wooded San Leandro Creek canyon.

Beyond a wooden bridge, a short walk brings you to San Leandro Creek; after crossing it, climb about 100 yards to a T-junction, marked with a trail post, and turn right. This is a lush and possibly muddy area, shaded by curving bay trees and home to hazelnut, creambush, and western sword fern. Now in Huckleberry Botanic Regional Preserve, you turn sharply left at the next junction and follow the Huckleberry Path, a self-guiding nature trail described elsewhere in this book, on a moderate uphill course. The route traces the indentations of a steep, northeast-facing ridge, more or less maintaining a steady elevation. After passing junctions, about 0.4 mile apart, with the Huckleberry Path and Huckleberry Trail, right, the route enters a eucalyptus grove and soon emerges in civilization—Oakland's Montclair neighborhood—where Skyline Blvd. and Pinehurst, Shepherd Canyon, and Manzanita roads all converge.

Pinehurst Road is the paved road you reach first. After carefully crossing it, look left and uphill for a trail leading to a fence marked with the East Bay Skyline Trail and Bay Area Ridge Trail emblems. After passing through the fence, follow a dirt trail uphill across a clearing that opens toward Mt. Diablo, with private homes on your right. Now back in trees, the route levels and then descends to meet the East Ridge Trail, a dirt road in Redwood Regional Park. Here you turn right, and perhaps in the company of bicyclists, dog-walkers, and other hikers, proceed a short distance, the last bit of it paved, to Skyline Gate.

Skyline Gate to MacDonald Gate

Length: 5 miles

Time: 3 to 4 hours

Rating: Moderate

Regulations: EBRPD; no bicycles on the Golden Spike or MacDonald trails. Bicyclists must follow the West Ridge Trail to the Fishway Interpretive Site, then take the park entrance road south to Redwood Road, turning right to reach MacDonald Gate.

Facilities: Water and toilets are available at Skyline Gate and Redwood Bowl; there are picnic tables at Redwood Bowl, and phones at Skyline Gate and in the parking area near the archery range; horse staging at MacDonald Gate.

Directions: This is a car shuttle trip, starting at **Skyline Gate** in Redwood Regional Park, and ending at **MacDonald Gate** in Anthony Chabot Regional Park. Drive first to MacDonald Gate, leave a car there, and proceed to Skyline Gate.

To reach **MacDonald Gate:** From Interstate 580 eastbound in Oakland, take the 35th Ave. exit, turn left and follow 35th Ave. east into the hills. After 0.8 mile 35th Ave. becomes Redwood Road, and at 2.4 miles it crosses Skyline Blvd., where you stay in the left lane and go straight. At 4.3 miles from Interstate 580 you reach MacDonald Gate, right. (If you see the entrance to Redwood Park, left, you have gone too far.)

From Interstate 580 westbound in Oakland, take the Warren Freeway/Berkeley/Highway 13 exit and go 0.9 mile to the Carson St./Redwood Road exit. From the stop sign at the end of the exit ramp, continue straight, now on Mountain Blvd., 0.2 mile, and bear right onto Redwood Road. Go 2.9 miles to MacDonald Gate, right.

From Highway 13 southbound, take the Redwood Road/Carson St. exit, turn left onto Redwood Road and follow the directions above.

To reach **Skyline Gate:** From MacDonald Gate, return on Redwood Road to the junction of Redwood Road and Skyline Blvd. and turn right. At the 0.6-mile point, Skyline Blvd. makes a sudden right turn. Follow Skyline Blvd. for a total of 3.7 miles to Skyline Gate, right. The trailhead is at the south side of Skyline Gate parking area.

This section of the East Bay Skyline National Recreation Trail, here part of the Bay Area Ridge Trail, follows the West Ridge Trail through Redwood Regional

Park for almost that trail's entire length, then uses the Golden Spike and MacDonald trails to reach the northern edge of Anthony Chabot Regional Park. While not particularly scenic, this point-to-point trip gives you an opportunity to see a wide variety of trees and shrubs, including impressive coast redwoods, and, in spring, songbirds and butterflies. The West Ridge Trail spends much time in the open, a consideration on a hot day, but is considerably less strenuous than the alternate East Bay Skyline route, the well-shaded French Trail.

Three of Redwood Regional Park's many trails—East Ridge, West Ridge, and Stream—can be found at Skyline Gate. Your route is the West Ridge Trail, a dirt road that heads south from the parking area and follows a level course past stands of California bay, coast live oak, coast redwood, eucalyptus, and Monterey pine. (This route is very popular with dog walkers, and while most clean up after their pets, as required, the few who do not can make hiking here an unpleasant experience for everyone.) Butterflies are the prime attraction in late spring along this part of the hike, filling the air with moving patches of color and landing on thistle that borders the road. This is also a good spot to listen for birds: you may hear the chestnut-backed chickadee saying its name, the wrentit giving a staccato trill, or the mourning dove making its sad call.

The variety of trees and shrubs here makes this an ideal place to learn about the plants of the East Bay. Besides the common trees already mentioned, you are likely to find blue elderberry, hazelnut, and madrone, along with shrubs such as creambush, evergreen huckleberry, snowberry, and toyon. Coyote brush and poison oak, present throughout the East Bay, are here too. Where the road makes a sharp right-hand bend, at about 0.6 mile, you pass the French Trail, left, an alternate and considerably more challenging—but less busy—East Bay Skyline route that is closed to bicycles. (The French Trail is described elsewhere in this book.)

Staying on the West Ridge Trail, you enter a shady corridor of redwoods, then emerge to find a rest bench with a view east toward Las Trampas Wilderness. Now the road climbs slightly; where it crests and starts to descend, you pass an unsigned trail, right, and then a junction, left, with the Tres Sendas Trail. As the trail bends left, several houses come into view, and a short distance ahead is a path to Moon Gate, right, beside busy Skyline Blvd. Here your route swings left and climbs in the open, with views of Mt. Diablo and soon your first, albeit small, glimpse of San Francisco Bay. It is said that early mariners entering the Bay would steer a safe course between Yerba Buena and Alcatraz islands by sighting on two of the tallest redwoods in these hills, some of which grew to more than 20 feet in diameter.

Those giants are long gone, felled by loggers from 1840 to 1860 to build the Bay Area's cities. Now redwoods and other native trees compete for survival with eucalyptus, a fast-growing import from Australia. A program to control the eucalyptus is underway in Redwood and Anthony Chabot regional parks, and you may see areas that have been logged.

About 0.5 mile past Moon Gate you come to a wood gate across the West Ridge Trail. Just beyond, the trail crosses a paved driveway into the Chabot Space and Science Center parking lot. Continue past another wood gate, and soon the center's buildings appear just to the left of the trail. A sign, left, points the way to the science center and parking lot. Shortly you reach still another wood gate and a cross-

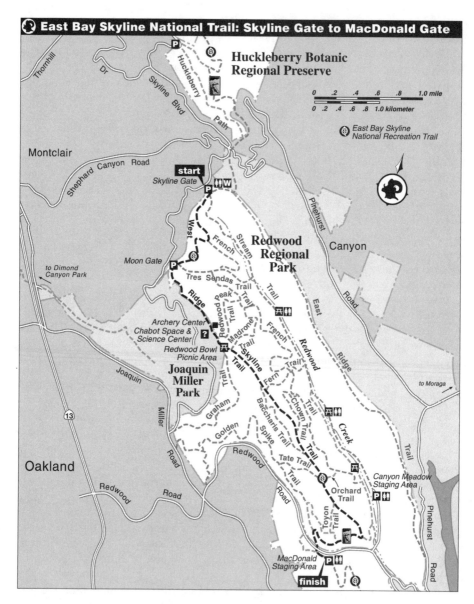

walk on another paved entrance to the parking area. (Use caution here, as the crosswalk is on a blind curve.)

The trail continues just past a metal gate, and in about a hundred yards, you reach a six-way junction. On the far left is a signpost for the Roberts Ridge Trail and the Archery Range. Also on the left is a sign for Redwood Bowl, next to a trail down to a meadow. To the right of that sign, the West Ridge and Roberts Ridge trails merge; continue straight here, descending gently downhill to the far end of the Redwood Bowl picnic area, a convenient rest stop with water, picnic tables, and toilets.

Just past the picnic area, at about the 2-mile point, you turn left and follow the West Ridge Trail downhill, soon meeting a dirt road, left, and then a fork. Here the Graham Trail heads right, but you bear left, still on the West Ridge Trail, heading southeast. Several hundred yards past the fork, you pass a short connector trail, left, to the Redwood Peak and Madrone trails. (A short side-trip from here climbs Redwood Peak, at 1619 feet the park's highest point.)

Continuing straight through a corridor of Monterey cypress, you soon reach an open, brushy area bordered by eucalyptus and acacia, and begin a descent over rocky and eroded ground. The view southward skims across the nearby uplands toward the Coyote Hills and the shores of San Francisco Bay. Where the Baccharis Trail branches right, you stay on the West Ridge Trail by bearing left.

Soon you pass the Fern Trail, left, and continue to descend, sometimes over bare rock. Near the end of a large clearing, you pass the Chown Trail, left, and, after more bare rock, meet the other end of the Baccharis Trail merging from the right. Now you enter a corridor of eucalyptus, then emerge into an area of chaparral, mostly chamise and manzanita. Here you pass junctions with the Tate Trail, right, and the Orchard Trail, left. (If you are using the French Trail as an alternate route, you will arrive at the West Ridge Trail via the Orchard Trail.)

As you enter a wooded area, the route descends past the Toyon Trail, right, and soon steepens, following a big S-bend down through bay, coast live oak, eucalyptus, and madrone. Use caution here: the eucalyptus capsules scattered beneath your feet are like ball-bearings and can cause a fall, as can slippery leaves. Watch also for descending bicyclists.

As the grade eases and the route begins to bend left, at about the 4-mile point, look for a trail post with emblems for the East Bay Skyline and Bay Area Ridge trails. Here you turn right onto a short connector trail, and in a few hundred feet come to a T-junction with the Golden Spike Trail. Turning right on this single-track trail, you descend into a heavily wooded canyon filled with redwood and bay. After leveling, the route begins to climb on a gentle and then moderate grade, hugging the edge of a steep hillside that falls away left.

Now the route begins to descend, bringing you to a brushy area of coyote brush, blue bush lupine, canyon gooseberry, and bush monkeyflower. Passing a closed trail, right, your route bends sharply right, then climbs gently through a lovely, open stretch decorated with paintbrush and California sagebrush. This is a hidden corner of Redwood Regional Park, less traveled and more like a wilderness, with an intimate feel.

Soon you reach a junction, marked by a trail post, where the Golden Spike Trail continues straight, and your route turns left at a sign pointing toward Redwood Road. The trail then drops to a flat area, surrounded by bigleaf maple, next to Redwood Road. After crossing a bridge over a tributary of Redwood Creek, carefully cross Redwood Road, walk through the Big Bear Gate parking area, and find the MacDonald Trail, and overgrown single-track, heading southeast. The creek you just crossed comes under the road through a culvert, merges with another that flows under the trail, and now is to your left as you walk downstream. About 100 yards past the Big Bear Gate parking area, you pass the Big Bear Loop Trail, right, and after several hundred more yards reach MacDonald Gate.

MacDonald Gate
to Proctor Gate

Length: 9.3 miles

Time: 4 to 6 hours

Rating: Difficult

Regulations: EBRPD

Facilities: Water is available at the Chabot Marksmanship Range, a little east of the trail, and at the Willow Park Golf Course, near the southern end of the trail. Toilets are at the marksmanship range, the junction of the Brandon Trail and Marciel Road, the golf course, and Proctor Gate. There are a phone and cold beer at the golf course. Horse staging at MacDonald Gate, Bort Meadow, the golf course, and Proctor Gate. The only overnight campground currently available for individuals and groups using the Skyline Trail is located on Marciel Road, near Lake Chabot; for information call (510) 562-2267.

Directions: This is a car shuttle trip, starting at **MacDonald Gate** and ending at **Proctor Gate**. Drive first to Proctor Gate, leave a car there, and proceed to MacDonald Gate.

To reach **Proctor Gate:** From Interstate 580 eastbound in Castro Valley, take the Redwood Road exit and go north 2.3 miles to a small unsigned parking area, left.

From Interstate 580 westbound in Castro Valley, take the Castro Valley exit, turn left onto E. Castro Valley Blvd. (which soon becomes Castro Valley Blvd.) and go 1.1 miles to Redwood Road. Turn right and go 1.8 miles to a small unsigned parking area, left.

To reach **MacDonald Gate:** From Proctor Gate, go north on Redwood Road 8.6 miles to a parking area, left, just beyond the entrance to Redwood Regional Park. The trailhead is at the east side of MacDonald Gate parking area.

This lengthwise exploration of Anthony Chabot Regional Park is the southernmost leg of the East Bay Skyline National Recreation Trail, using the MacDonald, Grass Valley, and Brandon trails. The Bay Area Ridge Trail also uses most of this route, leaving it near the end via the Willow View Trail. The beginning and end of this point-to-point route are mostly on open ridgetops, and the middle third passes through open Grass Valley and then enters mixed woodland on the slopes above Grass Valley Creek and Lake Chabot. In spring, wildflowers add color to the grasslands, and birds, especially hummingbirds, are everywhere.

From the east side of the parking area, you follow the MacDonald Trail, a dirt road shaded here by California bay and willow, and in about 100 yards pass a trail post and the Bird Trail, right. Just ahead, you cross a creek that flows under the road through a culvert, and begin to climb on a gentle and then moderate grade. Trees and shrubs in this beautiful, lush area include coast live oak, madrone, California sagebrush, creambush, and toyon. The route alternates between open and wooded areas as it winds uphill to the top of a ridge. French broom, bush monkeyflower, and blue bush lupine add color in spring and summer.

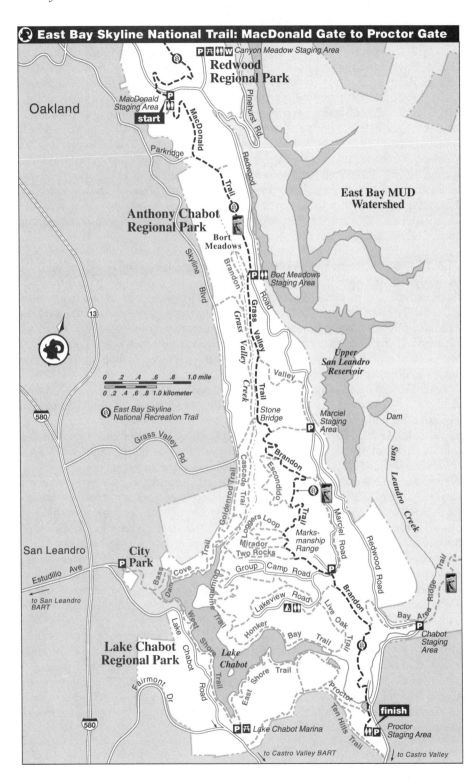

East Bay Skyline National Trail: MacDonald Gate to Proctor Gate

P A W Canyon Meadow Staging Area

Redwood Regional Park

Oakland

MacDonald Staging Area
start

Parkridge

MacDonald

Pinehurst Rd.

Redwood

East Bay MUD Watershed

Trail

Anthony Chabot Regional Park

Bort Meadows

Skyline Blvd

Brandon

P Bort Meadows Staging Area

13

Grass Valley

Grass Valley Creek

Valley

Trail

Road

Upper San Leandro Reservoir

0 .2 .4 .6 .8 1.0 mile
0 .2 .4 .6 .8 1.0 kilometer

East Bay Skyline National Recreation Trail

Stone Bridge

Marciel Staging Area

Dam

580

Grass Valley Rd.

Brandon

San Leandro Creek

Cascade Trail

Goldenrod Trail

Escondido

Trail

Marciel Road

Redwood Road

Loggers Loop

Marksmanship Range

San Leandro

City Park

Mirador
Two Rocks

Group Camp Road

P

Brandon

Estudillo Ave

Bass Cove

Columbine Trail

Lakeview Road

Live Oak Trail

Bay Area Ridge Trail

to San Leandro BART

West Shore Trail

Honker Bay Trail

P Chabot Staging Area

Lake Chabot Regional Park

Lake Chabot Road

Lake Chabot

East Shore Trail

Fairmont Dr

580

P A Lake Chabot Marina

Proctor

Ten Hills Trail

finish

Proctor Staging Area

to Castro Valley BART

to Castro Valley

Just before the ridgetop, a short, unsigned trail, left, leads to a bench, with a view of the hills above the Upper San Leandro Reservoir and a glimpse of Mount Diablo. Once atop the ridge the route maintains a mostly level course above a deep canyon, right, beyond which rises a forested slope dotted with private homes. At about the 1-mile point, you pass a road, right, leading to a residential area along Parkridge Road, off Skyline Blvd. Now the view improves dramatically, taking in the rest of this regional park and extending southeast all the way to the Sunol/Ohlone Wilderness, Mission Peak, and the Santa Cruz Mountains. Tall Monterey pines nearby make ideal perches for birds of prey such as the American kestrel, the smallest North American falcon. The route here is in the open, crossing rolling grassland studded with clumps of coyote brush. Soon you pass a path, left, that climbs a grassy hill to a viewpoint; continuing straight, you enjoy a superb vista that now includes EBMUD lands to the east and the high ground around Rocky Ridge.

Passing the Brittleleaf Trail, left, a short trail to a high point with a bench, you begin to descend over easy ground, soon reaching a gate. Along this route you will see unsigned paths leaving the main trail: ignore them. Passing through the gate, you now have a view of the Upper San Leandro Reservoir, left, nestled in a narrow valley. The route continues its descent via several sweeping bends, still along the crest of a ridge. You may be visited here by hummingbirds, especially if you are wearing red, and you may hear California quail calling from a valley, right. (You may also hear the annoying sound of rifle fire from the Chabot Marksmanship Range, which, thankfully, is closed Tuesday–Thursday.)

Reaching a sparsely wooded area—coast live oak, eucalyptus—you pass a grove of acacia trees, fragrant when in bloom, and then reach a gate. About 100 feet past the gate is a junction marked by a trail post. Here the MacDonald Trail, signed with emblems for the East Bay Skyline and Bay Area Ridge trails, continues straight. But your route, similarly signed, turns right, toward Bort Meadow and Grass Valley. Descend an eroded single-track trail a hundred yards or so to a junction, then turn left and follow the trail a short distance to reach a gravel road. Once on the road, turn left, toward Grass Valley, and in about 50 feet you reach a potentially confusing intersection, where one road heads left and uphill to the Bort Meadow staging area off Redwood Road, and another goes right, to a parking area and the Brandon Trail.

Continue straight across the intersection to a gate. Your route, the Grass Valley Trail, heads southeast past the gate and through Grass Valley, staying east of willow-lined Grass Valley Creek. (On a hot day, consider taking the Brandon Trail, a shaded route west of the creek; the two trails merge in about 1.5 miles at the Stone Bridge.)

Grass Valley, being wide and open, is a good place to observe birds that might otherwise stay hidden in trees. Depending on time of year, you may see gold-crowned sparrow, northern flicker, California towhee, and western scrub-jay. Listen for the repeated staccato call of the wrentit, often heard but seldom seen. After passing a cattle gate—Grass Valley is a grazing area—you begin to see a forest of tall eucalyptus, right; an occasional coast live oak gives the trail some much-needed shade on a hot day.

Passing the Redtail Trail, left, you soon enter a forest of eucalyptus, coast redwood, bigleaf maple, bay, and willow, with a tangled understory of poison oak and blackberry vines. Going through another gate and past a possibly muddy area, you reach a T-junction with the Brandon Trail, just a few feet east of the Stone Bridge, a shady rest stop at about the 4.3-mile point. Here you turn left on the Brandon Trail, part of the Lake Chabot Bicycle Loop (a circuit of either 12.42 or 14.41 miles, depending on choice of route).

Now on a moderate uphill grade, your route alternates between open areas and eucalyptus forest, some of which is being thinned to reduce fire danger and allow other species to thrive. Most of Chabot's eucalyptus trees were planted beginning in 1910 by People's Water Company, precursor to the East Bay Water Company, which was later incorporated into EBMUD. On a breezy day, you may enjoy the rustling of the eucalyptus leaves and the strange groaning sounds the trunks make when they rub against each other.

After its climb from the Stone Bridge, the Brandon Trail levels and tries to maintain a contour as it follows the indentations of a hillside above Grass Valley Creek. On this part of the route, you will pass a number of trails, including the Cottontail Trail and the unsigned start of the Escondido Trail. Stay on the obvious main road, which takes you from time to time past lovely patches of spring wildflowers, mostly California buttercup and blue-eyed grass, complimented by colorful clumps of bush monkeyflower, paintbrush, and lupine.

After the Brandon Trail turns uphill again, you pass the Deer Canyon Trail, left, a connector to the Redtail Trail. Here the Brandon Trail continues straight for a short level stretch, makes a sharp bend right, and then begins a gentle climb, giving you the first view so far of San Francisco and the Bay Bridge. Just before the 6-mile point, you pass the other end of the Escondido Trail, right, then walk through a heavily logged area where all the eucalyptus has been removed. The route swings sharply right, enters a wooded area, and soon passes a path, left, to the marksmanship range. (A sign here reads CAUTION DO NOT ENTER RIFLE RANGE; if the range is open, you will hear plenty of loud gunfire.)

Next you pass a road to the marksmanship range, clearly marked, and in 100 feet or so come to twin entrances, about 100 feet apart, to the Loggers Loop Trail, right. Staying on the Brandon Trail, you veer left and descend, crossing a creek, perhaps seasonal, over a culvert and reentering shade. In about 0.2 mile, you pass the other end of the Loggers Loop Trail and the Mirador Trail, both on the right. Another 0.2 mile brings you to the Two Rocks Trail and a fine vantage point for a view of San Francisco Bay. Here the Brandon Trail turns left and heads east across an open, grassy field speckled with California poppies.

Reaching a gate, you go through it and then cross paved Marciel Road, which runs from Marciel Gate on Redwood Road to Anthony Chabot Campground. Once across the road, continue straight through a paved parking area, past two information boards and a toilet, and onto a dirt path. About 30 feet farther you pass the Redtail Trail, left, and in another 40 feet or so reach a fenced dirt road, the continuation of the Brandon Trail. Pass through an opening in the fence and follow the road southeast on a mostly level grade, past coast live oak and bigleaf maple, to a junction, right, with the Towhee Trail.

Continuing straight, the Brandon Trail begins to lose elevation, and crosses an open area where spectacular views extend south to Hayward and the Coyote Hills, and east to Mt. Diablo. At about the 8-mile point, where a rest bench beckons from beneath a coast live oak, the Willow View Trail, part of the Bay Area Ridge Trail, heads left, and your route, the Brandon Trail, swings right.

The route continues to descend, mostly in the open, and now you can see down to Redwood Road and Willow Park Golf Course. To your right, beyond a steep drop-off, are the waters of Lake Chabot. Nearing the end of a ridge, the route makes gentle S-bends downhill, taking its time to reach the golf course. (The golf course, where you will find a restaurant, coffee shop, and bar, is the only place in the East Bay where you can get a cold beer a few paces off the trail.)

The Brandon Trail ends at the golf course parking area. To reach Proctor Gate, follow a dirt path that runs just left of and parallel to the golf course entrance road. Before reaching Redwood Road, cross the entrance road, and in about 50 feet you will pass a wooden shed and then come to a fork. Here you bear left and walk parallel to Redwood Road, which is left and just beyond a barbed-wire fence. In several hundred yards you pass an unsigned trail, right, but you continue straight, soon reaching the Proctor Gate entrance road. Turn right and walk about 200 feet to the parking area.

◆ Wildcat Canyon Regional Park ◆

SAN PABLO RIDGE

Length: 7 miles

Time: 3 to 4 hours

Rating: Difficult

Regulations: EBRPD; Havey Canyon is closed to bicycles and horses during wet weather.

Facilities: Toilets; at Alvarado Area are picnic tables and water, northwest of parking area.

Directions: From Interstate 80 eastbound in Richmond, take the Solano Ave. exit, which puts you on Amador St. Turn left and go 0.4 mile to McBryde Ave. Turn right and follow McBryde Ave. 0.2 mile, staying in the left lane as you approach a stop sign. (Use caution at this intersection; traffic from the right does not stop.) Continue straight, now on Park Ave., for 0.1 mile to the Alvarado staging area, left. The trailhead is at the east end of parking area.

From Interstate 80 westbound in San Pablo, take the McBryde Ave. exit, turn left onto McBryde Ave., go over the freeway and, from the intersection of McBryde Ave. and Amador St., follow the directions above.

This loop takes you from the lowlands of Wildcat Creek to the high, open slopes of San Pablo Ridge, using the Wildcat Creek, Havey Canyon, San Pablo Ridge, and Belgum trails, and Nimitz Way. You are rewarded for your efforts by

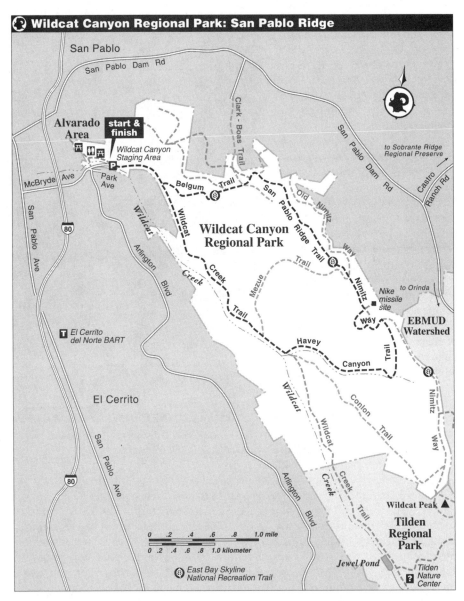

Wildcat Canyon Regional Park: San Pablo Ridge

some of the best views in the East Bay, including a 360-degree panorama from an old Nike missile site. Exposed to sun and wind for much of the way, this hike is best done when spring wildflowers bloom or after summer's heat has abated, when the hills are golden brown.

From the east end of the parking area, continue past a gate on pavement, the remnant of Wildcat Canyon Road, closed in the early 1980s by landslides. Renamed the Wildcat Creek Trail, the road, paved here and later dirt, runs southeast to the Environmental Education Center in Tilden Regional Park. Stay to the right and be alert for bikes. Parts of your loop—the Wildcat Creek, Belgum, and San Pablo Ridge trails and Nimitz Way—are used by the East Bay Skyline National Recreation Trail, a 31-mile route that starts here and ends in Anthony Chabot Regional Park.

The grasslands of the Berkeley Hills, which at one time supported large herds of cattle, horses, and sheep, have now been invaded by cardoon, a nonnative thistle related to the artichoke. A program is underway by EBRPD to control this pest, which is particularly rampant in this park. Other nonnatives flourishing by the side of the road include eucalyptus, cotoneaster, and French broom. Even the tall Monterey pines, planted throughout the East Bay hills, are not true natives, growing in the wild only on California's central coast, around Monterey, Año Nuevo, and Cambria.

As you make a gentle climb past coast live oak and willow, you reach a junction with the Belgum Trail, left, which you will

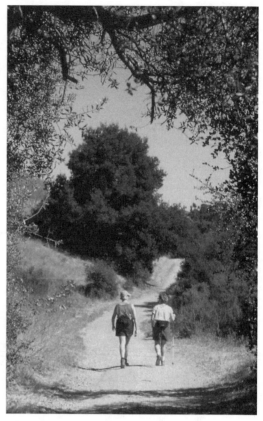

The Wildcat Creek Trail runs between Wildcat Canyon and Tilden regional parks.

use later to return. Continue straight, alternating on dirt and pavement, parallel to Wildcat Creek, right. The creek gets its start high on Tilden's Vollmer Peak, is interrupted by the impoundment that forms Lake Anza, and empties into San Pablo Bay north of the Richmond–San Rafael Bridge. Other trees and shrubs, objects of interest in an otherwise boring stretch of the route, include California bay, blue elderberry, coffeeberry, toyon, and evergreen huckleberry. Soon the pavement ends and you are walking on a dirt road between the tree-lined creek bed, right, and steep, open hills, left. At one point the route passes through a tunnel of overhanging coast live oak limbs, offering welcome shade on a hot day.

When the newly formed East Bay Regional Park District in 1935 acquired the southern part of Wildcat Canyon, which soon became Tilden Regional Park, from EBMUD, it left the northern part in the Utility District's hands, and in 1952 ownership of the land passed to private interests; there was even exploratory drilling by Standard Oil in 1966, which fortunately proved fruitless. In 1967 EBRPD bought a nucleus of 400 acres, and in the years that followed further acquisitions expanded the park to its current 2431-acre size.

At about the 2-mile point, you reach a junction with the Mezue Trail, climbing left. There is a drinking fountain here, and a watering trough for animals. Your route continues straight, but if you want a lovely glimpse of Wildcat Creek, shaded here by bay trees, turn right and walk downhill about 100 yards on a dirt path. Back on the Wildcat Creek Trail, you follow the line of willow, white alder, and western sycamore bordering the creek and soon pass Rifle Range Road, which leads right and crosses the creek on a bridge.

Now the route starts to climb, arriving soon at a junction with the Havey Canyon and Conlon trails. Here your route turns left up Havey Canyon, the farthest left of the trails at this junction. Now you follow a tributary of Wildcat Creek, left, into a shady area lush with bigleaf maple, California buckeye, and hazelnut. An understory of western creek dogwood, snowberry, vine honeysuckle, blackberry, and ferns gives a wild, almost jungle-like aspect to this dark, wooded canyon. You traverse an eroded section of trail, cross the tributary, and then go through a cattle gate. On a hot day the air here is fragrant with bay and eucalyptus.

As the route abruptly breaks into the open, you see the open slopes of San Pablo Ridge ahead, dotted with coyote brush and stunted coast live oak. As the route, now a dirt road, turns north, power lines ahead traverse your field of view, but to the west, on a clear day, Mt. Tamalpais is engraved on the unobstructed skyline. Redtailed hawks, aerial hunters looking for prey in the fields below, cruise overhead, while oblivious cows graze nearby. Passing through another cattle gate, you soon reach a T-junction, where you make a left turn on paved Nimitz Way, a popular route shared by hikers, horseback riders, bicyclists, in-line skaters, and joggers.

Now you get your first view of Mt. Diablo, east, and the Santa Cruz Mountains, south. As you wind uphill on a gentle grade toward an unnamed peak, the high points in Tilden Regional Park, topped by Vollmer Peak (1905'), appear to the southeast. San Francisco Bay, shimmering perhaps in late afternoon sunlight, leads your eye southwest to the Golden Gate Bridge. Colorful wildflowers decorate the grassy hillsides here in spring. As you near the summit, just over 1000 feet in elevation, you begin to see north toward San Pablo Bay, the Carquinez Strait, and Mt. St. Helena, a high peak on the border of Lake, Napa, and Sonoma counties.

When you reach a junction with a road heading right and uphill, take a few minutes to make the climb to an abandoned Nike missile site, a relic of the Cold War, which is perched above. You will be rewarded with a rest bench, 360-degree views, and a chance to reflect on the fact that, for most people, Nike is a name no longer associated with the fear of nuclear war. Now return to Nimitz Way, named for Chester W. Nimitz, the admiral who commanded the Pacific Fleet during World War II. After the war he lived in Berkeley and became a regent of the University of California, taking time to hike and sprinkle wildflower seeds along this road, according to Mimi Stein, author of EBRPD's official history, *A Vision Achieved*.

Now the pavement ends, and Nimitz Way continues as a dirt-and-gravel road. You go through a gate and have a view of San Pablo Reservoir, right and far below. At about the 4.5-mile point, you come to a cattle pen and a choice of three dirt paths. The right-hand path is Old Nimitz Way. The left-hand path is the Mezue Trail. The middle path, unnamed, rejoins the Mezue Trail a few hundred feet ahead. Bear left on the Mezue Trail, and after about 100 yards or so, bear right at a fork, where the Mezue Trail heads left and the San Pablo Ridge Trail goes right and uphill.

Now the route climbs up and over a series of high points on San Pablo Ridge, then plunges very steeply northwest to a junction with the Belgum Trail, a dirt road. A watering trough for animals is ahead. Turning left and leaving the San Pablo Ridge Trail, you climb past an active ground-squirrel colony, whose members may stand up to get a better look at the tired hikers marching past. Soon you pass the Clark–Boas Trail, right, and then an unsigned road cutting sharply left.

Now you climb to an unsigned fork, where you bear left, still following the Belgum Trail, a dirt road. The route now makes a well-graded descent, via S-bends, to a forest of coast live oak, bay, and eucalyptus, with a few palm trees and agaves thrown in for good measure. Nearby is the site of the former Belgum Grand Vista Sanitarium, named for its founder, Dr. Belgum. The facility, established in 1914, featured an elegant mansion with a farm, and was used to treat people with "nervous disorders." A gate ushers you onto a paved section, which you follow downhill to the junction with the Wildcat Creek Trail you passed earlier. (The Belgum mansion sat on a rise above this junction.) Turn right and retrace your route to the parking area.

◆ Tilden Regional Park ◆

One of EBRPD's original three holdings, this park is named for District founding father and first board president Major Charles Lee Tilden, a prominent civic leader, businessman, law-school graduate, and Spanish-American War veteran. The name was changed from Wildcat Canyon Park on Major Tilden's 79th birthday in 1936. As leader of EBRPD, Tilden had two goals: to acquire parklands before they were lost to development, and to do so without floating bond measures. To this end, he even advanced the District money to pay expenses until tax revenues arrived, and to purchase 60 acres of private land in Redwood Canyon, the nucleus of a future Redwood Regional Park. Tilden's 93rd birthday in 1950, like nine previous ones, was celebrated in the park's Brazil Building, a WPA stone building whose interior came from the 1939 World's Fair held on Treasure Island. On that occasion, a bronze bust of Major Tilden was unveiled, commemorating his public service.

The 2000 acres of rolling hills and forested ravines that became Tilden Regional Park had been used by ranchers and dairy farmers in bygone days. In the Depression, New Deal work projects brought roads, trails, and picnic sites to the new park. An old military tractor was used to construct an 18-hole championship golf course. During World War II, Tilden Regional Park, like Redwood, was used by the military: the Army ran survival training in the woods for its troops, and the Air Force used a windowless blockhouse in what is now the Tilden Service Yard as the "nerve center" for 15 radar stations. The Army returned the favor by maintaining trails, cutting trees, building bridges, and putting up signs. During the Cold War the Army returned, bringing Nike missiles via Nimitz Way to a site atop San Pablo Ridge.

In addition to its many miles of trails, Tilden Regional Park has other wonderful attractions. One of California's finest native plant gardens, Regional Parks Botanic Garden, is set on a 10-acre site at the junction of Wildcat Canyon Road and South Park Dr. Lake Anza, located in the middle of the park off Central Park Dr., is an artificial impoundment on Wildcat Creek with a public swimming beach and a lovely trail around its perimeter. Scattered throughout the park are several dozen picnic sites, many suitable for large groups and available by reservation.

At the north end of the park, in the Tilden Nature Area, are the Environmental Education Center, Little Farm, and Jewel Lake, reached by a self-guiding nature trail—all great places to take children. The Environmental Education Center has a display of Wildcat Creek ecology plus books, maps, and pamphlets. A separate map is available for the Tilden Nature Area, including the Jewel Lake, Pack Rat, Sylvan, Peak, Pine Tree, Laurel Canyon, and Memory trails. There is also a brochure for the self-guiding Jewel Lake Nature Trail, which may be borrowed or purchased for a small fee.

Bicycles in Tilden are allowed on these trails: Big Springs, Curran, Golf Course, Meadows Canyon, Nimitz, Quarry, Redwood, and Sea View. Bicycles are not allowed on these trails: Arroyo, Grizzly Peak, Lake Anza, Lupine, National, Selby, and Tower.

Bicycles in Tilden are allowed on the East Bay Skyline Trail, except between the Sea View Trail and the Steam Trains overflow parking lot. Bicycles are allowed on the Vollmer Peak Trail, except between the Steam Trains overflow parking lot and the north end of Tilden Corporation Yard. Bicycles are allowed on the Wildcat Gorge Trail from Lone Oak Road to the Curran Trail only during dry weather, and are not allowed on the Wildcat Gorge Trail from the Curran Trail to Anza View Road.

Botanic Garden: (510) 841-8732; 8:30 A.M. to 5 P.M. daily.

Environmental Education Center: (510) 525-2233; 10 A.M. to 5 P.M., closed Mondays, Thanksgiving, Christmas and New Year's Day.

Lake Anza: (510) 848-3028; open for swimming May through October.

Picnic reservations: (510) 636-1684

LAKE ANZA

Length: 1.4 miles

Time: 1 hour

Rating: Easy, but involves some scrambling over rocks.

Regulations: EBRPD

Facilities: Swimming, bath house, water, toilets, phone.

Directions: From Interstate 80 in Berkeley, take the University Ave. exit and go east 2.1 miles to Oxford St. Turn left and go 0.7 mile to Rose St. Turn right and go one block to Spruce St. Turn left and follow Spruce St. 1.8 miles to an intersection with Grizzly Peak Blvd. and Wildcat Canyon Road. Cross the intersection and immediately turn left from Wildcat Canyon Dr. onto Canon Dr. There is a sign here

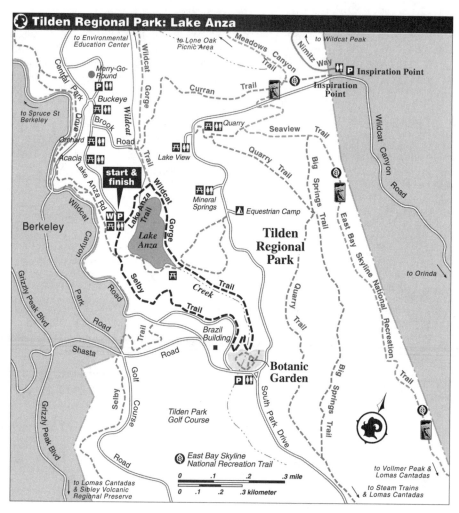

Tilden Regional Park: Lake Anza

for NATURE AREA, PONY RIDE, WILDCAT CANYON. Go downhill 0.3 mile to a junction with Central Park Dr., then turn right and go southeast 0.7 mile to Lake Anza Road. Turn left and go 0.3 mile to a large parking area. The trailhead is on the east side of the parking area, facing the lake.

From Highway 24 just east of the Caldecott Tunnel, take the Fish Ranch Road exit and go 1 mile uphill to a junction with Grizzly Peak Blvd. Turn right and go 5.4 miles to the intersection with Wildcat Canyon Road and Spruce St. mentioned above. Turn right onto Wildcat Canyon Road, then immediately left onto Canon Dr. From here follow the directions above.

Crowded with swimmers on warm weekends, Lake Anza and the surrounding woodlands can also offer a sample of East Bay solitude, provided you pick a quiet time to visit. This easy loop uses the Lake Anza, Wildcat Gorge, and Selby trails.

From the parking area, walk east and downhill on a paved path toward Lake Anza. Where the path branches to the bath house, right, turn left on the Lake Anza Trail, here a paved path that borders the lake, and walk north under coast redwood, white alder, willow, and coast live oak. At the next junction, turn right and cross a bridge over Wildcat Creek, home to native rainbow trout and California newts. The creek, which empties into San Pablo Bay north of the Richmond–San Rafael Bridge, gets its start high on the northwest flank of Vollmer Peak, then flows through Tilden's Botanic Garden into Lake Anza.

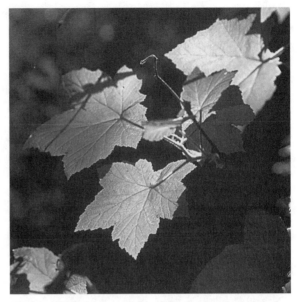

The broad, lobed leaves of thimbleberry identify this shade-loving shrub.

Now follow a wide dirt path on top of the dam that forms Lake Anza. Once across the dam, you meet two trails, one rising steeply uphill, the other turning right and hugging the lake shore. You turn right. Your route stays by the water's edge, crosses a narrow, rocky section beneath a steep cliff, left, and then enters a eucalyptus grove from where you can look across the lake to the popular swimming beach.

California bay trees form the next grove, where the route passes up and over the first of several rocky ribs jutting into the lake. Near the southeast corner of the lake, you scramble through a notch in the final rib and step down over some rock ledges near where Wildcat Creek flows into the lake. Here the Lake Anza Trail veers right, and the Wildcat Gorge Trail goes straight. (To shorten the trip, turn right, cross a bridge, and follow the lake shore back to the parking area.)

Stay on the creek's left side and walk upstream on the narrow and rocky Wildcat Gorge Trail, a shady route that rises abruptly to avoid rock outcrops and large bay trees, then drops steeply to the creek. This small canyon, where the sound of running water accompanies your footfalls, is home to shrubs such as thimbleberry, snowberry, and western creek dogwood, and its shaded slopes provide fertile ground for ferns.

After crossing the creek on a wooden bridge, the route begins to climb across a steep hillside and head west, past a sign for the Brazil Building, which is left and uphill. Now in the realm of bays, their trunks curved and twisted, you begin a gradual descent and soon come to a level clearing with picnic tables and a trail post. Here, at about the 1-mile point, the Wildcat Gorge Trail ends and you join the

Selby Trail by going straight. (The Selby Trail also climbs left from here to Wildcat Canyon and Shasta roads.)

On a wide dirt path littered with eucalyptus leaves and strips of bark, you pass through a shrubby area of coyote brush, hazelnut, rose bushes, and blackberry vines. Descending on a moderate grade, you soon you come to a flat spot under a tall Monterey pine, near Lake Anza's beach area, which is just behind a fence. Turn right on a dirt path, then left on the Lake Anza Trail, heading for the bath house and keeping the fence close on your right. Beyond a grove of redwoods you come to the bath house. Now follow the paved path to the parking area.

WILDCAT PEAK

Length: 3.3 miles

Time: 1.5 to 2 hours

Rating: Moderate

Regulations: EBRPD; no horses, bicycles, or dogs.

Facilities: Visitor center with displays, books, maps, guided walks, helpful staff; picnic tables, water, restrooms, phone.

Directions: From Interstate 80 in Berkeley, take the University Ave. exit and go east 2.1 miles to Oxford St. Turn left and go 0.7 mile to Rose St. Turn right and go one block to Spruce St. Turn left and follow Spruce St. 1.8 miles to an intersection with Grizzly Peak Blvd. and Wildcat Canyon Road. Cross the intersection and immediately turn left from Wildcat Canyon Road onto Canon Dr. There is a sign here for NATURE AREA, PONY RIDE, WILDCAT CANYON. Go downhill 0.3 mile to a junction with Central Park Dr. Turn left and go 0.1 mile to a large parking area. The trail begins at the Environmental Education Center, which is a short walk north from the parking area on a paved path.

From Highway 24 just east of the Caldecott Tunnel, take the Fish Ranch Road exit and go 1 mile uphill to a junction with Grizzly Peak Blvd. Turn right and go 5.4 miles to the intersection with Wildcat Canyon Road and Spruce St. Turn right onto Wildcat Canyon Road, then immediately left onto Canon Dr. There is a sign here for NATURE AREA, PONY RIDE, WILDCAT CANYON. Go downhill 0.3 mile to a junction with Central Park Dr. Turn left and go 0.1 mile to a large parking area. The trail begins at the Environmental Education Center, which is a short walk north from the parking area on a paved path.

This scenic loop hike takes you from the Tilden Park Environmental Education Center to the summit of Wildcat Peak via the Jewel Lake, Sylvan, Peak, and Laurel Canyon trails. Terrific views of the Bay Area and a variety of plants and birds keep this route interesting throughout. This route may be very muddy in wet weather.

Go through the Environmental Education Center and from its back deck walk north across the lawn, following a sign for the Jewel Lake Nature Trail and a trail post with the Jewel Lake emblem, a duck with upraised wings. Around you are stands of Monterey pine, coast live oak, eucalyptus, and California bay. After following the Jewel Lake Trail, a single track, for about 100 yards, you come to a dirt road. Cross it and walk ahead about 50 yards on a wide dirt path until you come to a trail post and a trail veering left. This post has the Jewel Lake emblem, and also emblems for other trails in the Nature Area—Sylvan (three trees), Laurel Canyon (a leaf), and Pine (a single conifer). Both the Jewel Lake and Sylvan trails are left; the Laurel Canyon and Pine Tree trails are right.

Turn left and follow the Jewel Lake Trail as it crosses two small streambeds on wooden planks, and then a larger streambed on a wooden bridge. If the trail is muddy, you may see animal tracks here, especially deer. Just after the bridge, you walk up a few wooden steps and reach a junction marked by another trail post. From here the Jewel Lake Trail climbs steeply on more wooden steps to the left, but your route, the Sylvan Trail, heads right. The trail post also has the emblem for the Peak Trail (a rounded hill), which you will reach in a few minutes.

Turn right and follow the Sylvan Trail as it makes an easy climb through groves of eucalyptus, bay, and coast live oak, with underbrush of coyote brush and poison oak. The route begins to switchback uphill, in places climbing steps made of railroad ties. After about 0.3 mile you come to Loop Road. Crossing this dirt road, you find the continuation of the Sylvan Trail heading northwest: a trail post here has emblems for the Sylvan and Peak trails. Follow the trail as it crosses an open hillside, then returns to eucalyptus forest.

This forest is a good place to study eucalyptus, an Australian tree introduced to the Bay Area in the 1850s and planted extensively in the East Bay at the turn of the century as part of an ill-fated timber scheme. Although fast growing, the species most commonly planted here proved worthless unless seasoned and dried carefully over a long time, thus dashing the hopes of would-be timber barons for a quick profit on their investments. But the trees thrived, despite fires and frost, and are now considered, at best, a mixed blessing.

Blue gum and red gum eucalyptus, the two most common species in California, shed strips and flakes of bark to allow for a rapid increase in trunk diameter. Notice the difference between the blue-gray leaves on young eucalyptus and the green leaves on adult trees. Leaves on the young, short trees are broad and flat, perfect for absorbing sunlight in dense shade; but leaves on tall adult trees, exposed to the hot sun, are narrow and hang vertically to minimize evaporation and conserve water. If it's breezy, listen to the rustle of the adult leaves in the wind, and the weird groaning sounds the trees make as they rub against each other.

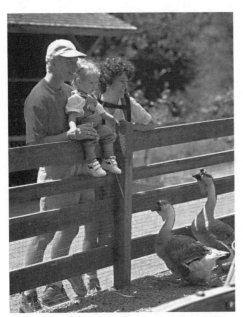

The Little Farm, sure to please children, is near the Tilden Environmental Education Center.

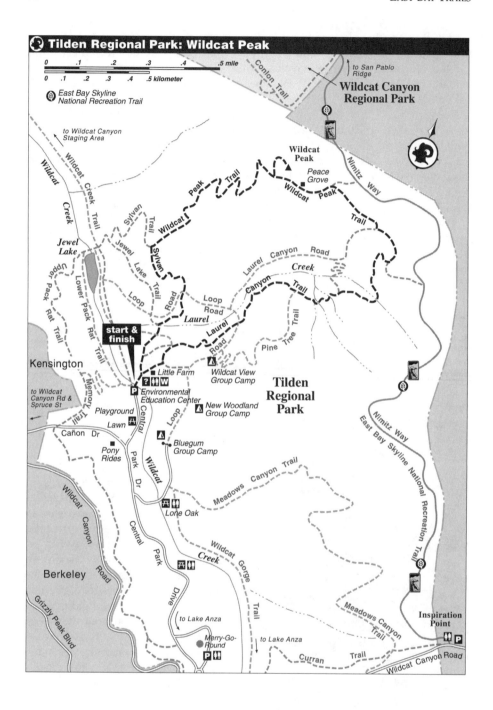

Tilden Regional Park: Wildcat Peak

0   .1   .2   .3   .4   .5 mile
0   .1   .2   .3   .4   .5 kilometer

East Bay Skyline
National Recreation Trail

to San Pablo
Ridge

**Wildcat Canyon
Regional Park**

to Wildcat Canyon
Staging Area

Conlon Trail

Wildcat Creek Trail

Wildcat Creek

Jewel Lake

Sylvan Trail

Jewel Lake Loop

Upper Pack Rat Trail

Lower Pack Rat Trail

Wildcat Peak Trail

Wildcat Peak

Peace Grove

Nimitz Way

Sylvan Trail

Sylvan Road

Loop Road

Laurel Canyon Road

Laurel Canyon Creek Trail

Creek

start & finish

Laurel Road

Pine Tree Trail

Kensington

to Wildcat
Canyon Rd &
Spruce St

Memory Trail

Little Farm

Environmental
Education Center

Wildcat View
Group Camp

**Tilden
Regional
Park**

Central Park Dr

Loop

New Woodland
Group Camp

Playground

Cañon Dr

Lawn

Pony Rides

Bluegum
Group Camp

Wildcat

Wildcat Canyon Road

Berkeley

Grizzly Peak Blvd

Central Park Drive

Meadows Canyon Trail

Lone Oak

Wildcat Creek

Wildcat Gorge Trail

Meadows Canyon Trail

Nimitz Way
East Bay Skyline National Recreation Trail

to Lake Anza

Merry-Go-Round

to Lake Anza

Curran Trail

**Inspiration
Point**

After about 0.5 mile you reach a junction, where the Sylvan Trail swings left. Your route, the Peak Trail, heads right and uphill, through groves of eucalyptus and twisted coast live oaks. In late summer or early fall you may find California fuchsia, a bright red wildflower that attracts hummingbirds, in bloom here beside the trail. Although you are climbing steadily, the grade is easy. The trail narrows as it passes under power lines, then breaks into an open area where willow, blue elderberry, and coffeeberry grow beside the trail, along with thickets of blackberry, coyote brush, and poison oak. In summer and fall the nearby slopes are decorated with asters, bush monkeyflower, California poppies, and lupine in bloom. You may see red-tailed and red-shouldered hawks overhead or hear their plaintive cries, and western scrub-jays, guardians of the forest, are sure to sound their raucous alarms if they detect your presence.

Each switchback brings better views, rewarding your uphill effort. Northeast is your goal for today, Wildcat Peak. West and southwest, most of the Bay Area is revealed: San Francisco, Oakland, Alcatraz and Angel islands, the Golden Gate, Bay, and Richmond–San Rafael bridges, and Mt. Tamalpais. In places the trail hugs a hillside of steep cliffs, with a steep drop to your left. Soon an unsigned trail merges from the left, but you follow the Peak Trail as it bends right and climbs toward Wildcat Peak.

At about the 1.4-mile point you reach a T-junction. Here you turn left and climb a short distance to the summit of Wildcat Peak (1250') and the Rotary Peace Monument, a circular stone wall. To the east are San Pablo and Briones reservoirs, along with the hulking form of Mt. Diablo on the horizon. Southeast is Vollmer Peak, at 1913 feet the high point in Tilden Regional Park. Northwest are the high hills of San Pablo Ridge in Wildcat Canyon Regional Park, linked to Tilden by several routes, including paved Nimitz Way.

A grove of young giant sequoias, called the Rotary Peace Grove, sits directly below and east of Wildcat Peak's summit, but the metal plaque describing this grove is, for some reason, on the west side of the summit's stone monument. Because these trees are out of their habitat, they will never attain giant status like their cousins in Yosemite and Sequoia parks. More sequoias, along with Monterey pines and eucalyptus, have been planted along Nimitz Way. After spending time on the summit, retrace your steps to the last junction, then continue straight and downhill on the Peak Trail, here a dirt road.

Soon you pass the Rotary Peace Grove, left, and reach a junction, just before Nimitz Way, where the Peak Trail turns sharply right and downhill. This junction is marked by a trail post which has the Peak Trail emblem on its downhill side. Here you turn right and follow Peak Trail, now a single track, as it winds east through stands of eucalyptus, pines, and coyote brush. After a short steep section the route levels, takes you across an open hillside, and then brings you via a few short switchbacks to unsigned Laurel Canyon Road. (The Laurel Canyon Trail, which you reach at the next junction, may be difficult in wet weather. For an alternate descent, turn right on Laurel Canyon Road, go downhill to Loop Road, and follow the directions below.)

Turn left on Laurel Canyon Road and go about 0.1 mile to the edge of a large pine grove, at about the 2-mile point. Here you turn right on the Laurel Canyon Trail, a shady single track that descends through a beautiful forested canyon, where blackberry vines and thimbleberry clog the hillsides, giving color in the fall.

The trail hangs on the steep edge of Laurel Canyon: use caution! The summit of Wildcat Peak, where you stood just a few minutes ago, is visible west across the canyon. Stop and listen—you may hear the "dee dee dee" call of a chickadee or the rustling sound that betrays a towhee scraping in the dry leaves.

Soon you come to a small bridge that takes you across Laurel Creek. Ferns are abundant in this cool, shady area, along with blue elderberry and snowberry. You are now on the south side of Laurel Canyon, which drops steeply right, walking west on a level trail. This is one of the prettiest sections of Tilden Park, away from the hustle and bustle of the more popular areas. Here you may find bush monkeyflower, hazelnut, and beautiful, big, twisted coast live oaks.

Now passing a trail to Laurel Canyon Road, right, you follow the Laurel Canyon Trail as it turns left and continues downhill on a moderate grade. After about 100 yards, the route bends sharply right at a trail post, dips twice to cross tributaries of Laurel Creek, and then emerges from forest into a clearing overgrown with grasses and blackberry vines. Where the Pine Tree Trail heads uphill to the left, you continue straight and descend on an eroded section of trail through a dense stands of bay and coast live oak. Here you can enjoy a solitude that belies the park's proximity to a large, metropolitan area. Several downhill switchbacks followed by a climb on wooden steps bring you to another small wooden bridge. On a sunny day, notice the dappled effect the light makes as it filters through the trees.

At Loop Road, you turn left and walk uphill. After about 100 feet, look for the continuation of the Laurel Canyon Trail, marked by a trail post, heading right and downhill. Here you begin an easy descent through eucalyptus and coast live oak, enjoying the fragrance of the trees and perhaps a serenade from twittering flocks of dark-eyed juncos. In fall, poison oak brightens this area with its yellow and red leaves. Soon you cross a streambed and descend via wooden steps to several small wooden bridges. When you reach a dirt road, turn left and walk uphill, past an unsigned trail heading right. Just ahead is the fence at the corner of Little Farm. When you reach the fence, turn right and go downhill for about 0.2 mile to the visitor center.

◆ Sibley Volcanic Regional Preserve ◆

ROUND TOP LOOP

Length: 1.6 miles

Time: 1 to 2 hours

Rating: Easy

Regulations: EBRPD; no bicycles on the Round Top Loop Trail between the quarry pit and the visitor center.

Facilities: Visitor center with exhibits explaining the area's volcanic past, as well as its plant and wildlife communities; water, toilets.

Directions: From Highway 24 just east of the Caldecott Tunnel, take the Fish Ranch Road exit and go uphill 1 mile to Grizzly Peak Blvd. Turn left and go 2.5

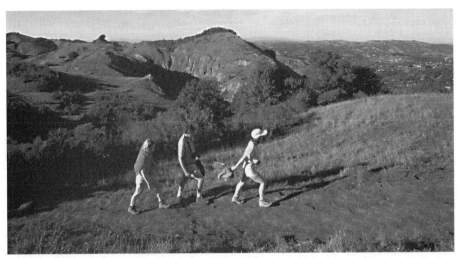

The Round Top Loop Trail explores part of Sibley Volcanic Regional Preserve.

miles to Skyline Blvd. Turn left and go 0.1 mile to the preserve entrance, left. The trailhead is at the north side of parking area.

This delightful loop circles Round Top, an extinct volcano and one of the highest peaks in the Oakland and Berkeley hills, and also provides access to a volcanic area that will be of interest to geology buffs. The preserve, named for Robert Sibley, director and president of EBRPD from 1948 to 1958, is one of the oldest East Bay regional parks. Originally called Roundtop, it was dedicated in 1936, just two years after the District was formed. The preserve was enlarged to its present size by additions of old Kaiser Sand and Gravel quarry sites. The Sibley Volcanic Regional Preserve brochure and map, available free at the visitor center, has descriptions that correspond to numbered posts on the self-guiding Volcanic Trail. Because this is a short and easy hike, you may also have time to visit nearby Huckleberry Botanic Regional Preserve, just 0.4 mile south on Skyline Blvd.

Although the terms "rock solid" and "on firm ground" are common figures of speech, anyone who has spent much time in California knows that the terra here can sometimes be less than firma. As you hike this enjoyable loop around Round Top (1763'), remember that it once was an active volcano—there are three other former volcanoes nearby—and that the surrounding hills were created by unimaginable forces acting along nearby fault lines. The volcanic activity took place approximately 10 million years ago, but occasional moving and shaking, sometimes violent, continues to this day.

The trailhead here serves several trails: the Round Top Loop and Volcanic trails, joined as one at first; and the East Bay Skyline/Bay Area Ridge Trail. As you approach the visitor center from the parking area, there is a paved road, right, which goes to the summit of Round Top, and another, left, that goes around the west side of the center. Follow the left-hand road to a junction just past the center and just before a gate across the road. Here a single-track trail heads right and uphill, marked by a trail post reading TO ROUNDTOP LOOP TRAIL, TO VOLCANIC TRAIL,

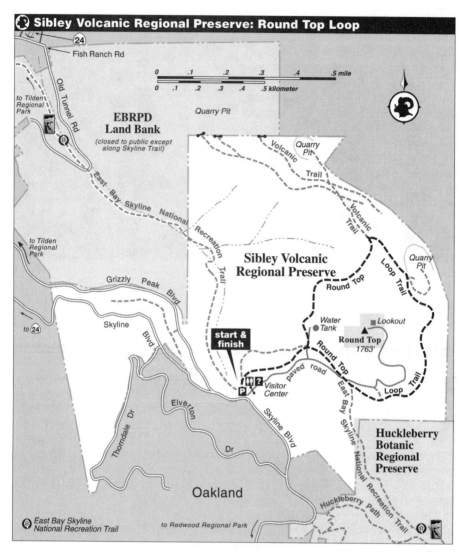

and a sign indicating that this trail, which reaches Redwood Regional Park in 2.9 miles, is part of the East Bay Skyline/Bay Area Ridge Trail.

Bear right and climb through a wooded area with stands of California bay, Monterey pine, and eucalyptus. As you contour along a steep embankment, past coyote brush, toyon, poison oak, and coffeeberry, the paved road to Round Top's antenna-topped summit is right and downhill. Just before coming to a clearing, you pass a junction, left, with a trail that leads back to the visitor center. In another 100 feet or so, you reach a four-way junction, marked by a trail post, where you turn left onto a wide dirt-and-gravel road that heads north and then northeast into the volcanic area.

Ahead are grassy hills, deep valleys, and rolling ridges, a tranquil scene that masks this area's violent volcanic birth. A mostly level walk over rocky ground takes you around the west and north sides of Round Top to a T-junction, where the Volcanic Trail heads left, and the Round Top Loop Trail continues right. Turning right and walking uphill, you soon come to a wonderful viewpoint above a quarry pit, 4, left, with Mt. Diablo looming on the eastern skyline. Quarry operations here from the 1930s to the 1960s dug into the side of Round Top, exposing the basalt lava interior of the volcano, to the delight of geologists. Because of its bulk and shape, Mt. Diablo could be mistaken for a volcano as well, but it is not, having been formed instead by a mass of rock pushing upward through sedimentary layers.

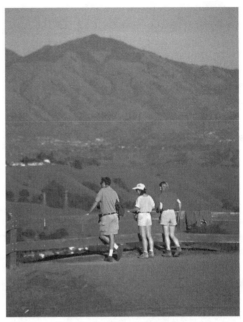

Hikers enjoy view of Mt. Diablo from quarry pit overlook on Round Top Loop Trail.

Just past the viewpoint, the continuation of the Round Top Loop Trail, here a dirt path, leaves the road, heads right and uphill, and makes a rising traverse across the grassy east side of Round Top. As you follow the trail into an area dense with bay, pine, blue elderberry, and coffeeberry, you soon reach the crest of a low ridge, where a side trail, left, offers access to another east-facing viewpoint. Continuing on the main trail, you descend to a cattle gate, and now enjoy the shade of a pine, madrone, and eucalyptus forest, where, on a sunny day, golden light filters through the trees.

The route swings west and comes to an open area, then reaches an unsigned fork where you bear left. (If instead you go right, you reach Round Top Road, the route to the peak's summit.) Soon you pass a grove of oneseed hawthorn, a beautiful tree with smooth gray bark, thorny branches, and deeply lobed leaves. This hawthorn, which flowers white in the spring and produces red berries in the fall, is originally from Europe, North Africa, and western Asia, but was brought to America as a cultivated species.

The trail next passes through a corridor of stately pines, meeting the East Bay Skyline/Bay Area Ridge Trail, a trail that goes left to Huckleberry Regional Preserve and beyond. Continue straight, and in about 125 feet, you arrive at Round Top Road. Cross the paved road and follow the Round Top Loop Trail as it reenters the pines, here joined by madrone, coast live oak, and eucalyptus. Coming to a clearing, you now cross the paved road leading uphill to the EBMUD water tank, and, in about 25 feet, reach the four-way junction with the dirt-and-gravel road to the volcanic area. From this junction, continue straight—staying left at an upcoming fork—and retrace your steps to the parking area.

◆Huckleberry Botanic Regional Preserve ◆

HUCKLEBERRY NATURE PATH

Length: 1.9 miles

Time: 1 to 2 hours

Rating: Easy

Regulations: EBRPD; no bicycles, dogs, or horses.
Facilities: Toilet.
Directions: From Highway 24 just east of the Caldecott Tunnel, take the Fish Ranch Road exit and go uphill 1 mile to a junction with Grizzly Peak Blvd. Turn left and go 2.5 miles to a junction with Skyline Blvd. Turn left and go 0.5 mile to a parking area, left. The trailhead is on the southeast side of parking area.

This easy, self-guiding loop through a 240-acre botanical treasure trove is simply not to be missed, especially from late winter through spring, when its shrubs and flowers are in bloom. Among the highlights are two rare plants: western leatherwood, which is hard to find elsewhere in the East Bay; and pallid, or Alameda, manzanita, found only here and in Sobrante Ridge Botanic Regional Preserve, near El Sobrante. **Boldface** numbers in the route description refer to numbered markers along the trail and plant descriptions in "Huckleberry Self-Guided Nature Path," an interpretive pamphlet available at the trailhead. Because this is a short and easy hike, you may also have time to visit nearby Sibley Volcanic Regional Preserve, just 0.4 mile north on Skyline Blvd.

While a walk in the woods is always enjoyable, Huckleberry Botanic Regional Preserve offers much more: a chance to see and learn about a wide variety of native plants, some only found in a few areas of the East Bay. The soil in parts of the preserve is rocky and lacks nutrition for all but the hardiest chaparral species, such as manzanita. Establishing itself on "barrens," manzanita helps create soil that is then hospitable to other shrubs and trees, a process called "plant succession." As you start out on the dirt hiking trail, pick up a copy of the pamphlet, "Huckleberry Self-Guided Nature Path," published by EBRPD. Keyed to the numbered posts along the trail, this pamphlet will help you identify more than a dozen native plants.

About 100 yards past the trailhead, the Huckleberry Path forks: descend left on a series of switchbacks through a fragrant forest of California bay and coast live oak. Evergreen huckleberry, the plant that gives this park its name, is here, along with two other berry producers, blackberry and blue elderberry. Soon you come to a large madrone, **1**, an evergreen tree with smooth, reddish bark and finely-toothed elliptical leaves. Related to and sometimes mistaken for manzanita, madrone in spring produces lovely white flowers and in fall red berries which are eaten by birds. Also in this area are toyon, vine honeysuckle, and bush monkeyflower.

A short walk brings you to hazelnut, **2**, a relative of the commercial filbert. The bright green leaves of this shrub, renewed each spring, feel like pieces of soft felt. When you come to the next fork, bear right and begin to climb; here the

Huckleberry Path joins the East Bay Skyline/Bay Area Ridge Trail, on its way between Sibley Volcanic Regional Preserve and Redwood Regional Park. Be sure to scan the ground for spring wildflowers, such as columbine, as you walk.

Thriving in damp areas beneath California bay and coast live oak is western sword fern, **3**. Long, pointed fronds give this fern its name and distinguish it from wood fern, **4**. To compare the two, find the wood fern, then look across the trail for western sword fern growing on the downhill slope. Now the route swings left to contour around a bulge in a ridge, then continues its southeast course and arrives at a grove of large bay trees, **5**. Here the towering bays have established dominance by depriving their would-be competitors of sunlight. Just past this grove is a junction; here the East Bay Skyline/Bay Area Ridge Trail continues straight, but your route, the Huckleberry Path, climbs steeply right via wooden steps and switchbacks.

At about the 1-mile point, after a short climb, you reach a T-junction with the upper segment of the Huckleberry Path. Turn right, and almost immediately come to a junction, **6**. Turn right again and climb a rocky path to a manzanita barren—a dry, gravelly plateau in the early stage of succession from manzanita to huckleberry. Also here are canyon live oak and chinquapin, two plants described in the brochure as numbers 10 and 13. From this perch your views range northwest to Round Top, one of the highest summits in the Oakland and Berkeley hills, and east to Mt. Diablo, the highest peak in the East Bay.

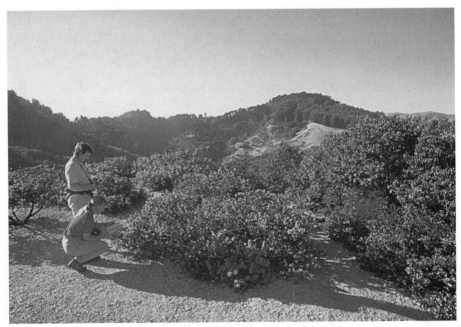

This botanic preserve is an excellent place to study native East Bay plants, including some that are rare and extremely localized. Here, hikers examine manzanita and other shrubs growing on one of the area's manzanita "barrens," which are dry, rocky areas of poor soil.

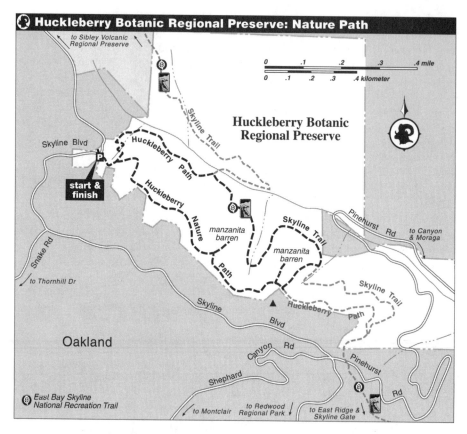

Huckleberry Botanic Regional Preserve: Nature Path

Back at the main path, you turn right and continue on a shady, rolling course to search for the lavender-to-blue flowers of Douglas iris, **7,** a spring bloomer. At about the 1.3-mile point, turn right at a junction and descend on a side trail through the woods to find markers **8, 9,** and **10.** As you begin walking on this trail, look for a short path leading right and downhill to a rare shrub called western leatherwood, **8.** The yellow flowers of this shrub, which gets its name from the flexibility of the wood, appear in the winter, when its branches are still bare. Climb back to the side trail, turn right, and walk to another manzanita barren, where you will find jim-brush, **9,** and canyon live oak, **10.**

Now retrace your steps to the main trail, where you turn right. Walking past stands of huckleberry, **11,** you soon reach an area, **12,** where the plants are in an intermediate stage of succession. Here manzanitas are being replaced by other, faster-growing plants, such as huckleberry and chinquapin, **13.** Two types of manzanita grow along this exposed stretch of trail: brittleleaf, **14,** and pallid, **15.** Pallid manzanita is rare, growing only in this preserve and Sobrante Ridge Botanic Regional Preserve, an area described elsewhere in this book. Brittleleaf manzanita is a small shrub with a burl, or knot, at its base and stiff-pointy leaves with stems. Pallid manzanita is a large shrub whose gray-green leaves tightly clasp its reddish branches, attaching with hardly any stem.

In addition to its notable plants, this preserve is home to many birds. Two species here are often heard rather than seen—wrentit and bushtit. The wrentit's song, given year-round, sounds like someone trying, without luck, to start a car: a series of sharp notes and then a trill. This sparrow-sized brown bird, a member of the thrush family, is usually alone or with a mate. Bushtits, tiny gray birds belonging to their own family, travel in swarms and make high-pitched twittering sounds from the tree limbs where they feed.

A bit farther, you come to coast silk tassel, **16,** a shrub with stiff, curly leaves that are shiny green on top, gray-green underneath. The tassel in its name refers to the flower clusters hanging in winter from male plants. The route now descends via wooden steps into a dense bay forest, where you may hear a spotted towhee rustling in the leaf litter, and then levels in an area where you can see pinkflower currant, **17.** This beautiful shrub dangles its delicate flowers from bare branches in the winter, then produces fresh green leaves that are somewhat sticky. Just past marker 17 you reach a junction; here you continue straight and retrace your route to the parking area.

⬥ Redwood Regional Park ⬥

Redwood Regional Park is a land of ghosts. The stately trees that tower over the park's steep hillsides and shady canyons are second-growth descendants of a vanished race of giants, *Sequoia sempervirens*, or coast redwood, originally found along the coast of Oregon and California. In their prime, if allowed to grow undisturbed for hundreds of years, redwoods become the tallest trees on Earth, reaching skyward more than 300 feet and growing to a diameter of 10 to 15 feet, sometimes larger. Ring counts have found trees more than 2000 years old, and when a redwood dies or is cut, new trees sprout in a circle around their ancestor. European settlers coming to the West Coast nearly wiped out the redwoods, and today only isolated pockets of virgin forest remain on federal, state, and private lands.

But there are other ghosts here too, shades of rough and rowdy loggers who, in the years from 1840 to 1860, managed to fell nearly every old-growth tree in the East Bay's redwood forest, including two trees so prominent they were used as points of reference by mariners entering the Golden Gate, 16 miles away. At least 10 sawmills operated in the area, including four within or near the park's current boundaries, supplying lumber to fuel the building boom that followed California's gold rush. After the loggers had done their work, an Alameda physician and botanist, Dr. William Gibbons, found 2000 redwood stumps, some of them 20 feet in diameter, the remains, he wrote, of what "must have constituted the most magnificent forest on the continent." Another visitor to this scene of devastation was John Muir.

This 1831-acre park has been the hub of much other human activity as well. After the loggers came woodcutters, who removed redwood stumps and even roots for firewood. After the 1906 earthquake, young redwood trees were cut for timber to rebuild San Francisco. Farming and ranching took place here, and as you walk the trails you may see fruit trees, remnants of old orchards. At the end of the

Depression, WPA workers built roads, trails, and four stone huts near the banks of Redwood Creek. During World War II the park was used by Naval Air Cadets for survival training and by a grave-registration training battalion as a practice cemetery. The line between Alameda and Contra Costa counties neatly bisects Redwood Park, attesting to the importance each county placed, when they split in 1853, on getting an equal share of the valuable trees.

Although Redwood Regional Park, dedicated in 1939, was officially the fourth member of the East Bay Regional Park District's fledgling system, in some ways it was actually the first. During the difficult negotiations that took place in the mid-1930s to acquire EBMUD's surplus land, the District's first board president, civic leader and businessman Major Charles Lee Tilden, advanced his own money to buy 60 acres of private land in Redwood Canyon for $35 per acre, a Depression-era bargain price. This helped get the ball rolling for the 1936 purchase of the first three regional parks—Lake Temescal, Roundtop (now Sibley Volcanic Regional Preserve), and Wildcat Canyon, soon renamed Tilden Regional Park.

EAST RIDGE

Length: 6 miles

Time: 3 to 4 hours

Rating: Moderate

Regulations: EBRPD; fees for parking and dogs when entrance kiosk is attended; no bicycles on Stream Trail from Skyline Gate to Trail's End picnic area.

Facilities: Picnic tables, water, toilet, phone near the trailhead; water, toilet, phone at Skyline Gate; water, toilets, and picnic tables along the Stream Trail; horse staging at the Wayside parking area, about 0.3 mile before the Canyon Meadow staging area.

Directions: From Interstate 580 eastbound in Oakland, take the 35th Ave. exit, turn left and follow 35th Ave. east into the hills. After 0.8 mile 35th Ave. becomes Redwood Road, and at 2.4 miles it crosses Skyline Blvd., where you stay in the left lane and go straight. At 4.6 miles from Interstate 580 you reach the park entrance; turn left and go 0.5 mile to the Canyon Meadow staging area. The trailhead is at the northwest end of the parking area.

From Interstate 580 westbound in Oakland, take the Warren Freeway/Berkeley/Highway 13 exit and go 0.9 mile to the Carson St./Redwood Road exit. From the stop sign at the end of the exit ramp, continue straight, now on Mountain Blvd., 0.2 mile, and bear right onto Redwood Road. Go 3.2 miles to the park entrance; turn left and go 0.5 mile to the Canyon Meadow staging area. The trailhead is at the northwest end of the parking area.

From Highway 13 southbound, take the Redwood Road/Carson St. exit, turn left onto Redwood Road and follow the directions above.

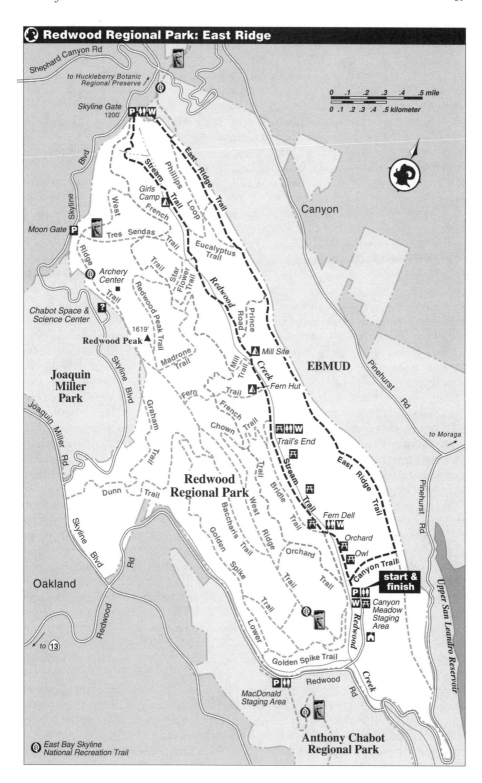

Redwood Regional Park: East Ridge

Shephard Canyon Rd

to Huckleberry Botanic
Regional Preserve

Skyline Gate
1200'

0   .1   .2   .3   .4   .5 mile

0   .1   .2   .3   .4   .5 kilometer

Skyline Blvd

Phillips Loop Trail

East Ridge Trail

Girls
Camp

French Trail

Canyon

Moon Gate

Tres Sendas

Eucalyptus Trail

Skyline Ridge Trail

West Ridge Trail

Redwood Road

Prince Road

Archery
Center

Star Flower Trail

Chabot Space &
Science Center

Redwood Peak Trail

1619'

Redwood Peak

Mill Site

Fern Hut

EBMUD

Pinehurst Rd

**Joaquin
Miller
Park**

Madrone
Trail

Mill Trail

Creek

Fern Trail

French Trail

Trail's End

to Moraga

Joaquin Miller Rd

Graham Trail

Chown Trail

Stream Trail

East Ridge Trail

Pinehurst Rd

**Redwood
Regional Park**

Dunn Trail

West Ridge Trail

Bridle Trail

Fern Dell

Orchard

Owl

Baccharis Trail

Orchard Trail

Canyon Trail

**start &
finish**

Oakland

Skyline Blvd

Redwood Rd

Golden Spike Trail

Canyon
Meadow
Staging
Area

Upper San Leandro Reservoir

to ⑬

Lower Trail

Golden Spike Trail

Redwood Creek

Redwood Rd

MacDonald
Staging Area

Redwood

**Anthony Chabot
Regional Park**

East Bay Skyline
National Recreation Trail

This loop, using the East Ridge and Stream trails, pairs a vigorous hike along an exposed ridge with a secluded downhill ramble in the shade of tall redwoods, an unbeatable combination. Views from the East Ridge Trail, especially of the surrounding East Bay parklands, are superb, and the redwood forest along Redwood Creek, though merely a shadow of its former old-growth self, is nevertheless majestic. As an extra bonus, water is available not only at the trailhead, but also at Skyline Gate and various points along the Stream Trail.

Before leaving the Canyon Meadow parking area, take a moment to notice the variety of trees here—coast redwood, California bay, coast live oak, bigleaf maple, willow, black walnut—a preview of what you will see on this wonderful hike. From the parking area, walk northwest, past a gate marked FIRE TRAIL, on a paved path, reaching a junction with the Canyon Trail, a dirt-and-gravel road heading right and uphill. You may see a red-tailed hawk circling overhead or hear one giving its "keeer, keeer" call.

Turning right on the Canyon Trail, a dirt road, you pass picnic tables at the edge of an open field, then merge with another dirt road joining from the right. Soon you are climbing on a moderate grade in the shade of coast live oak, California bay, willow, Monterey pine, and blue elderberry. A few small redwoods, the tree for which this park is named, have taken root under the canopy of bay and oak. You will see their much larger cousins later along the Stream Trail, your return route.

Now in the open, the route bends left just before merging with the East Ridge Trail, a wide dirt road, where you bear left. Western scrub-jays may loudly announce your arrival on the ridgetop, where you have a great view east to Mt. Diablo and west across Redwood Creek to the high ground near Skyline Blvd. Invasive plants such as coyote brush, French broom, and pampas grass have taken hold here, but you will also see oak, bay, madrone, and more small redwoods. The route follows a rolling course along the ridgeline, passing EBMUD's Redwood Trail, right, and climbs above 1000 feet to a rest bench. Now you can pick out other prominent East Bay summits, including Round Top, northwest, and Rocky Ridge, east, both topped with communication towers.

Just past the 2-mile point, Prince Road leads left and downhill, but your route stays straight and climbs past a large pine grove, soon reaching a fork with the Phillips Loop, left. Here you bear right, and continue climbing through pines, grateful for shade on a hot day. Dark-eyed juncos and nuthatches thrive in wooded areas, and you may see them here. Now heading through a corridor of pine, eucalyptus, and madrone, the route passes a junction with the Eucalyptus Trail, left, and begins to bend west. Red-tailed hawks and turkey vultures may be seen high above the trees, riding the wind.

With the Skyline Gate parking area in view, you pass the Phillips Loop, left, and the East Bay Skyline/Bay Area Ridge Trail, right, on its way north to the Huckleberry Botanic and Sibley Volcanic regional preserves. Just before reaching the parking area, where water, toilets, a rest bench, and a phone are available, the route becomes paved. At the southeast end of the parking area you meet the Stream and West Ridge trails. The West Ridge Trail, straight, is the continuation of the East Bay Skyline/Bay Area Ridge Trail, and is open to bicycles all the way to Canyon Meadow, making a round trip on bicycle possible. The Stream Trail, left, is closed to bicycles from Skyline Gate to the Trail's End picnic area.

Turn left and begin a moderate downhill walk on a dirt road, past willow, hazelnut, and tangles of vine honeysuckle. You soon come to Girls Camp, a lovely picnic area with a large wood hut, water, a restroom, and picnic tables shaded by black walnut trees. Now on a gentle descent beside Redwood Creek, you pass the Eucalyptus Trail, heading left and uphill. Here, at about the 4-mile point, the vegetation changes dramatically, and you now walk in a shady forest of magnificent redwoods growing straight and tall, towering overhead. (Redwood seedlings are so spindly that it is hard to imagine them reaching such statuesque proportions.)

Redwood Creek is in a deep ravine, right, and a moderate descent soon brings you to a rest bench and a junction with the Tres Sendas Trail, right. Your route continues straight. A unique strain of rainbow trout lives in Redwood Creek, prompting park officials to develop a creek-restoration program to protect spawning areas. Signs here ask you not to climb on creek banks and to keep dogs and horses from doing so.

If you are here in the fall, you may be in for a treat. I did this hike in September, and was puzzled by what appeared to be reddish growths covering the hazelnut, blackberry vines, and sword ferns beside the Stream Trail. To my amazement, I discovered thousands of breeding ladybugs clustered on the foliage, with others flying through the air and soon covering me as well. I had seen a similar display in Muir Woods, but never with this quantity of bugs.

With Redwood Creek on your right, continue on the Stream Trail through deep forest, where only ferns, lovers of the dark and damp, grow in soil littered with bay leaves and redwood twigs. Now you cross several bridges, as the creek meanders back and forth under the road. Beyond a junction with Prince Road, left, you emerge into an open area surrounded by coast live oak, walnut, and willow. Now back in redwoods, you pass two stone shelters at the Mill Site picnic area, left, just before a bridge over the creek.

As you continue your level walk on the road, you pass the Fern Hut picnic area, right. At about the 5-mile point, the Fern Trail heads right and uphill. Continue straight, and if

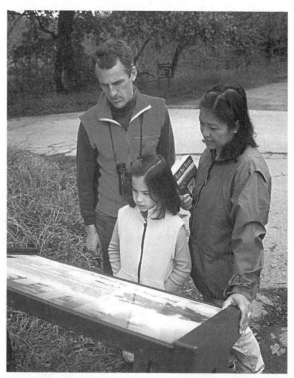

Interpretive panels along the Stream Trail describe the ecology of a coast redwood forest.

you look up here, you may notice that the redwoods grow straight and tall, but the bay trees arch over the road. Especially on the steep hillside to your right, the bays start out growing straight, then begin to curve. Because they cannot compete with the redwoods in height, bays choose this devious strategy to seek sunlight.

Soon you reach a junction with the Chown Trail, right, which connects with the Bridle Trail. Continuing straight, you reach pavement at the Trail's End picnic area, and after a short walk, leave the forest near the Fern Dell picnic area, a lovely meadow with white alder, bigleaf maple, box elder, and walnut. At a four-way junction with the Bridle Trail, where a sign, right, points to the camper exit (used by drive-in camping groups), you follow the Stream Trail as it bends left to cross Redwood Creek. Beyond the Orchard picnic area, you meet the Canyon Trail, left. From here, retrace your route to the parking area.

FRENCH TRAIL

Length: 8.1 miles

Time: 4 to 6 hours

Rating: Difficult

Regulations: EBRPD; fees for parking and dogs when entrance kiosk is attended; no bicycles; no horses on park entrance road, on the Stream Trail south of Trail's End picnic area, or in picnic areas except Trail's End.

Facilities: Picnic tables, water, toilet, phone near the trailhead; water, toilet, phone at Skyline Gate; water, toilets, and picnic tables along the Stream Trail; horse staging at the Wayside parking area, about 0.3 mile before the Canyon Meadow staging area.

Directions: From Interstate 580 eastbound in Oakland, take the 35th Ave. exit, turn left and follow 35th Ave. east into the hills. After 0.8 mile 35th Ave. becomes Redwood Road, and at 2.4 miles it crosses Skyline Blvd., where you stay in the left lane and go straight. At 4.6 miles from Interstate 580 you reach the park entrance; turn left and go 0.5 mile to the Canyon Meadow staging area. The trailhead is at the northwest end of the parking area.

From Interstate 580 westbound in Oakland, take the Warren Freeway/Berkeley/Highway 13 exit and go 0.9 mile to the Carson St./Redwood Road exit. From the stop sign at the end of the exit ramp, continue straight, now on Mountain Blvd., 0.2 mile, and bear right onto Redwood Road. Go 3.2 miles to the park entrance; turn left and go 0.5 mile to the Canyon Meadow staging area. The trailhead is at the northwest end of the parking area.

From Highway 13 southbound, take the Redwood Road/Carson St. exit, turn left onto Redwood Road and follow the directions above.

This loop, combining the Stream, West Ridge, French, Orchard, and Bridle trails, takes you into the heart of this unique regional park, the only one in the East Bay where coast redwoods, heavily logged in the mid-1800s, have been preserved to such an extent. The climb along the Stream Trail to Skyline Gate is easy, steepening only at the very end, and the rolling, meandering return through the redwoods via the French Trail, an alternate segment of the East Bay Skyline/Bay Area Ridge Trail, although strenuous, is not to be missed.

Walking northwest from the parking area on a paved road, you soon pass a junction with the Canyon Trail, right. Water and toilets are available here, at Skyline Gate, and at various points on the Stream Trail. Beyond this junction, the route enters the shade of a beautiful redwood grove, a taste of things to come, then emerges into the open at the Orchard picnic area, a large grassy meadow with a children's play area.

Now the trail bends left to cross Redwood Creek near the Fern Dell picnic area. Across the creek is a four-way junction with the Bridle Trail, where a sign, left, points to the camper exit (used by drive-in camping groups). Here you stay on the Stream Trail by angling right. You pass five more picnic areas along the Stream Trail before leaving the pavement at Trail's End. Steller's jays—blue birds with a black, crested head—may give you a raucous welcome as you walk through their forest home, and you may see a black phoebe, also black-headed, a member of the tyrant flycatcher family.

After the pavement ends, continue on the Stream Trail, now a dirt road, along the banks of Redwood Creek, with steep hillsides rising up on either side. The air here may be fragrant with the smell of California bay, a relative of the Mediterranean tree whose leaves are used in cooking, and at times the only sounds reaching your ears will be bird song and the trickle of water in the creek.

Soon you meet the Chown Trail, left, which connects to the Bridle Trail. Here continue straight. At the Fern Hut picnic area you pass the Fern Trail, left, and a water fountain presented to the park by the California Federation of Women's Clubs, Alameda District. Now veer right to cross the creek near the Mill Site picnic area. A restoration project to protect a unique species of rainbow trout that inhabits Redwood Creek is in progress here; signs ask you to stay off the creek banks and make sure your dogs and horses do too.

Continue straight to an open area surrounded by hazelnut, bay, and willow. Thimbleberry, a shrub with white flowers, red berries, and large, fuzzy leaves—a relative of blackberry and raspberry—grows here. You may also see periwinkle, a nonnative ground cover with dark green leaves and blue, five-petaled flowers, blooming year-round. Overhead, watch for turkey vultures, soaring on uplifted wings. Back in the shade of tall redwoods, the route passes a junction with Prince Road, heading right and steeply uphill, and you continue straight on a carpet of bay leaves and redwood twigs. A steep hillside, left, is covered with similar litter, fertile ground for sword ferns, which thrive in dense forest.

The route crosses Redwood Creek over small bridges in several places; with it now on your left you reach a clearing in a large grove of redwoods and a junction, left, with the Tres Sendas Trail. Here the Stream Trail, your route, bends right and begins a moderate climb, then levels in an open area lined with French broom and poison oak, where the Eucalyptus Trail branches right, steeply uphill. Eucalyptus, madrone, toyon, coyote brush, and bush monkeyflower are crowded together here, taking advantage of a break in the forest canopy to bask in sunlight.

At about the 2.4-mile point, after crossing the creek, you reach Girls Camp, a lovely picnic area with a large wood hut, water, a restroom, and picnic tables shaded by black walnut trees. As the route, still a dirt road, begins to climb again, you

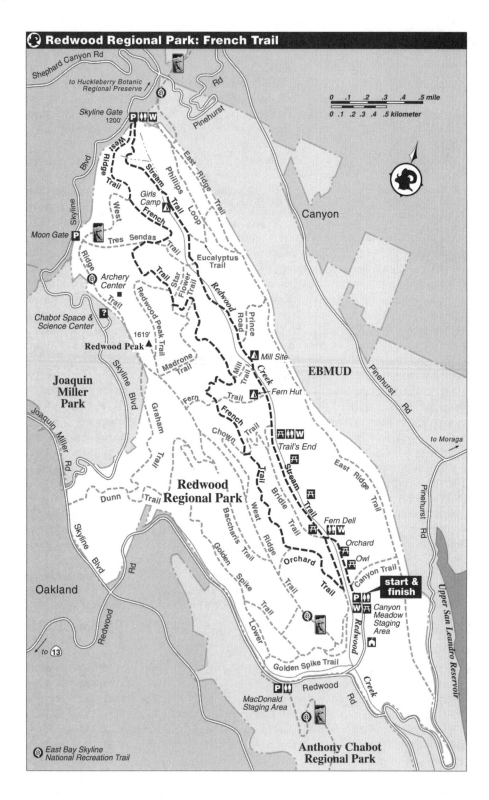

Redwood Regional Park: French Trail

pass stands of willow and coast live oak lining the upper reaches of Redwood Creek. Flowering currant and California buttercup bloom here from late winter through spring, and vine honeysuckle and columbine continue the colorful show into summer. Uphill and right, a large forest of eucalyptus and Monterey pine graces a ridgetop, not far from Skyline Gate, the high point of this route. As you pass a small stream flowing under the road, the grade steepens, and you climb via S-bends to Skyline Gate, where water, toilets, phone, and a rest bench await.

After stopping to rest for perhaps a few minutes, head south on the West Ridge Trail, a dirt road that is part of the East Bay Skyline/Bay Area Ridge Trail. Savor the long-distance views from this stretch of trail, because you will soon descend into forest. Along this part of the route you may see large thistles with purple flowers and crinkled, white-veined leaves—nonnative milk thistle. The East Bay parks host several varieties of nonnative thistles, one of which, cardoon, an invasive relative of the artichoke, is the subject of an eradication program run by the park district. Two birds often heard but not seen, California quail, whose call sounds like "chi-ca-go," and wrentit, which may remind you of someone trying to start a reluctant car, may let you know of their nearby presence.

At about the 3.3-mile point, where the West Ridge Trail bends sharply right, find the single-track French Trail heading left and downhill through a forest of bay, madrone, hazelnut, and pine. (The French Trail is an alternate and more scenic leg of the East Bay Skyline/Bay Area Ridge Trail.) Despite the shade, this route, sheltered from any sea breeze, may be hot. It is also narrow and overgrown in places, with lots of poison oak. The trail switchbacks down to a tributary of Redwood Creek, nestled in the bottom of a heavily wooded canyon, and arrives at a junction, left, with the Tres Sendas Trail, a wide dirt road. Continuing straight—for the next 0.1 mile or so the French and Tres Sendas trails are combined—you begin a moderate climb to the next junction, where the Tres Sendas Trail continues straight, and your route, the French Trail, turns left. The redwoods here, despite being second growth, grow tall, some reaching neck-craning heights.

After crossing the creek on a stone bridge, you climb steeply on a wide dirt path littered with redwood cones and needles. If the air is hazy or foggy, you should be able to see shafts of sunlight filtering through the giant trees. While not a true wilderness, given the area's history as a timber center in the mid-1800s, Redwood Regional Park, especially this section, has many wilderness attributes, including natural beauty, seclusion, and tranquility. At the same time, it is one of the East Bay's most accessible and enjoyable parks.

The French Trail is a rolling route, mostly moderate or steep, with occasional level areas where you can catch your breath and admire the scenery. Now the route narrows and climbs over rocky, rutted ground, past sword fern and huckleberry, to a junction, right, with the Redwood Peak Trail. Continue straight, and make a moderate descent past some fire-scarred redwoods to a four-way junction with the Star Flower Trail, which you cross. The French Trail, here a wide dirt road, climbs in shade to the top of a ridge and soon reaches a junction with the Madrone Trail. Turn left and follow the French Trail, now a single track, as it makes a gradual, then steep descent.

At about the 5.3-mile point, you come to a junction with the Mill Trail, left, heading downhill to the Stream Trail and Mill Site picnic area; here you continue straight on the French Trail. For a short distance, the redwoods are replaced by bay and coast live oak, and there is much more light reaching the ground. But soon the tall trees resume, and where they grow the only other trees usually found are bay and hazelnut. As you are about to climb over a rise, you pass on your left the Fern Trail; about 20 feet farther are a trail post and the continuation of the Fern Trail, right. Continue straight, passing a break in the redwoods that allows enough light for madrone trees to establish a foothold.

At the next junction, as the Chown Trail heads straight and climbs, you bear left and descend. In about 100 yards the continuation of the Chown Trail goes left. Here you stay right, still on a rolling, single-track trail, through forest that alternates between redwood, bay, and, in clearings, madrone. At about the 7.3-mile point, in a grove of madrone, the French Trail ends at a junction with the Orchard Trail, a wide dirt path. (If you are using the French Trail as an alternate East Bay Skyline/Bay Area Ridge Trail route, turn right here, follow the Orchard Trail 0.2 mile uphill on a moderate grade, and join the West Ridge Trail. Then follow the route description in "Skyline Gate to MacDonald Gate" elsewhere in this book.) Turn left here and begin descending on a moderate grade, via S-bends, to the Bridle Trail, a dirt road. Turn left on the Bridle Trail and go 0.2 mile to the bridge across Redwood Creek at Fern Dell. Turn right and retrace your route on the Stream Trail to the parking area.

◆ Joaquin Miller Park ◆

REDWOOD FOREST

Length: 3.6 miles

Time: 1.5 to 2 hours

Rating: Moderate

Regulations: City of Oakland, Office of Parks, Recreation, and Cultural Affairs; no dogs in picnic areas; dogs on leash at all times elsewhere; bicycles not allowed on the Wild Rose, Fern, and Ravine trails, or on the Palos Colorados Trail between Sinawik Cabin and Joaquin Miller Court.

Facilities: Ranger station, with maps, brochures, and displays on the geology and trees of the park, open 9 A.M. to 5 P.M. seven days a week; toilets; water; picnic tables.

Directions: From Highway 13 northbound in Oakland, take the Joaquin Miller Road/Lincoln Ave. exit, bear right onto Joaquin Miller Road, and go 0.8 mile to Sanborn Dr., the park entrance. Turn left and go 0.1 to the ranger-station parking area, left. The trailhead is in front of the ranger station.

From Highway 13 southbound in Oakland, take the Joaquin Miller Road/Lincoln Ave. exit, stay left, and at a stop sign turn left onto Monterey Blvd. Go several hundred feet to Lincoln Ave., turn left and cross over Highway 13. Now on Joaquin Miller Road, follow the directions above.

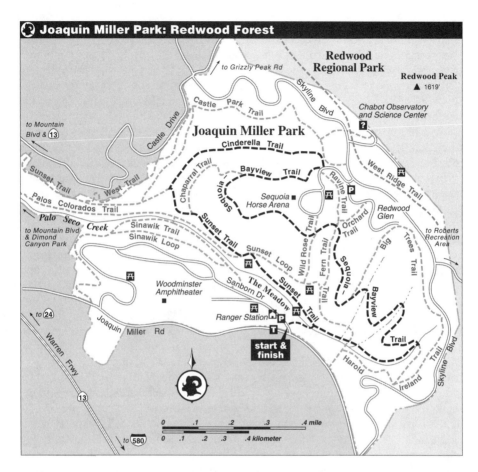

Joaquin Miller Park: Redwood Forest

This park, adjacent to Redwood Regional Park, offers many of its neighbor's attractions in a more intimate and less crowded setting. Using the Sunset, Cinderella, and Sequoia–Bayview trails, this loop explores forests of redwood, Monterey cypress, eucalyptus, and acacia, and offers a fine view of Oakland and San Francisco. The park is named for Joaquin Miller (1841–1913), a colorful figure best known as a poet and an arborist. He settled in the hills above Oakland, where he planted thousands of trees and built monuments to his heroes—Moses, explorer John C. Frémont, and poets Robert and Elizabeth Barrett Browning.

From the front of the ranger station, leave the parking area and walk south along Sanborn Dr., in a corridor of California bay, coast live oak, madrone, and pine, toward the park entrance. After about 0.1 mile, just before you reach Joaquin Miller Road, you come to a yellow gate, left. Past the gate, go straight on a dirt-and-gravel road toward the Upper Meadow and Greenwood picnic areas.

After a short distance, you reach a flat area where Palo Seco Creek flows under the road. Just past the creek is a T-junction with the Sunset Trail, as well as two paths—one left, the other right—leading to open, grassy meadows. Turn left at the junction and follow the Sunset Trail, a dirt road, northwest past stands of bay and coast redwood, which tower over a tangled understory of ferns, blackberry vines, and woodland strawberry. With a meadow on your left, you enjoy a level walk on a well-maintained road carpeted with pine needles and leaf litter, passing a path going right and uphill to a picnic area, and another joining your road from the left.

Following Palo Seco Creek, left, you descend gradually, and soon pass the Sinawik Trail, a dirt path that crosses the creek on a small stone bridge. About 100 feet farther, you come to a junction where the Sunset Loop heads right and steeply uphill. Continue straight on the Sunset Trail, and in another 100 feet or so, you pass a junction, left, with the Palos Colorados Trail. Soon the surrounding dense forest ends, and you emerge into a more open area, where bay and redwood are joined by bigleaf maple, blue elderberry, pine, and toyon. Two nonnative plants that thrive along this section of the route are French broom, an invasive member of the pea family with bright yellow flowers, and cotoneaster, a bushy shrub with small oval leaves and bright red berries.

With Palo Seco Creek now in a deep ravine, left, you pass the Chaparral Trail, unsigned, heading right and uphill; here your route narrows to a single track as it crosses a slope prone to landslides. Ahead on a ridge is a forest of eucalyptus, and soon you reach a tributary of Palo Seco Creek, flowing under the trail through a culvert. Where the Sunset Trail swings sharply left, you turn right onto the Cinderella Trail at an unsigned junction and begin climbing steeply uphill. The trail, rocky and eroded, follows a beautiful ravine lined with willows, right, that holds the tributary creek. The grade eases somewhat as you climb mostly in the open, past hillsides of French broom, California sagebrush, and a few bushes of California barberry, a holly-like shrub rarely seen in the East Bay parklands.

This section of the route may be muddy; in one place water may be flowing across the trail from a pipe on the left. As you gain elevation, the eucalyptus on the ridge above and left give way to pines, while closer at hand, blackberry vines replace the French broom. Crossing the creek, which flows under the trail, you begin a series of alternately steep and level sections, past stands of pinkflower currant and thimbleberry. At about the 1.4-mile point, just before you reach Pine View Flat, a level clearing carpeted with wood chips, look for an unsigned junction. Here you turn sharply right and follow the Sequoia–Bayview Trail, a single track, as it skirts below a parking and picnic area, with a restroom above and left.

After several hundred yards you come to a junction marked by a trail post; here you turn right and walk about 100 feet to a T-junction, also marked, with a path that is paved to your left and dirt to your right. Turn right and follow the Sequoia–Bayview Trail on a level course, past an overgrown area of evergreen huckleberry, creambush, and gooseberry. Soon you pass a path, left, leading uphill to the Sequoia Arena, an equestrian facility. A bit farther, you come to a sign on the right side of the trail that reads NATURE TRAIL CONTINUES, and then reach a junction where your route, the Sequoia–Bayview Trail, turns left, and the Chaparral Trail continues straight.

Climbing from the junction on a moderate grade, the route then levels and enters a magical forest—cool, quiet, and secluded—of Monterey cypress, pine, and, farther along, acacia, an import from Australia. At about the 2-mile point, you pass a junction with a trail that heads left and uphill to the horse arena. Now the route maintains a contour as it follows the indentations in a steep, southwest-facing ridge that dominates this park, leading you through a eucalyptus forest and then into the domain of coast redwood, a true East Bay native.

Once in the redwoods, you pass a four-way intersection with the Wild Rose Trail, and then, at the head of a ravine where a stream flows under the trail, junctions with two branches of the Fern Ravine Trail. Where the Sequoia–Bayview Trail swings sharply right, one branch of the Fern Ravine Trail goes left and uphill. About 75 feet farther, the other branch veers right and downhill. Continuing on a level course, you soon pass a junction, left, with the Big Trees Trail, and also with an unsigned path heading right and downhill. Hazelnut, with fuzzy, toothed leaves, and snowberry, with small round leaves, some of which are irregularly indented, thrive here. Passing another unsigned path, right, you now reach a clearing

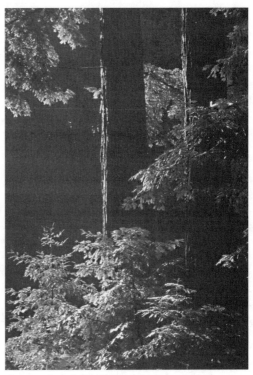

Coast redwoods in the East Bay were heavily logged, but fine second-growth forests remain.

where a view west across San Francisco Bay allows the trail to live up to its name: From this vantage point, the skylines of San Francisco and Oakland are aligned one behind the other.

As the route finishes a right-hand bend at the head of a little canyon, at about the 3-mile point, where water may spill across the trail in wet weather, you will find a sign marking a junction, right, with the Sunset Trail, your return route downhill to the meadow area. On this trail the grade is moderate at first, then gentle, and the ground is rough and rocky in places, with magnificent redwoods towering overhead. As you near the end of the descent, you pass a trail post, right, signed for the Sunset and Palos Colorados trails. There are also several paths here joining on the left. About 200 feet past the trail post is a sign, which you must face uphill to read, commemorating Harold Ireland, a nature lover and mountain climber who for more than 60 years led hikes in the Bay Area, and especially on this trail. Resuming your downhill course, you pass two paths heading right and uphill, the first unsigned, and the second signed as the Sunset Loop.

Continuing straight on the Sunset Trail over level ground, you pass the Greenwood picnic area, left, a grassy meadow, and another unsigned path, right. Look for common star lily—spikes of six-petaled white flowers held upright on tall triangular stems—beside the trail here in spring. Soon you close the loop beside Palo Seco Creek; now retrace your route uphill to the parking area by the ranger station.

◆ Lake Chabot Regional Park ◆

LAKE LOOP

Length: 9 miles

Time: 4 to 6 hours

Rating: Difficult

Regulations: EBRPD; fees for parking and dogs; no bicycles on the Columbine Trail. During periods of extreme wet weather the Columbine Trail may be closed where it crosses Grass Valley Creek, making it impossible to complete the loop: call (510) 635-0138 to check.

Facilities: Picnic tables, water, toilets, snack bar; boat rentals and fishing licenses. A lake shuttle/tour boat makes stops at various points along the shoreline; see the EBRPD Lake Chabot brochure for more details. For more information about the history of Lake Chabot and its dam, pick up a copy of the brochure "History Walk At Lake Chabot," available at the Marina Cafe. Year-round camping is available at the Anthony Chabot Family Campground; call (510) 562-2267 for information and reservations.

Directions: From Interstate 580 eastbound in San Leandro, take the 150th Ave./Fairmont Dr. exit. Go through the first light at 150th Ave. and at the next light turn left onto Fairmont Dr. After 1.8 miles, Fairmont Dr. becomes Lake Chabot Road. Continue 0.1 mile and turn left into the Lake Chabot Marina parking area. The trailhead is at the northeast side of parking area.

From Interstate 580 westbound in San Leandro, take the 150th Ave./Fairmont Dr. exit, turn right onto Fairmont Dr. and follow the directions above.

From Castro Valley Blvd. in Castro Valley, go north 1.8 miles on Lake Chabot Road to the Lake Chabot Marina parking area. The trailhead is at the northeast side of parking area.

This loop, combining the East Shore, Honker Bay, Columbine, Bass Cove, and West Shore trails, takes you around the 315-acre lake that forms the heart of Lake Chabot Regional Park. A wide variety of plant and bird life, along with ever-changing terrain, makes this a rewarding trip. A surprising degree of solitude can be found here, especially on the Columbine Trail. Length, not terrain, earns this trip its "difficult" rating. The East and West Shore trails may be hiked separately for shorter, less strenuous out-and-back trips.

As you leave the parking area, walk downhill on the East Shore Trail, a paved road, and immediately come to a four-way intersection with a paved path. To your left are the marina and a launch site for boats, canoes, and kayaks. A signboard with a map and park information is on your right. Continue straight, cross a small creek, and where a dirt path joins from the right, follow the paved road as it swings left, and, in about 50 feet, passes a paved path leading uphill to the Mallard picnic site. Continue straight, passing a small pond on your left, and in another 50 feet or

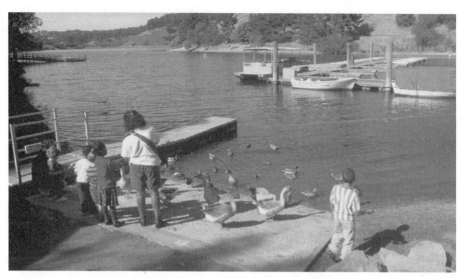

Feeding the waterfowl is a popular pastime for children visiting the Lake Chabot Marina.

so you reach an intersection with a paved path that leads left and downhill, past the Willow picnic site, to the marina and cafe.

Continue straight and walk northwest through a wooded area of willow, poplar, coast live oak, walnut, and white alder. The East Shore Trail, paved and relatively flat, is very popular with hikers, dog-walkers, joggers, and exercise walkers; as part of the Lake Chabot Bicycle Loop it is used by bicyclists as well. (Bike loop distance: 12.42 miles via the Live Oak Trail; 14.41 miles via the Honker Bay Trail.) Soon you can see the marina across the water, left. You may also see and hear a large flock of geese on the lawn next to snack bar, begging passersby for food. The route climbs gently, past stands of Monterey and Coulter pine, and turns northeast as it follows the contour of the lake.

In sunny areas, you may see blue elderberry, California sagebrush, toyon, coyote brush, poison oak, and bush monkeyflower. But as soon as the route enters shade, following indentations in the shoreline, the vegetation changes abruptly, and you find yourself in a cool, dark forest of coast live oak and California bay, with ferns, creambush, and blackberry vines clinging to the damp hillsides. The route repeats this transition many times as it circles the lake. As you come into the open again, there is a view of Live Oak Island (restricted access) in the middle of the lake, left. Nearby, a wooden staircase leads from the East Shore Trail down to the water's edge.

You may see a plump black bird floating on the water, with white bill and large yellow lobed feet. This is the American coot, a common bird related to rails and gallinules. Another black waterbird—larger than a coot, and with a snake-like neck—is the double-crested cormorant. You will often see cormorants perched on rocks or snags, drying their outstretched wings. Unlike many other waterbirds, cormorants have no waterproofing oil in their feathers. After diving for fish, they must dry out. You also may see or hear Anna's hummingbird, tiny and gray-green, with males displaying a bright ruby-red throat.

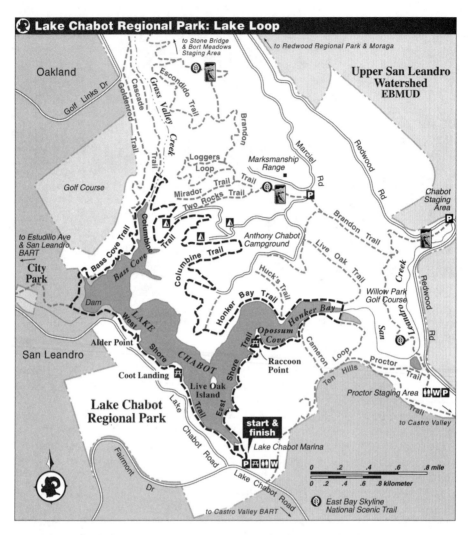

Lake Chabot Regional Park: Lake Loop

At about the 1.3-mile point, you reach a trail post and a trail leading left and downhill to Raccoon Point, a spit of land that marks the entrance to Opossum Cove and Honker Bay. Here the East Shore Trail swings right and begins a moderate climb in the shade of large bay trees. You may also find coffeeberry and snowberry in this shady section. The route descends, then begins a series of ups and downs. Soon you pass a ravine, right, filled with a jumble of rocks and large boulders, possibly dry in summer. In wet weather, however, water cascading down this ravine flows under the road through a large metal culvert. Steller's jays and western scrub-jays favor this area, and your passage may set off their raucous alarms. Look here also for the diminutive ruby-crowned kinglet, a nervous bird about the size of a chickadee, dull yellow-green with white wing bars.

The lake, left, is here shallow and marshy, filled with cattails and bulrushes, also called tule. Great blue herons and great egrets often wade in these shallows or stand on low islands, hunting for small fish. At the other end of the size scale, gold-crowned sparrows may be seen feeding in flocks on the ground beside the road. Small birds that feed in the open need the protection from predators that is provided by a flock. But other small ground feeders who feed while hidden in dense thickets, like the spotted towhee, can safely feed alone.

At about 1.7 miles, the paved East Shore Trail ends at a metal gate. Here you join the Cameron Loop Trail, a wide dirt road heading sharply right but also straight ahead. Continue straight and climb a gentle grade in dense forest, past stands of willow and bigleaf maple. After about 0.1 mile, you leave the Cameron Loop Trail by turning left, walking down a few wooden steps, and crossing a 200-foot wooden bridge over San Leandro Creek. From the bridge, stop and look for birds in this marshy, wooded area and listen for their calls—the sharp "klee-yer" of the northern flicker, or the plaintive "keeer" of the red-tailed hawk.

Once across the bridge, you are back on a dirt path, with underbrush and trees on either side. About 100 yards from the end of bridge, just as you begin to emerge from the marshy area, you come to a four-way junction. Your route is the Honker Bay Trail, a wide dirt road heading left. A dirt road, right, leads to a restricted area. The Live Oak Trail goes straight and heads uphill; cyclists can choose this route or go left on the Honker Bay Trail. Turn left and walk on a level grade past a brushy area with coyote brush, California sagebrush, fennel, and cotoneaster, a nonnative shrub with red berries. This area may be muddy in wet weather. A large expanse of marsh is to your left, and a steep, rocky hillside rises on your right.

At about the 2.3-mile point, you pass a junction with Huck's Trail, a steep path for hikers only, heading right and uphill. (There is a toilet on the left here.) As you round a point, Honker Bay is left, and a large eucalyptus forest graces the ridge ahead and also right. Closer at hand are coast live oak, willow, and white alder. Keep a sharp eye out for deer lurking in the shade. You may be startled by a loud scratching in the underbrush: this may be a California towhee or perhaps a spotted towhee searching for food. Look high in the tree branches to find yellow-rumped warblers.

The sight of small boat dock (and another toilet) indicates you've reached the start of the route's hilly section. Here the Honker Bay Trail turns right, away from the lake, and begins to climb on a moderate grade, passing coast live oak, bay, and blue elderberry along the way. The grade levels, then climbs steeply to an area of low shrubs, including coyote brush, toyon, bush monkeyflower, and California sagebrush. Ahead on a ridge, you will see a large eucalyptus forest, perhaps with hawks or vultures soaring above. Views of the lake, looking back toward the marina, are soon left behind, but with the trees comes shade, welcome on a warm day. The route switches back and continues to climb, soon reaching a junction with the Columbine Trail.

From here the Honker Bay Trail continues its climb to the Anthony Chabot Family Campground, at the end of Marciel Road, but your route, the single-track Columbine Trail, closed to bicycles, heads left around the lake. The air here on a warm day is wonderfully fragrant with the smell of eucalyptus and bay. The route now meanders, mostly maintaining a contour as it follows ridges and inlets along the lake's indented east shore. Hazelnut and vine honeysuckle can be added to your list of today's plants.

At about the 4-mile point, you reach a junction with fenced-off trail leading left and downhill. Your route goes right and stays level, then drops on a series of switchbacks to a streambed, which may be dry in summer. In an area overgrown with blackberry vines and poison oak, cross the streambed and climb on a gentle grade, soon reaching open terrain on the side of a ridge. Farther along this ridge, you can look northwest, across an arm of the lake, to Chabot Municipal Golf Course. As you round the ridge, you pass the trail to Lost Ridge Group Campground, taking off sharply right. If you look southwest, you get a good look at the dam that formed Lake Chabot.

After walking almost another mile, you reach an unsigned fork in the trail; here you stay left, now enjoying the shade of coast live oak and bay. Soon you pass the Hawk Ridge Group Camp Trail, leading right and uphill via several sets of wooden steps. The Columbine Trail continues straight, then bends right to cross a streambed, and swings left toward a junction with the Cascade Trail. At about the 6-mile point, you reach a sandy, brushy area, sometimes dry, where Grass Valley Creek flows into Lake Chabot. In extreme wet weather the Columbine Trail may be closed here. After crossing the creek bed, you come to a T-junction and several trail signs. From here the Cascade Trail goes right, but your route, the Bass Cove Trail, goes left and continues around the lake to the dam. The signs at this junction list mileages to various points around the lake, but the figures do not exactly match mileages given on the EBRPD or Olmsted maps.

Following a line of willow and bay, you turn left onto the Bass Cove Trail, a dirt road, and walk south, past a rest bench, soon leaving the trees and coming into the open. The lake is to your left, and soon the road swings back to the shade of an oak and bay enclave. Now in the sun again, the route starts a short, moderate climb, passes a junction, right, with the Goldenrod Trail, and then another with an unsigned dirt road to a restricted area going right and uphill. As you descend toward the lake, you get good views of the dam, and to its left, forested Fairmont Ridge, topped by a communication tower. Just downhill is a toilet.

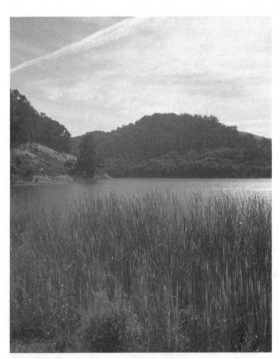

Cattails line the shore near Bass Cove, as seen from the Bass Cove Trail.

The route meanders in and out of little coves as it contours and climbs along the lakeshore. At one point, with the dam in sight, a hidden inlet forces you to jog north, then south. Soon, in an area where large pines and coast redwoods reach for the sky, you reach a junction with a road heading left. Veer right, and almost at once you come to another junction, this time with a paved road. Here you will find a trail post with a sign for the Bass Cove Trail, and a toilet. Veer left and walk downhill on pavement, which leads you across the dam. (To the right the West Shore Trail continues to the city of San Leandro's Chabot Park, the entrance to which is off Estudillo Ave.)

The earthen dam you are crossing was built in 1874–75 by Anthony Chabot, founder of the Contra Costa Water Company. With Oakland and surrounding cities facing a water shortage, Chabot decided to dam San Leandro Creek, which flows west from here and empties into San Leandro Bay at the Martin Luther King, Jr. Regional Shoreline. According to Malcolm Margolin, author of *East Bay Out*, Chabot used hydraulic techniques developed for California gold mining. Chabot's crews, which included around 800 Chinese laborers, used high-pressure streams of water to wash thousands of tons of dirt into San Leandro Creek, and then brought in herds of wild horses to compact the dirt into a dam. Construction began in 1874, and in 1876 the first water entered the reservoir's pipelines. A filter plant was added in 1890. The dam, originally called San Leandro Dam, was acquired along with the reservoir and filter plant in 1928 by EBMUD, which renamed the facilities to honor Chabot. The lake was opened to recreation in the 1960s and now serves as an emergency water supply for the East Bay.

Just after crossing the dam, now on the West Shore Trail, you can visit an observation deck, left, with fine views of the lake and dam, a California historic civil-engineering landmark. Note, too, Diana's Temple (built in 1917), which tops a tunnel at the far end of the dam. Proceeding southeast, you come to a wonderful, shady part of the route, thick with all the now-familiar trees and shrubs. Here you may see a gray sparrow-like bird with a black head, pink bill, and white along the outer edges of its tail. This is the dark-eyed junco, usually found in flocks in wooded areas or at backyard bird feeders, where it comes readily. A highly variable bird found across the United States and Canada, the dark-eyed junco was formerly divided into four species; our variety was known as the Oregon junco.

At about the 7.5-mile point, you come to an unsigned junction; here the West Shore Trail turns left and goes downhill, and another path continues straight to Lake Chabot Road. When you reach the lake shore, your route bends right, passing a dirt trail that heads left to Alder Point. Soon you pass another trail going left, this one to Coot Landing; a nearby rest bench beckons from beneath a coast live oak. From here you can glimpse your goal, the marina, ahead and left. Before you reach it, however, the route climbs until it is high above the lake. From a vantage point, you can see familiar landmarks—Live Oak Island, the East Shore Trail, and Honker Bay.

Just before reaching the marina, the route crosses a ledge cut from the steep hillside, exposing layers of rock. When you reach the marina, you may be surrounded by ducks and geese begging for food. Among the domestic geese may be Canada geese, large gray-brown birds with a black head and neck, and a white throat patch. These "honkers" are often seen during spring and fall migration, flying in a classic V-formation over wetlands and marshes. From the marina, follow the West Shore Trail as it passes right of the cafe on its way to the parking area.

◆Upper San Leandro Reservoir ◆

KING CANYON LOOP

Length: 6.1 miles

Time: 3 to 4 hours

Rating: Moderate

Regulations: EBMUD; Trail Use Permit required; no bicycles, no dogs, no smoking.

Facilities: Toilet.

Directions: From Highway 24 in Orinda, take the Orinda/Moraga exit and go southeast on Camino Pablo—which soon becomes Moraga Way—4.6 miles to Canyon Road. Turn right, and go 1.1 miles to EBMUD's Valle Vista parking area, left. The trail begins at the EBMUD trail register, just southwest of the parking area.

This loop, combining the Rocky Ridge and King Canyon Loop trails, explores two narrow canyons at the northern end of EBMUD's Upper San Leandro Reservoir. Birders will enjoy the variety of habitats visible from this route, from open water to secluded forest, and those out for exercise will profit from many ups and downs. Parts of this route have steep ground, and parts are extremely muddy in wet weather.

From the parking area, go through a cattle gate and sign the EBMUD register, then turn left and walk downhill on the Rocky Ridge Trail, a gravel path that crosses an open field of coyote brush and blackberry vines. (Another EBMUD route that starts here, the Redwood Trail, goes right and climbs to the East Ridge Trail in Redwood Regional Park.) The northernmost finger of Upper San Leandro Reservoir, which you will soon cross, is visible from here. After about 150 feet you reach a dirt road coming from the parking lot and joining on your left. Here you angle right on the road. When you reach the remains of an orchard, left, bordered by Monterey pines and eucalyptus, find a gravel turnout, also left. (This turnout is opposite a trail post marking the Riche Loop Trail.)

Turn left at the turnout and follow the Rocky Ridge Trail, a dirt-and-gravel path, through an old plum orchard—in summer, these trees produce several varieties of edible plums. Now go past a fence and over several small creeks flowing through culverts. When I hiked this route in mid-January, there was a pair of red-shouldered hawks here, perhaps getting ready to nest, calling from the treetops. The marshy area here provides excellent cover for towhees, both California and spotted, and the tree branches offer lookout posts for western scrub-jays, sentinels of the forest.

With Canyon Road just left, turn right at a T-junction and cross a bridge spanning a narrow, shallow part of the reservoir, just below the inflow of Moraga Creek. On the other side of the bridge, the Rimer Creek Trail, a path that starts behind a fence, goes left, but your route, the Rocky Ridge Trail, marked by a trail post, veers right. Continue south on the trail, here a level dirt road, which passes through a

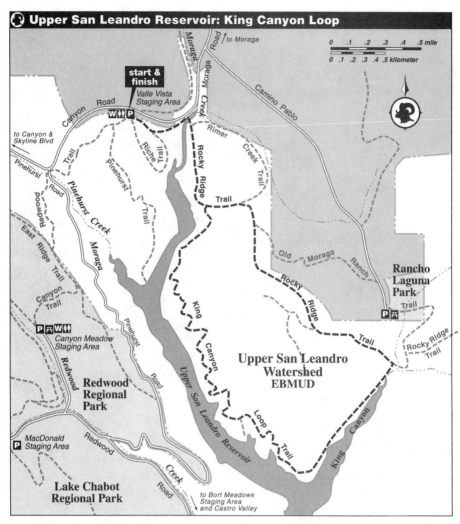

Upper San Leandro Reservoir: King Canyon Loop

wooded area of large coast live oak, pine, and acacia. Large groups of birders often frequent this route, searching for ducks, geese, wading birds, songbirds, and raptors. The large wooden bird houses high on pine trunks near the water are designed for wood ducks.

Passing a large row of pines, you follow the road as it bends east, away from the reservoir, and, in about 250 feet, come to a cattle gate. Continue straight, past a creek flowing under the road, and in about 150 feet you reach a junction. Here the Rocky Ridge Trail, the return part of your loop, climbs left, but you follow the King Canyon Loop Trail, also called the George Wagnon Memorial Trail to honor a local horseman who loved to ride EBMUD trails and share them with his friends. Climbing a dirt road through a forest of California bay, coast live oak, and eucalyptus, the route passes over a creek flowing through a culvert, and begins a rolling, zigzag course that traces the wrinkled shape of the hillside above the reservoir.

Where the lush, dense forest gives way to open areas, you may find sun-loving shrubs such as bush monkeyflower, blue bush lupine, California sagebrush, and even an occasional madrone. Back in shade, ferns form the ground cover. Eroded sections of the hillside, left, reveal layers of rock tipped 90 degrees, an indication of the geologic forces at work in the East Bay hills. Power-line towers interfere with the view from time to time, as you look across the reservoir to Anthony Chabot and Redwood regional parks, but provide convenient perches for raptors such as red-tailed hawks.

As you climb to a grassy clearing at about the 2.5-mile point and leave the power lines to their run across open water, look for an unsigned junction, where you bear left and downhill on a moderate and then steep grade. After reaching the

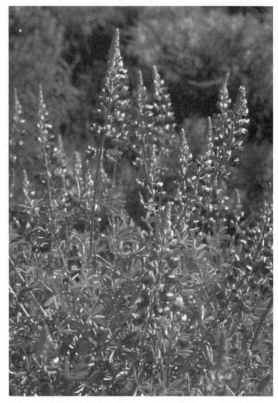

Blue bush lupine.

bottom of a gully, where a stream runs under the road through a culvert, you begin an up-and-down course, alternating between open grassland and oak-and-bay forest, and cross several more streams, one of which may have a small waterfall. This is a charming part of the route, with views that take in steep, forested ridges and an expanse of sun-brightened waters. As the road turns northeast around the end of a ridge, you begin to follow an arm of the reservoir filling King Canyon.

The route descends almost to the shore, and here you may see a flock of Canada geese floating on the water, joined perhaps by mallards. Canada geese come in a variety of sizes, the smallest subspecies breeding in western Alaska, and the more familiar form breeding on the Pacific Coast, including the Bay Area. Their V-formation flight and their honking calls are a joy to see and hear.

Continuing northeast on an open and mostly level course, you soon reach a marshy area near the inflow of King Canyon Creek. A short walk brings you to a large EBMUD trail sign, at about 4 miles, marking the end of the King Canyon Loop/George Wagnon Memorial Trail and its junction with the Rocky Ridge Trail. Here, one branch of the Rocky Ridge Trail goes right, through a gate, and crosses Camino Pablo, a dirt-and-gravel road. Your branch of the trail, however, stays left of the road, continues straight, and climbs gradually across a grassy hillside, with a fence on the right.

Now the single-track trail goes across a streambed lined with bay and California buckeye. Here the fence takes a sharp right and your route turns left, beginning to climb on a moderate grade. Turning north, you emerge from dense forest into open grassland, where you have a good view east of the rolling hills that rise up to Rocky Ridge, topped by a single communication tower, on the border of Las Trampas Wilderness. At an unsigned T-junction, follow the arrow on a trail post and turn left on a dirt road. Continue moderately uphill, soon reaching a fork where you bear left. Now comes the steepest part of the route, as you climb a rocky dirt road that winds back and forth through an oak-and-bay forest as it gains elevation, giving you a view north to Moraga Valley. At the next junction, marked by a trail post, bear right and go slightly downhill on a dirt road, past a shrubby area of coffeeberry, coyote brush, and poison oak.

Passing a gate, right, you follow the road as it swings left and makes a moderate descent, levels, and then climbs. If the ground is muddy, you may see the tracks of deer or other animals. The route finally reaches a cool, dark forest and tries to hold a contour there before breaking into the open and beginning to descend. The horse pastures and housing subdivisions that greet your eye here are apt symbols of the pressures put on open space by population growth and suburban sprawl. A steep downhill section that soon relents brings you to a junction, right, with the Old Moraga Ranch Trail. Continue straight, with open grassland on your left sweeping down to the reservoir. Now veer sharply left and follow the road as it descends moderately past the Rimer Creek Trail, right, to close the loop at the King Canyon Loop Trail. From here, turn right and retrace your route to the parking area.

RAMAGE PEAK

Length: 10.6 miles

Time: 6 to 8 hours

Rating: Very difficult

Regulations: EBMUD; Trail Use Permit required; no bicycles, no dogs, no smoking.

Facilities: Toilet at the Chabot staging area; Las Trampas Wilderness parking area has picnic tables, toilet, and water (may not be available at certain times of year).

Directions: This is a car shuttle trip, starting at EBMUD's **Chabot staging area** and ending at **Las Trampas Wilderness.** Drive first to Las Trampas Wilderness, leave a car there (with plenty of water, snacks, and a change of footwear), then proceed to the Chabot staging area.

To reach **Las Trampas Wilderness:** From Interstate 680 in San Ramon, take the Crow Canyon Road/San Ramon exit and go west 1.1 miles on Crow Canyon Road to Bollinger Canyon Road. Turn right and go 4.5 miles to the end of the road, past the first Las Trampas Wilderness entrance, and turn left into the parking area.

From Interstate 580 eastbound in Castro Valley, take the Center St./Crow Canyon Road exit, go left over the freeway, then right on Castro Valley Blvd.,

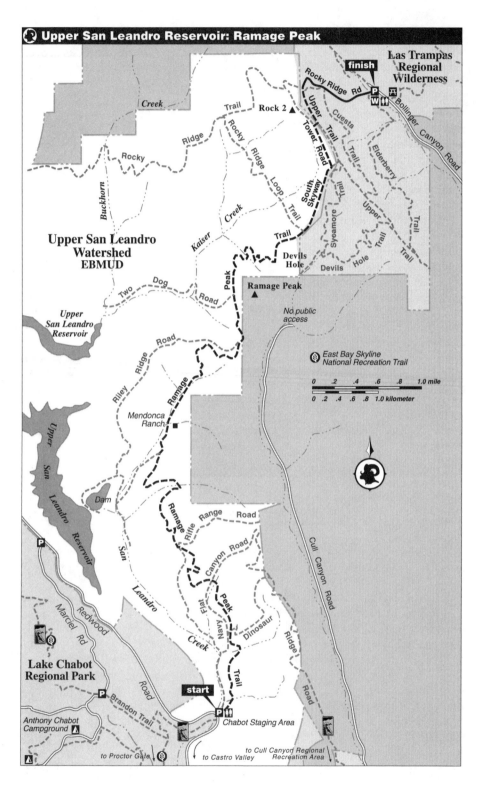

Upper San Leandro Reservoir: Ramage Peak

finish

Las Trampas
Regional
Wilderness

Rocky Ridge Rd

Creek

Trail

Rock 2

Ridge

Rocky

Buckhorn

Rocky Ridge Loop Trail

Cuesta Trail

Elderberry Trail

Upper Trail

Tower Road

South Skyway

Sycamore Trail

Upper Trail

Trail

Bollinger Canyon Road

Kaiser Creek

Upper San Leandro
Watershed
EBMUD

Trail

Devils
Hole

Devils Hole

Peak

Two

Dog

Road

Ramage Peak

No public
access

Upper
San Leandro
Reservoir

Riley

Ridge

Road

Ramage

East Bay Skyline
National Recreation Trail

0   .2   .4   .6   .8   1.0 mile

0   .2   .4   .6   .8   1.0 kilometer

Mendonca
Ranch

Upper

San

Leandro

Reservoir

Dam

Ramage

Rifle Range

Road

San

Leandro

Peak

Cull Canyon Road

Redwood

Marcel Rd

Flat

Navy

Dinosaur

Ridge

Road

Lake Chabot
Regional Park

Creek

Trail

start

Anthony Chabot
Campground

Brandon Trail

Road

Chabot Staging Area

to Proctor Gate   to Cull Canyon Regional
            to Castro Valley   Recreation Area

which soon becomes E. Castro Valley Blvd., 0.7 mile to Crow Canyon Road. Turn left and go 7.5 miles to Bollinger Canyon Road, then follow the directions above.

From Interstate 580 westbound in Castro Valley, take the Castro Valley exit, turn left onto E. Castro Valley Blvd. and go 0.1 mile to Crow Canyon Road. Turn right and follow the directions above.

To reach the **Chabot staging area:** From the Las Trampas Wilderness parking area at the end of Bollinger Canyon Road, return to Crow Canyon Road, turn right and go 7.5 miles to E. Castro Valley Blvd. Turn right and go 1.1 miles on E. Castro Valley Blvd., which soon becomes Castro Valley Blvd., to Redwood Road. Turn right and go 3.2 miles north to Chabot staging area, right, at a sharp bend in the road. The trailhead is at the east corner of parking area.

This is one of the most adventurous hikes in the East Bay, combining beautiful scenery, rugged terrain, and a sense of isolation found in few other East Bay parks, most notably the Ohlone Wilderness. Yet the point-to-point Ramage Peak Trail can be completed in a day, albeit a long one, whereas visiting the Ohlone Wilderness requires backpacking for several days at least. Ramage Peak should be reserved for cool weather: although much of the route stays in the shade, the open stretches can be blisteringly hot. Finally, remember to bring plenty of water and food, and get an early start. (Road names in parentheses in the route description are from the Olmsted map, *Trails of the East Bay Hills, Central Section.*)

A journey of 1000 miles starts with the first step, and although your destination is not quite that far away, this hike is a big undertaking, leading you over some of the most remote and rugged terrain in the East Bay. As you take your first steps from the east corner of the parking area, you pass through a gate next to a Bay Area Ridge Trail sign, and turn left onto a dirt-and-gravel road. About 100 feet ahead you come to an EBMUD trail sign, left, and a trail register, right. After signing in, go through another gate, right, and follow the Ramage Peak Trail, a dirt path, heading northeast and uphill on a gentle grade. The emblem for the Ramage Peak Trail, which you will see on trail posts along the way, is a black arrow on a beige disk. A trail post, right, gives the distance to the Rocky Ridge Loop Trail as 7.4 miles, but this is suspect: the actual distance is almost a mile more. The first 0.9 mile of this hike, which is also part of the Bay Area Ridge Trail, heads northeast and then north past a Christmas-tree farm on a mostly level grade. Along the way you pass an unsigned road with a cattle gate, left, and a cattle pen, also left. The trail then crosses two tree-lined streambeds on wooden bridges, and meets a gated road joining from the left.

The route forks just past the junction. The wide road heading right and uphill is the unsigned Chabot-to-Garin Regional Trail (Dinosaur Ridge Road), the continuation of the Bay Area Ridge Trail. Your route, the Ramage Peak Trail, is the path leading slightly left and downhill, past several watering troughs, left. As you descend, the path crosses a gully, then climbs steeply up an embankment, the air fragrant with the smell of California bay. Soon you are out in the open, traversing a grassy hillside under power lines, then following a gully gently uphill through bay, coast live oak, and blue elderberry.

The route switchbacks and crosses the gully, then climbs in the open, where swallows and red-tailed hawks may circle overhead, to a junction under a power-line tower. Here, at about the 1.5-mile point, a dirt road joins from the right, but you continue straight and slightly downhill, through a forest of oak and bay, past a watering trough, to a four-way junction with an unsigned dirt road (Navy Flat Canyon Road).

Continue straight and begin climbing a gravelly dirt path that makes long, steep switchbacks across an open hillside under power lines. After crossing another dirt road (Rifle Range Road), continue straight and uphill through an area of chaparral, mostly chamise, and then descend over loose ground past a watering trough to a streambed where coast live oak, bay, and bigleaf maple provide welcome shade.

After crossing the streambed, the route again climbs steeply in the open, levels in a wooded area, then descends through a sandy, dusty area, where you get your first view of Upper San Leandro Reservoir, left. On a hot day, its water looks inviting. Now the route descends through dense forest, where large ferns thrive in the shade, into a small ravine that holds a tributary of San Leandro Creek. Climbing out of the ravine, you pass a large stand of eucalyptus on your way to a junction with a closed dirt road, right.

Now descending in the shade on a dirt road, you soon come to a rest bench and a junction with another dirt road joining from the left. Bearing right, you emerge onto an open, eroded hillside above Miller Creek, which is left and downhill. When you reach a wooden fence, turn left and walk downhill, following the route as it passes through an old orchard and the site of a dairy ranch owned by J.B. Mendonca, whose name first appears on land records in 1915.

After passing through a gap in a fence and leaving the ranch area, you begin to climb on well-graded switchbacks, first in forest, then in the open, where California sagebrush, coyote brush, and bush monkeyflower thrive in full sun. At about the 6-mile point, you reach a rest bench and a T-junction with a dirt road (Riley Ridge Road). Turn right and go through a cattle gate.

You are now climbing above 1000 feet for the first time on this trip, and your effort is rewarded by terrific views in all directions, especially west to Upper San Leandro Reservoir and Anthony Chabot Regional Park, and northeast to Ramage Peak (1401') and Rocky Ridge, 2000 feet in elevation, capped by a communication tower, guarding Bollinger Canyon.

Now the route levels and contours around a hill, then climbs to a junction, left, with an unsigned dirt road (Two Dog Road). You are now just west of Ramage Peak, which sits on private land. Veering right, you pass a watering trough and a large water tank, then climb north via a series of switchbacks to a saddle in the ridge running northwest from Ramage Peak. Once over the saddle, you descend a steep and narrow trail, lined with poison oak, that quickly reaches a shady, secluded forest. After crossing a creek, the trail becomes indistinct as it passes north through an abandoned pear orchard, then swings east to switchback up a grassy hillside overgrown with star thistle.

As you near a high point, look for a wooden rail used to tether horses. Here the trail turns north again and soon comes to a T-junction with a dirt road, where you turn left. Now you are walking on top of the world, or so it seems, with 360-degree views. Ahead is Rocky Ridge, a last obstacle between you and trail's end. At about 8.3 miles the Ramage Peak Trail ends at a junction with the Rocky Ridge Loop Trail. Here you turn right, pass through a gate, and climb steeply on a dirt road. When you soon reach the next gate, do not go through it; instead, turn left, stay on the dirt road (South Skyway), and begin a long, steep climb through chaparral, with a barbed-wire fence—the boundary between EBMUD lands and Las Trampas Wilderness—on your right.

Near the top of Rocky Ridge, the route levels, giving you a chance to enjoy the scenery and your achievement. Just behind you is Ramage Peak, already shrinking in size; in the distance, southwest, are Upper San Leandro Reservoir and the start of today's trip. Beyond lie San Francisco Bay, the towns of Hayward and Fremont, and the Santa Cruz Mountains. Late in the afternoon, if the moon is near full, look east to see it rise. A final steep push on loose dirt brings you, at about the 9-mile point, to a fence and a gate, where a trail to Rock 2 (2024'), the summit of Rocky Ridge, heads left. Enjoy the appropriately placed rest bench here. Continue straight through the gate and follow the road as it bends northwest, passing another junction, right, with a dirt road coming through a locked gate in a fence.

You are now walking on a level grade (Tower Road), directly toward the communication tower on the summit of Rocky Ridge. Just before the route begins to climb to the tower, you reach a gate, right, and a path leading through it to the Upper Trail, in the Las Trampas Wilderness. Once on the Upper Trail, turn left and follow it downhill, across a steep hillside falling away northeast into Bollinger Canyon, to paved Rocky Ridge Road. Turn right and follow the road down to the parking area, where, if it is near dusk, you may hear a great horned owl giving you a well-deserved welcome.

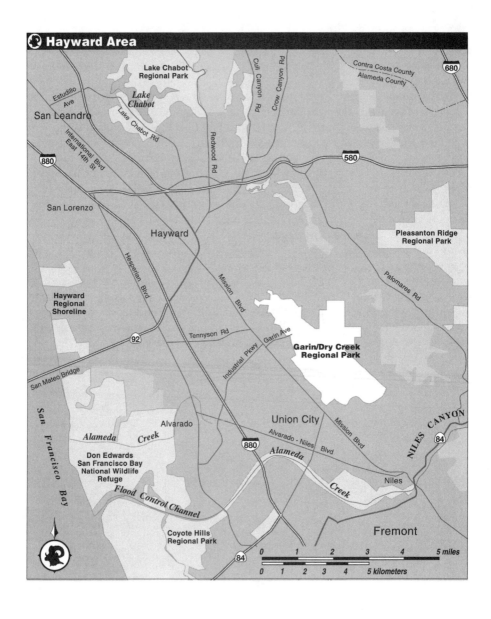

Hayward Area

◆ Hayward Area ◆

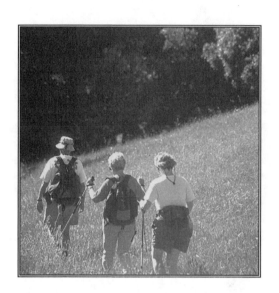

✦Garin Regional Park ✦

GARIN PEAK

Length: 3.3 miles

Time: 2 to 3 hours

Rating: Moderate

Regulations: EBRPD; fees for parking and dogs when entrance kiosk is attended.

Facilities: The visitor center in a restored barn has displays of antique farm equipment and information about Hayward's ranching and farming history; toilets nearby in a separate building; picnic tables, water, phone.

Directions: From Interstate 580 eastbound in Castro Valley, take the Hayward/Route 238 exit and follow signs for Hayward. From the first traffic light, continue straight, now on Foothill Blvd., for 1.7 miles to Mission Blvd., staying in the left lanes as you approach Mission Blvd. Bear left onto Mission Blvd. and go 3.5 miles to Garin Ave. Turn left and go 0.9 mile uphill to the entrance kiosk. At the kiosk bear left, find the parking area farthest left, and enter by turning right. The trailhead is at the northeast end of parking area.

From Interstate 580 westbound in Castro Valley, take the Strobridge exit and go 0.2 mile to the first stop sign. Turn right, go 0.1 mile to Castro Valley Blvd., and turn left. Follow Castro Valley Blvd. 0.5 mile to Foothill Blvd., turn left, and follow the directions above.

A perfect introduction to the rolling hills, windy summits, and shaded creeks of Garin Regional Park, this trip uses the Vista Peak Loop Trail to take you past Vista and Garin peaks, from whose summits you will have most of San Francisco Bay displayed for your enjoyment.

From the end of the parking area, follow a paved, gated road northeast beside a creek, right, lined will willow and western sycamore. The visitor center and picnic areas are across the creek. Soon you pass through a shady corridor of Monterey pine, coast live oak, willow, and white alder. Two very different birds, the California quail and kestrel, may be heard and seen here. The quail, with its repetitive "chi-ca-go" call, is a ground-dweller and travels in flocks, taking flight when flushed. The kestrel, the smallest North American falcon, is a solo acrobat of the skies, hovering and diving on prey, and sometimes giving a shrill "killee, killee, killee" call.

At the end of the paved road you pass a junction with a road heading left to the Arroyo Flats picnic area. About 50 feet past this junction, you reach a cattle gate; now you are on a dirt road. Approximately 100 yards past the gate you reach another junction. From here, the road, shown on the park map as the Old Homestead Trail, continues straight, skirting the Newt Pond Wildlife Area. Your route, the Vista Peak Loop Trail, goes left.

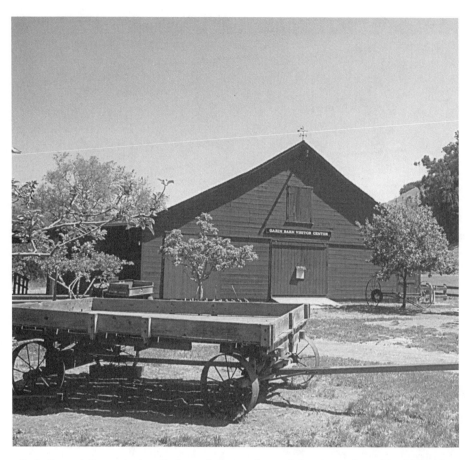

Garin Barn visitor center has displays relating to the area's farming and ranching history.

Now you climb a dirt-and-gravel road on a moderate grade toward a cattle pen, but before reaching it, you bear right on a dirt road and continue uphill to a junction with the return part of the Vista Peak Loop Trail, right. From here you continue climbing through an area of coast live oak and California bay, where a few eucalyptus and olive trees have been planted, and soon you are rewarded by wonderful views, if the day is clear, northwest to San Francisco, and south to the Coyote Hills and the Santa Cruz Mountains.

Garin Regional Park and its neighbor, Dry Creek Pioneer Regional Park, are a 3019-acre haven in the midst of bustling commercial and residential areas, some of which press right up to the parks' boundaries. But despite, or perhaps because of, the intense human activity nearby, wildlife, especially birds, finds refuge here. During your hike you may glimpse a small blue and orange bird—the western bluebird—darting out from the trees, hunting for insects. Also here is the western meadowlark, another colorful songbird, with a bright yellow breast, black breast band, and white outside tail feathers.

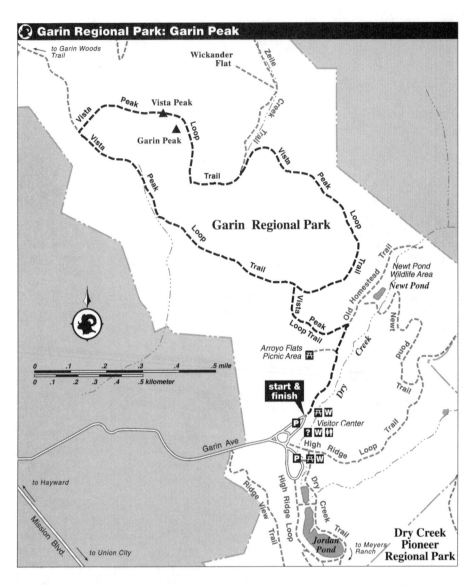

At about the 1.3-mile point, you reach a junction. Turn right and climb east over open ground, still on the Vista Peak Loop Trail. After 150 feet or so, you pass a shortcut, right, that traverses the southwest side of Garin and Vista peaks. Bush monkeyflower and California sagebrush are among the shrubs growing on the high ground around the peaks. As the road reaches the ridgetop just north of Vista Peak (934'), it bends right and heads for the summit of Garin Peak. To reach that peak's 948-foot summit, you leave the road before it starts to descend and walk uphill across a gentle, grassy slope.

From the summit, you have 360-degree views of the Bay Area landmarks, including Mt. Tamalpais (northwest), Mission Peak (southeast), and Mt. Hamilton, the large peak east of and beyond Mission Peak. California poppy, Ithuriel's spear, and yarrow decorate the scene in spring. After admiring the view, return to the road and descend through a gap between Garin Peak and an unnamed peak to the left. As the road makes a gentle descent through open country, the shortcut you passed earlier appears on your right. Now the descent steepens as the route drops into a small valley. Overhead, turkey vultures may be catching thermal updrafts or soaring on the breeze.

At about the 2-mile point, in the bottom of the valley, you pass a junction with the Zeile Creek Trail, left. Here the Vista Peak Loop Trail continues straight, then bends right, climbing to a gap between two hills. This is a scenic, more remote section of the park, and the route charts a rolling course across grassy hillsides and through occasional groves of trees. Soon, as the route starts to bend west, you see Newt Pond through some big western sycamore trees, downhill and left. Ahead in the distance are the visitor center and parking areas. If the sun is about to set, listen carefully here for the "hoo, hoo, hoo-hoo" call of a great horned owl. Just before the 3-mile point, you reach the junction you passed at the start of this loop. Turn left and retrace your route to the parking area.

ZEILE CREEK

Length: 4.3 miles

Time: 2 to 3 hours

Rating: Moderate

Regulations: EBRPD; fees for parking and dogs when entrance kiosk is attended; no bicycles.

Facilities: The visitor center in a restored barn has displays of antique farm equipment and information about Hayward's ranching and farming history; toilets nearby in a separate building; picnic tables, water, phone.

Directions: From Interstate 580 eastbound in Castro Valley, take the Hayward/Route 238 exit and follow signs for Hayward. From the first traffic light, continue straight, now on Foothill Blvd., for 1.7 miles to Mission Blvd., staying in the left lanes as you approach Mission Blvd. Bear left onto Mission Blvd. and go 3.5 miles to Garin Ave. Turn left and go 0.9 mile uphill to the entrance kiosk. At the kiosk bear left, find the parking area farthest left, and enter by turning right. The trailhead is at the northeast end of parking area.

From Interstate 580 westbound in Castro Valley, take the Strobridge exit and go 0.2 mile to the first stop sign. Turn right, go 0.1 mile to Castro Valley Blvd., and turn left. Follow Castro Valley Blvd. 0.5 mile to Foothill Blvd., turn left, and follow the directions above.

This loop shares the same start and finish with "Garin Peak," but trades the views from Vista and Garin peaks for a quiet stroll along Zeile Creek through a botanically rich, secluded canyon on the park's northeast boundary.

From the end of the parking area, follow a paved, gated road northeast beside a creek, right, lined with willow and western sycamore. The visitor center and pic-

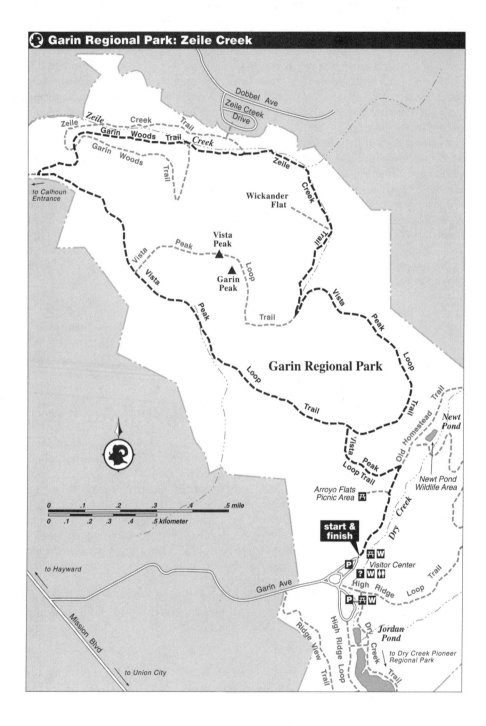

Garin Regional Park: Zeile Creek

Dobbel Ave

Zeile Creek Drive

Zeile   Creek   Trail
Zeile
Garin   Woods   Trail   Creek

Garin   Woods   Trail

to Calhoun Entrance

Zeile Creek

Wickander Flat

Vista Peak

Vista Peak

Vista
Peak

Vista

Garin Peak

Loop

Trail

Vista Peak Loop Trail

Peak

Loop

Trail

Garin Regional Park

Loop   Trail

Old Homestead Trail

Newt Pond

Newt Pond Wildlife Area

Vista Peak Loop Trail

Dry   Creek

Arroyo Flats Picnic Area

start & finish

P

Visitor Center

? High Ridge

P

Garin Ave

Loop   Trail

Jordan Pond

Ridge View Trail

High Ridge Loop

Dry Creek Trail

to Dry Creek Pioneer Regional Park

to Hayward

Mission Blvd

to Union City

0   .1   .2   .3   .4   .5 mile
0   .1   .2   .3   .4   .5 kilometer

nic areas are across the creek. Soon you pass through a shady corridor of Monterey pine, coast live oak, willow, and white alder. At the end of the paved road you pass a junction with a road heading left to the Arroyo Flats picnic area. About 50 feet past this junction, you reach a cattle gate; now you are on a dirt road. Approximately 100 yards past the gate, turn left on the Vista Peak Loop Trail.

Now you climb a dirt-and-gravel road on a moderate grade toward a cattle pen, but before reaching it, you bear right on a dirt road and continue uphill to a junction with the return part of the Vista Peak Loop Trail, right. From here you bear left, continue climbing, and, at about 1.3 miles, reach a junction. Go straight, descending just west of north on a dirt road, across open, rolling hills, with the CSU Hayward campus ahead in the distance. With a large barn, left, and a steep hillside dropping right, you pass through a gate and soon meet a road going right and downhill, signed for the Garin Woods and Zeile Creek trails.

Turn right and follow the road as it descends into a canyon via several long switchbacks. As the road bends left, you reach a junction with the Garin Woods Trail, a single track for hiking only, heading right. The Zeile Creek Trail, for horses and hikers, continues straight. The area you are about to enter, a botanical treasure trove, is owned by the California State Research Foundation and managed by EBRPD.

Turn right, and about 50 feet after leaving the road, pass a junction with a single-track trail climbing right. Continue downhill, and in another 50 feet you enter a cool, shady forest of California bay, with toyon, poison oak, blackberry vines, ferns, and mosses growing on the damp hillside. This hidden canyon, at about the 2-mile point, contrasts wonderfully with the open grassland you have been hiking across so far.

Zeile Creek is at the bottom of a steep ravine, left. Soon the route levels, then descends again on a gentle grade. You may notice a faint path coming up from the creek; about 200 feet farther, you come to a fence, with a housing development visible uphill on an open hillside, left. Just past the fence, another path comes in from the left, but you turn right and begin a gentle climb.

This area may be muddy in wet weather, and moisture stored year-round in the soil promotes a wide variety of plants, among them willow, bay, coast live oak, California buckeye, coffeeberry, vine honeysuckle, and canyon gooseberry. As you come over a rise, you pass an unsigned trail, right, and soon after, the Zeile Creek Trail joins from the left. The area you are now in, Wickander Flat, may be flooded during and after wet weather, because the trail is right beside the creek. Now you climb away from the creek on a moderate grade, past another fence, and soon come out of the trees, making an abrupt transition back to grassland.

After passing an unsigned road, right, the route, now a dirt road, bends left and continues uphill. Just before the 3-mile point, you reach a T-junction with the Vista Peak Loop Trail. Turn left and follow the trail as it bends right, climbing to a gap between two hills. Now the route follows a rolling course across grassy hillsides and through occasional groves of trees. Soon, as the route starts to bend west, you see Newt Pond through some big western sycamore trees, downhill and left. Ahead in the distance are the visitor center and parking areas. Closing the loop, you turn left and retrace your route to the parking area.

◆Dry Creek Pioneer Regional Park ◆

TOLMAN PEAK

Length: 9.6 miles

Time: 4 to 6 hours

Rating: Difficult

Regulations: EBRPD; fees for parking and dogs when entrance kiosk is attended; no bicycles on the South Fork or Dry Creek trails.

Facilities: The visitor center in a restored barn has displays of antique farm equipment and information about Hayward's ranching and farming history; toilets nearby in a separate building; picnic tables, fire grates, water, phone.

Directions: From Interstate 580 eastbound in Castro Valley, take the Hayward/Route 238 exit and follow signs for Hayward. From the first traffic light, continue straight, now on Foothill Blvd., for 1.7 miles to Mission Blvd., staying in the left lanes as you approach Mission Blvd. Bear left onto Mission Blvd. and go 3.5 miles to Garin Ave. Turn left and go 0.9 mile uphill to the entrance kiosk. At the kiosk bear right and proceed to parking areas; park in lowest one if space is available. The trailhead is at the northeast corner of the lower parking area.

From Interstate 580 westbound in Castro Valley, take the Strobridge exit and go 0.2 mile to the first stop sign. Turn right, go 0.1 mile to Castro Valley Blvd., and turn left. Follow Castro Valley Blvd. 0.5 mile to Foothill Blvd., turn left, and follow the directions above.

Combining the High Ridge Loop, Tolman Peak, South Fork, Meyers Ranch, and Dry Creek trails, this route—two loops attached by an out-and-back section— explores a regional park gem, an oasis in the middle of one of the East Bay's most heavily industrial and residential areas. Scenery, views, and variety of habitat combine to make hiking to Tolman Peak more than just a challenging workout. Mileage and commitment, rather than steepness of terrain, earn for this hike its "difficult" rating.

Go east and cross a bridged creek, then continue straight on a path into a picnic area. When you come to a gravel road, cross it, go through a cattle gate, and begin climbing the High Ridge Loop Trail. This dirt road ascends through an open area of tall grass and weeds, leaving behind the trees—sycamore, willow, fig, and California buckeye—that line the creek by the park's picnic area. Soon you pass the Newt Pond Trail, left, which connects this part of the High Ridge Loop Trail with the Newt Pond Wildlife Area.

As you gain elevation, turn around from time to time to appreciate the expanding view of San Francisco Bay. In spring, before the hills begin to turn brown, look for wildflowers such as California poppy, red maids, Ithuriel's spear, and Mariposa lily. Along the way uphill you may be accompanied by red-winged blackbirds, turkey vultures, or a kestrel hovering overhead.

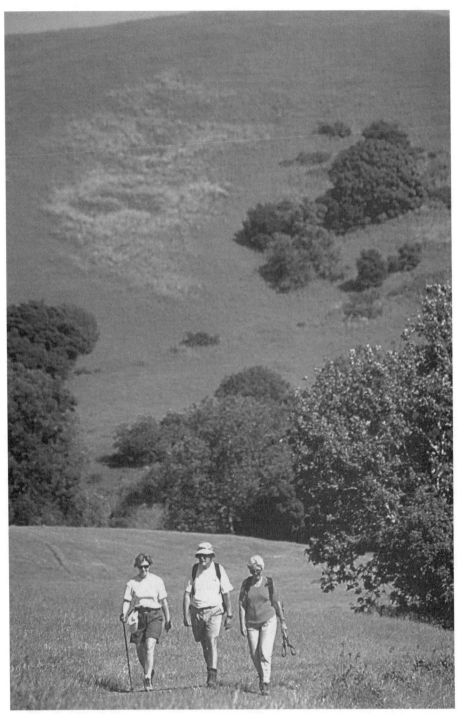

The high ground of Dry Creek Pioneer Regional Park features mostly open grasslands.

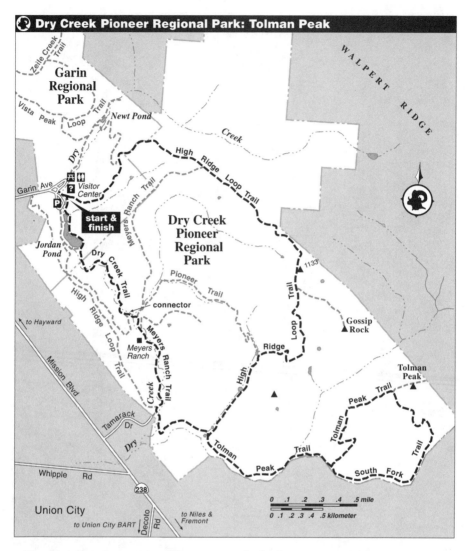

Dry Creek Pioneer Regional Park: Tolman Peak

The route levels, turns southeast, goes through a gate, and reaches a junction with the Meyers Ranch Trail, right. This area is used by cows, and you may notice several stock ponds along the way. Continuing straight, you are just east of and below the crest of a ridge that blocks your view of the Bay. But in a few minutes an expansive scene is revealed—San Francisco Bay National Wildlife Refuge, Coyote Hills, the Dumbarton and San Mateo bridges, Fremont, Newark, and Union City. A short climb to a notch between two low hills earns your first view of Mission Peak to the southeast, and the southern end of San Francisco Bay.

Just past the 2-mile point, you reach a junction with the Gossip Rock Trail, which heads left. There is a rest bench here, but on a hot day you may want to walk the short distance to Gossip Rock and enjoy the shade of the large California bay trees growing there. Western meadowlarks, western scrub-jays, wrentits, and horned larks are all possible sightings in this area. Keep your ears as well as your eyes alert: you will often hear birds before spotting them. Leaving the junction, the road descends through open grassland dotted with rocks and boulders. As the route steepens, notice the large western sycamore trees in a gully on your right. While the gully itself may be dry most of the year, there is enough moisture underground to support these large, water-loving trees. California sagebrush, a plant suited to dry areas, grows here on an east-facing slope above the gully.

Bear right at the next junction to stay on the High Ridge Loop Trail, and continue steeply downhill through a weedy area of thistle and poison hemlock. Soon you reach a shady stretch where bay, coast live oak, California buckeye, blue elderberry, snowberry, and vine honeysuckle thrive. The route descends to a lovely valley with a seasonal stream on the right. Just before the 3-mile point, the Pioneer Trail heads right, but your route continues straight. Bigleaf maple joins sycamore in a wet area on the right. Hear a scratching sound in the dry leaves? It could be a spotted towhee, or perhaps even a skunk.

At about 3.5 miles you reach a T-junction, with a stock pond just ahead. Here you turn left on the Tolman Peak Trail, a dirt-and-gravel road. (To shorten this route by omitting the hike to Tolman Peak, turn right to stay on the High Ridge Loop Trail and follow the directions below to the parking area.)

Now you skirt the pond and walk through Black Creek Valley, a lowland area of sycamore, eucalyptus, willow, bigleaf maple, coast live oak, and blue elderberry. While the grassy meadow bordering a creek on your right looks inviting, be careful: cows use this area and their pies are everywhere. A bit farther, past a cattle pen on the left, there is a place to sit and rest on handy stumps in a shady grove of tall eucalyptus.

Pass through a gate, and with a creek on your right, leave the eucalyptus grove behind. The route soon crosses the creek—here is lined with a few redwood trees—on a small bridge, then comes into the open. There is a bench, left, just after the bridge. Farther on, where the trail crosses the creek, you may have to hop from rock to rock if the creek is full. Soon the Tolman Peak Trail turns left, but you continue straight on the dirt road you have been following, here called the South Fork Trail. Just before reaching the regional park boundary, the South Fork Trail, now a single track, turns left and climbs across a steep hillside into a shady, overgrown area.

Gaining elevation in the shade of bay and coast live oak, the route veers left at about the 5-mile point and comes out of the forest to cross a grassy hillside. Here the trail may be completely overgrown and hard to spot: look for a line of matted grass as the trail curves right, following the hill's contour. As you continue to climb across the southwest slope of Tolman Peak, you have views to the southern end of San Francisco Bay and the Santa Cruz mountains; behind you looms Mission Peak.

Where the grade eases, you leave the single-track trail and regain a dirt road, heading northwest. A rest bench provides you with another opportunity to sit and admire the view of San Francisco Bay, and if you look northwest, you can see the trail to Gossip Rock you passed earlier. As you begin to descend, look for a trail post with a sign for the Tolman Peak Trail. From here, a faint path in the grass leads uphill to the right, heading for Tolman Peak, its summit topped by a grove of bay, buckeye, and bigleaf maple. (The 0.2-mile side trip to the summit is fun but does not gain you any better views.)

Bear left from the trail post and wind downhill on a moderate and then steep grade. Now you follow a small creek through an area of sycamore, coast live oak, and eucalyptus to a junction, where you turn right and retrace your route through Black Creek Valley, perhaps to the sound of a woodpecker drumming on a tree.

At about the 7.3-mile point, you return to the junction with the High Ridge Loop Trail. Here you continue straight, climbing in the open on a gentle grade, with a creek downhill and on the left. Soon an unsigned road heads left, but you turn sharply right and descend past stands of willow and coast live oak, which give shade that is welcome on a warm day.

About 0.5 mile past the previous junction, the route forks: a dirt road goes left to a fence at the end of Tamarack Dr., but you veer right toward a trail post. Here you leave the High Ridge Loop Trail, which curves left and climbs, and get on the Meyers Ranch Trail, which goes straight and slightly downhill. Dry Creek, which flows into San Francisco Bay via Alameda County's flood-control channel, is on your right, and you are walking upstream.

Meyers Ranch Trail, a dirt road, crosses Dry Creek on small bridges several times as the route ducks in and out of trees. Along the way you will notice many narrow paths diverging from the main road: ignore them.

If you hear a bird making a sound like a chickadee, you may glimpse instead its cousin, the oak titmouse, a small gray-brown bird with a small crest and a long tail. Chickadees and titmice belong to the same family (*Paridae*). Feeding mostly on insects, these lively birds are amusing to watch as they search branches and limbs, sometimes hanging upside down, for their supper.

Just past the 8-mile point, you come to a sign for Meyers Ranch; pieces of antique farm equipment, rusted, are lying in the grass to your right. Planted poplars and fruit trees show this was once a homestead. In fact, Garin and Dry Creek Pioneer regional parks were once occupied by two cattle ranches. Garin Ranch was obtained by EBRPD in the 1960s, and in 1978 the District received a gift of the 1200-acre Dry Creek Pioneer Ranch from the three Meyers sisters, grand-daughters of settlers who came here in 1884.

After passing a bench and leaving the Meyers Ranch site, look for a trail post on your left indicating the Dry Creek Trail. Turn left and descend a narrow path, which may be muddy in the spring. After about 100 feet, an unsigned path joins from the left, and just ahead is a narrow wooden bridge over Dry Creek.

Approximately 100 feet past the bridge, you come to a barbed-wire fence and cattle gate. Go through the gate and walk about 75 feet to a trail post and T-junction with the Dry Creek Trail, a single track. Turn right, toward Jordan Pond and the visitor center. Along the upcoming section of the Dry Creek Trail, you will see numbered markers for the park's self-guiding nature trail, a great excursion for children and parents. (A booklet keyed to the numbers can be bought or borrowed at the visitor center.)

Your route now winds through a shady area and crosses the creek on another wooden bridge. Ignore the unofficial trail branching right; it rejoins the main trail after 100 feet or so. Dark-eyed juncos frequent this area, and you may spot a western bluebird here, or get buzzed by a hummingbird.

After crossing a low ridge, you come to a grove of tall bay trees. Here one branch of the trail leads straight to a horse crossing at the creek, but you turn left and cross the creek on a wooden bridge. A dark shape gliding through the trees in this area may be a Cooper's hawk, a crow-sized raptor sporting a streaked breast—reddish in adult birds—and a long, black-and-white striped tail.

Once across the creek, turn right and, at a big rock, join the path coming from the horse crossing on your right. Now your route bends sharply left and soon reaches an open area, which may be muddy. Here a path heads left uphill, but you continue straight through a willow thicket, and in 150 feet reach a fork in the trail: right for horses, straight for hikers. Another bridge takes you over the creek, and now you pass the horse trail, which joins from the right. Where a path angles left, you go straight to a T-junction at artificial Jordan Pond.

Here you turn right and begin circling the pond on a dirt road, through an area of picnic tables and fire grates. Keep an eye out for birds in this part of the park too; songbirds, such as Bullock's oriole, favor the tree branches, with occasional forays into the open. As you near the end of the pond, you come to a fork: left to a picnic area, right to the visitor center and parking area. Bear right, go through a meadow, and just before reaching the visitor center, you meet the High Ridge Loop Trail, right. Turn left here and retrace your route to the parking area.

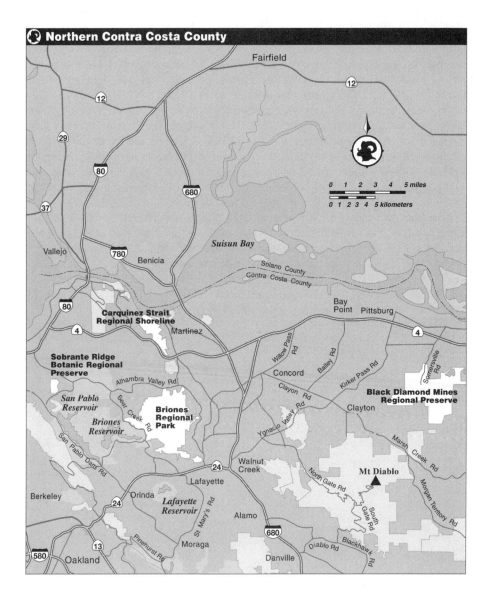

♦ Northern Contra Costa County ♦

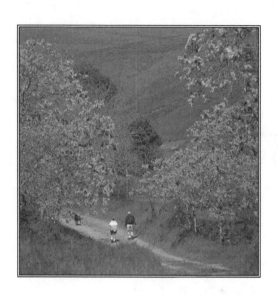

◆ Sobrante Ridge Botanic Regional Preserve ◆

MANZANITA GROVE

Length: 2.4 miles

Time: 1 to 2 hours

Rating: Easy

Regulations: EBRPD.

Facilities: Water, horse staging.

Directions: From Interstate 80 in San Pablo, take the San Pablo Dam Road exit and follow San Pablo Dam Road 3.9 miles north, east, then southeast to Castro Ranch Road. Turn left, go 1.2 miles to Conestoga Way, and turn left again. After 0.3 mile you reach Carriage Dr. Turn left, go 0.1 mile to Coach Dr., and turn right. After 0.3 mile Coach ends in a cul-de-sac, where a short driveway leads to the preserve parking area. The trailhead is on the west side of parking area.

There are two places in the East Bay to see rare and endangered pallid manzanita, also called Alameda manzanita: Huckleberry Botanic Regional Preserve, described elsewhere in this book, and here, a 277-acre preserve that was once part of a vast cattle ranch. This out-and-back route follows the Sobrante Ridge,

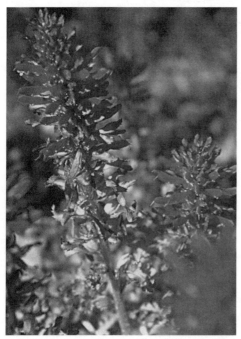

Heath warrior is often found growing near manzanita.

Manzanita, and Manzanita Loop trails. The Sobrante Ridge Trail, part of the Bay Area Ridge Trail, runs along a horseshoe-shaped ridge, with views of Mt. Diablo, Mt. Tamalpais, and San Pablo Ridge. The best time to hike here is winter, after the first rains, when the manzanitas are in flower.

From the west side of the parking area walk uphill past a gate on a paved road, and after several hundred feet you come to the Sobrante Ridge Trail, a dirt-and-gravel path. Turn left here and climb south toward a large power-line tower. From the suburban scene before you, it is hard to imagine that one of the East Bay's botanical treasures, a grove of rare and endangered pallid, or Alameda, manzanita lies only a few minutes away. The manzanita here owes its existence to two factors—poor, rocky soil and heat-tem-

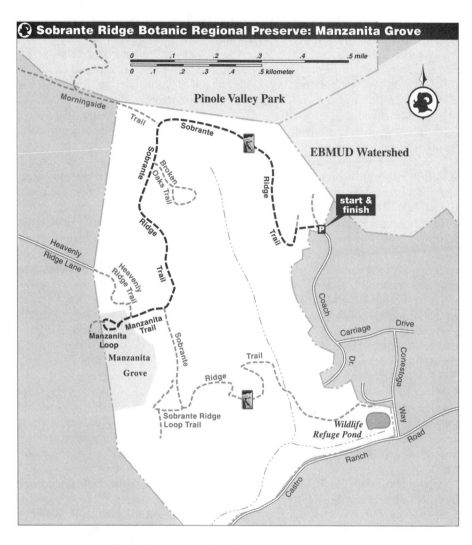

Sobrante Ridge Botanic Regional Preserve: Manzanita Grove

pering fog—that allow this species, also found in the Huckleberry Botanic Regional Preserve, to survive.

The housing developments nearby lay nestled in valleys, but beyond them rise high ridges—San Pablo, Sobrante, Oursan—in open space protected from development by EBRPD and EBMUD. Reaching the power-line tower, the route bends sharply right and continues its easy climb across a mostly open hillside where, in spring, California poppies dot the green grass with orange. Power-line towers, while an eyesore, provide perches for birds of prey in an otherwise treeless area, so you may see red-tailed hawks, red-shouldered hawks, or an American kestrel. As you head north, Mt. Diablo can be seen peeking over a ridge, right, and you have a steep forested canyon on your left.

As you come over the crest of a ridge, the view extends northwest, past the refineries that border San Pablo Bay, to the hills of Napa and Sonoma counties and

Mt. St. Helena. The route levels and turns left, taking you past stands of California bay and coast live oak, and brushy areas filled with coyote brush and poison oak. The call of a California quail, the buzz of a hummingbird's aerial display, or the medley of a mockingbird may be the only sound breaking the silence here. Where the route makes a left-hand bend, about the 0.6-mile point, you pass the Morningside Trail, right. Now you have a fine view west to Richmond, San Pablo Bay, and Mt. Tamalpais. Heading south, you soon reach a picnic table and a junction with the Broken Oaks Trail, left. The coast live oaks here are lovely, especially in spring when they flower.

Your route, the Sobrante Ridge Trail, descends through a wooded area decorated with spring wildflowers, then begins climbing to a clearing with another picnic table. Still on the rise, the route soon crests a ridge, turns sharply right, and drops to a junction. Here, at about the 1-mile point, a faint path heads right and uphill, and the Sobrante Ridge Trail turns left and goes about 100 yards to a picnic table. Continue straight, now the Manzanita Trail, a dirt road that descends on a gentle grade.

Approaching a stand of coast live oaks, the grade steepens and brings you to an unsigned and easily missed junction. Here the Heavenly Ridge Trail goes right, but you turn sharply left and walk in the shade of tall oaks, on a trail that may be overgrown with grass. Now you begin to see the pallid manzanita—red-barked shrubs with pointed, gray-green leaves, some tall, others low to the ground. A distinguishing feature of this species is the almost stemless leaves which attach directly to the shrub's branches.

Brittleleaf manzanita, which joins pallid manzanita in Huckleberry Botanic Regional Preserve, is here too. This small shrub has a basal burl—a large knot of wood at or just under ground level—and very stiff leaves with stems. (Manzanitas are hard to identify: they hybridize, and even experts disagree on how to classify certain varieties.) Where there is manzanita you are likely to find heath warrior, a curious parasitic plant with red and green leaves, related to owl's clover and paintbrush.

After a short, level walk you come to a trail post marking the Manzanita Loop Trail, left. Here a signboard describes this part of the preserve, where the soil is composed mostly of siliceous shale, as an "ecological island," unsuitable for most other plants but perfect for manzanita. Turning left onto the Manzanita Loop Trail, a single track, you begin walking uphill in a beautiful corridor of manzanitas, some of them holding their limbs high overhead, all with twisted dark-red trunks. Madrone, like manzanita a member of the heath family, is here too. Sharing some of its cousin's characteristics, madrone has reddish bark that turns scaly as the trees mature, larger, finely-toothed leaves, and differently shaped fruit.

After passing a clearing with a view of Mt. Tamalpais, the route descends and makes a sharp bend right, now near a housing development that borders the preserve: this juxtaposition of rare and endangered plants with suburban sprawl sends a strong message about the value of habitat preservation. Soon the route bends right and starts uphill, joining a path coming up from the housing development, left. At about the 1.33-mile point, you come back to the start of the Manzanita Loop Trail; from here retrace your steps to the parking area.

Carquinez Strait Regional Shoreline

FRANKLIN RIDGE

Length: 2.8 miles

Time: 1 to 2 hours

Rating: Moderate

Regulations: EBRPD.

Facilities: Picnic tables, toilets, horse staging.

Directions: From Highway 4 in Martinez, take the Alhambra Ave./Martinez exit and go north 2 miles to Escobar St. Turn left, go 0.1 mile to Talbart St. and turn right. Follow Talbart St. for 0.1 mile, veer left onto Carquinez Scenic Dr. and go 0.3 mile to the John A. Nejedly staging area, left. The lower parking area has some shade; the upper area has spaces for horse trailers. The trailhead is at the west end of upper parking area.

Circling a high ridge overlooking Carquinez Strait, this semi-loop has some steep sections, but your efforts are rewarded by terrific views of the strait, Suisun Bay, the west delta, Mt. Diablo, and the hills of Napa and Solano counties. Using the California Riding and Hiking Trail and the Franklin Ridge Loop Trail, your route explores open grassland, oak savanna, and shady, tree-lined ravines. Parts of this loop may be extremely muddy during and after wet weather.

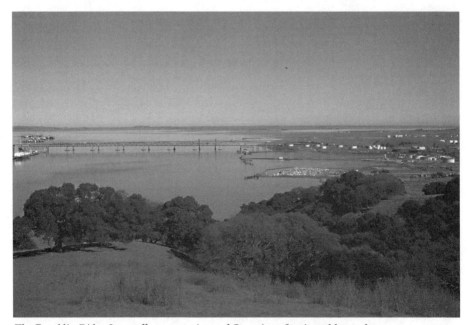

The Franklin Ridge Loop offers great views of Carquinez Strait and beyond.

From the west end of the upper parking area, go through a gate and walk west across a large, grassy field, coming after about 200 feet to a trail post. The emblems on the post indicate you are on the California Riding and Hiking Trail, which here is part of the Bay Area Ridge Trail. The Bay Area Ridge Trail is a proposed 500-mile multi-use trail—about half of which has been completed—that will pass through nine counties and completely circle the Bay Area.The California Riding and Hiking Trail was a similar idea on a state-wide scale, conceived in 1945, but only 16 miles of it are in use in the East Bay today.

Two other routes also begin here. The Rankin Park Trail leaves from the south side of the upper parking area, near picnic tables, and climbs west to the top of a ridge, joining the Bay Area Ridge/California Riding and Hiking Trail. And just past the gate, an unnamed dirt road heads right and steeply uphill, climbing to the top of the same ridge.

Continue straight past the trail post, following a single track through stands of California bay, California buckeye, coast live oak, and eucalyptus. There is a creek on your left, and this part of the route, in a cool, shady ravine, may be muddy. The trail widens and begins a moderate climb, soon turning away from the creek on a switchback and crossing an open, grassy hillside. Another switchback takes you through a wonderful area of blue elderberry, California sagebrush, and bush monkeyflower. As the trail heads back into the trees, a mourning dove's plaintive call may fool you into thinking you've heard an owl.

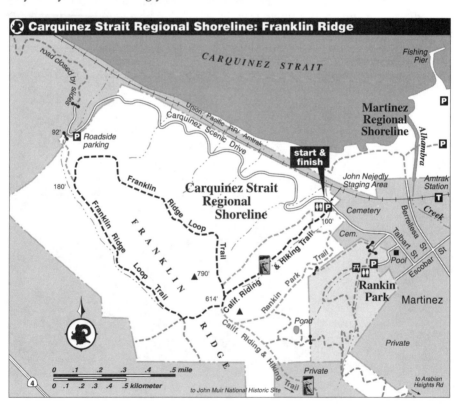

A steep climb in the shade of large bay trees, which soon give way to open grass-land, leads at last to a T-junction, marked by a trail post, at the summit of a ridge. Here you turn right onto the Franklin Ridge Loop Trail, a dirt road, and follow it north, enjoying magnificent views, right, of Martinez, Suisun Bay with its mothball fleet of World War II Navy ships, the west delta, and in the far distance, the Central Valley. From here you can even see all the way to the snow-capped peaks of the Sierra. Ahead are the housing developments that surround Benicia, and beyond are the hills of Napa and Solano counties. About 60 feet past the T-junction, you pass a road, right, leading to a viewpoint and a rest bench; this is the same steep dirt road you passed earlier as you left the parking area.

Enjoying a mostly level ridgetop walk, you enjoy splendid views of Mt. Diablo, southeast, and Mt. St. Helena, northwest. The Martinez Regional Shoreline, with its small lake and marshes, and the Martinez marina lie just in front of the Benicia–Martinez Bridge. As you round a bend in the trail, you can see ahead and below to the waters of Carquinez Strait, the narrow passage between Suisun and San Pablo bays. When you reach an unsigned fork, bear left, passing a rest bench where you can sit and enjoy the view, slightly marred by power lines. You may be visited by a hummingbird here, especially if you are wearing red. Now descend-ing northwest over eroded and perhaps muddy ground, you lose the dramatic vis-tas, and gain instead more intimate scenes of rolling hills and stately oaks, perhaps watched by a circling red-tailed hawk.

Passing another rest bench and a watering trough for animals, you get a good look at Carquinez Strait before the road drops off the ridge via a big S-bend. As you reach a saddle, you pass a path leading right and uphill to an oak-adorned summit. Below and right you can see the Carquinez Scenic Drive, which used to link Martinez and Port Costa until a 1982 landslide severed the road. Here your route bends left and continues to descend. At the next junction, an unsigned fork, bear right and enter an oak woodland—coast live oak, valley oak, and blue oak—where you may see or hear nuthatches and woodpeckers. A steep downhill pitch brings you, at about the 1.4-mile point, to a creek and a T-junction marked by a trail post.

Here you turn left, continuing on the Franklin Ridge Loop Trail, and begin a gentle climb on a dirt road, with a creek to your right. This is a peaceful area, with a mixture of bay and oak providing shade. In places you may find the road flood-ed by small rivulets running from a spring on the hillside, left, into the tree-lined creek. As the grade steepens you pass a fence and a restricted area, left, leaving the trees behind and coming again into open country. At a four-way junction marked by a trail post, just past the 2-mile point, you turn left and walk uphill, still on the Franklin Ridge Loop Trail. (The other two roads at this junction lead to the park boundary and private property.) At the end of a valley, right, you can see Highway 4, about 0.5 mile away.

Now you head northeast and, after a moderate climb, reach a flat spot and a T-junction marked by a trail post. Running left to right in front of you is the Bay Area Ridge/California Riding and Hiking Trail, a dirt road. To finish your loop, turn left and walk about 250 feet to the junction, marked by a trail post, with the trail com-ing from the parking area; here you turn right and retrace your steps.

◆ Briones Regional Park ◆

DIABLO VIEW

Length: 4.8 miles

Time: 3 to 4 hours

Rating: Moderate

Regulations: EBRPD.

Facilities: Toilet, water (may not be available due to contamination); horse staging.

Directions: From Highway 4 in Martinez, take the Alhambra Ave. exit and go 0.5 mile south on Alhambra Ave. to Alhambra Valley Road. Turn right and go 1.2 miles to Reliez Valley Road. Turn left and go 0.5 mile to the Alhambra Creek Valley entrance, marked by a sign. Turn right and follow the entrance road 0.8 mile to the parking area. The trailhead is at the southeast corner of the parking area.

This loop, which includes all or parts of the Diablo View, Spengler, Old Briones Road, Pine Tree, Orchard, and Alhambra Creek trails, gives you a chance to explore the East Bay's largest developed regional park, an area of deep wooded canyons, forested slopes, oak savannas, and open, grassy ridges. The varied habitat attracts a large variety of birds, from chickadees to golden eagles. The plant life along this route is equally diverse, with a wide range of trees, shrubs, and wildflowers.

From the southeast corner of the parking area, pass through a gate next to an information board, turn immediately left onto the Diablo View Trail, a dirt road, and follow it gently uphill. Another dirt road, heading straight from the gate, is the Alhambra Creek Trail, part of your return route. This is open, rolling country, the realm of grassland and oak savanna. Soon after leaving the parking area, you pass the Tavan Trail, left, and now the slope changes to moderate as you ascend via well-graded S-bends toward the top of a ridge, where a fine view of Mt. Diablo awaits. Along the way, you pass the Hidden Pond Trail, left, a dirt road. From the ridgetop you also can see Concord, Highway 4, and the west delta.

The oaks up here, mostly valley oaks, are full of large clumps of mistletoe, easy to see when the limbs are bare or just getting their beautiful yellow-green foliage in late winter. Other trees and shrubs here include California bay, California buckeye, blue elderberry, coffeeberry, and hillside gooseberry. In late winter and early spring, the surrounding hillsides are dotted with color from California buttercup, bluedicks, and shooting stars.

After about 0.5 mile you reach a fork marked by a trail post. Here you stay on the Diablo View Trail, now a dirt path, as it bends left and makes a gentle climb along a ridgetop that splits two deep valleys. The route enters the shade of coast live oak, valley oak, and blue oak, and begins a rolling course. Now in the open, you reach a fence with a gate; just beyond is a T-junction, where you turn right onto a dirt road.

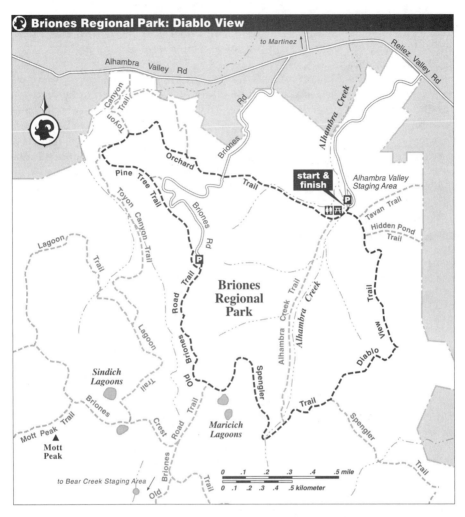

Briones Regional Park: Diablo View

Because of its diversity of habitat—shady canyons, oak savanna, open grass-land—this regional park attracts a wide variety of birds, each suited to a different environment. The tiny chestnut-backed chickadee, for example, is at home in the trees, where it often hangs upside-down on branches, picking off insects. Look in the trees also for woodpeckers, warblers, and dark-eyed juncos. The lark sparrow is a bird of open, grassy fields, sharing this terrain with the western meadowlark and the horned lark. Raptors—large birds of prey such as red-tailed hawks, red-shouldered hawks, and vultures—spend most of their time hunting from the air. The golden eagle, a raptor seldom seen in the East Bay, has been spotted here.

As you continue on a rolling course through the oaks, you pass an overgrown road leading left and downhill. From time to time you will also see dirt paths diverging from the main route; ignore these. Now the route breaks into the open, with a steep hillside dropping left, and a stunning view of Mt. Diablo, east. Soon you come to a four-way intersection and the end of the Diablo View Trail. Turn right on the Spengler Trail, an eroded dirt road, and descend moderately to a shady area of coast live oak and bay, where the forest floor is carpeted with miner's lettuce, whose tiny white flowers appear in late winter and last through May.

After passing through a gate, you continue to descend over easy and then moderate ground to the Alhambra Creek canyon. At the bottom of the canyon, two creeks merge on your left and flow as one through a culvert under the road. Just past the creek crossing is a junction. Here the Alhambra Creek Trail heads right and downhill, but your route, the Spengler Trail, bears left and begins its climb out of the canyon on a moderate grade. Bay limbs arch over the dirt-and-gravel road, giving shade to embankments where ferns and blackberry vines thrive. About 0.1 mile past the previous junction, your route swings sharply right. (An unsigned path continues straight, following the creek upstream past a lovely series of small waterfalls which tumble over large tree roots instead of rocks.)

Where the forest canopy—bays, bigleaf maples, buckeyes, and coast live oaks—gives way and allows sunlight to penetrate, shrubs such as black sage, bush monkeyflower, blue bush lupine, and toyon have taken hold. Just after the 2-mile point, you pass a dead-end road, right, and continue to climb through alternating sections of sun and shade. The route then breaks abruptly into the open, goes through a gate, and, in about 100 yards, reaches one of the two Maricich Lagoons.

At a T-junction here with the Old Briones Road Trail, turn right and walk downhill, coming in about 250 feet to another gate and a junction with an unsigned path, left. Stay right, go through the gate, and continue descending north on the Old Briones Road Trail, passing a rest bench on the left. Ignoring various unofficial trails, you soon reach the edge of a steep and wild-looking canyon, left. California sagebrush, lupine, paintbrush, and madrone cling to the canyon's sheer west-facing wall. A short while ago you were in a cool, shady canyon; now the route is open and exposed, a different environment entirely. Across the canyon rises the main crest of the Briones Hills, which you can explore another day by following the "Briones Crest" trip elsewhere in this book.

Following the road downhill, past clearings where you can see Concord and Mt. Diablo again, you eventually reach a parking area, right, at the end of Briones Road, with an information board and drinking fountain close by. Just past the information board is a gate, and beyond the gate, a paved area. Before reaching the gate, find the single-track trail that begins just left of the drinking fountain and skirts the left side of a wooden fence, which is next to paved Briones Road. Follow this trail for about 200 feet, pass through a gap in the fence, then turn left and walk along the fence until you reach a gate. Go through the gate and, with Briones Road on your right, climb past a power-line tower.

Now descending, at one point with a very steep drop on the left, you merge with the Pine Tree Trail, a dirt road, and bear left. Soon you pass the large grove of pines—Monterey and Coulter—that give this trail its name. Western bluebirds, hummingbirds, and western scrub-jays all frequent this area, and in the spring, red maids add patches of magenta, which complement the green grass. Shortly after merging with the Pine Tree Trail, the route passes another junction, where the Toyon Canyon Trail heads sharply left. Continuing straight, you pass an unsigned path on the right, and see ahead a fenced pond where you may catch a glimpse of a belted kingfisher, a compact blue-and-white bird with a long bill and a pronounced head crest. The kingfisher makes a dry, rattling sound as it flies from one perch to the next.

At the southeast corner of the pond is a junction. Here the Pine Tree Trail turns left and goes through a gate, but your route, the Orchard Trail, a dirt road, bends right and begins a rolling course over open terrain. The road skirts a barbed-wire fence, left, and enters a stand of eucalyptus and olive trees. Just before making a swing to the left, you pass a path, right, and then go through a gate and walk in the shade of eucalyptus, pine, and coast live oak.

At about the 4-mile point, you reach a junction where an unsigned trail merges sharply from the left. Here your route, the Orchard Trail, continues straight, passing a path, left, and a gate. This eroded section of the road, near the Rancho Briones Equestrian Facility, may be muddy in wet weather. Just after passing a stable, you cross Briones Road, go through a gate, and continue following the Orchard Trail, now a dirt path, as it leads directly toward Mt. Diablo, a perfect view marred by power lines.

You continue to walk southeast through a little valley, following a tributary of Alhambra Creek, left. At a place where the trail bends right and climbs slightly, you may see an entire hillside, left, full of ground squirrel holes—a squirrel condominium with a sunny, southwestern exposure. Just past the 5-mile point, you come to a large fenced picnic area, left, and a T-junction with the Alhambra Creek Trail. Turn left here, crossing Alhambra Creek, which flows under the road through a culvert, and walk a short distance to the parking area.

◆ Black Diamond Mines Regional Preserve ◆

This regional preserve, nestled in oak-studded foothills between Mt. Diablo and the west delta, was once the site of the largest coal-mining complex in California. From the 1860s to just after the turn of the century, the Mt. Diablo Coal Field yielded roughly four million tons of coal, or "black diamonds," to miners, mostly Welsh and Irish, wielding pick and shovel. Five mining towns were located nearby, and three of them—Nortonville, Somersville, and Stewartville—were within the current boundaries of the preserve. According to Malcolm Margolin, author of *East Bay Out*, the largest town, Nortonville, had in 1870 three general stores, three hotels, four boarding houses, six saloons, and a livery stable. Roads and railroad lines carried the coal north to river landings near present-day Antioch and Pittsburg, where it was shipped to San Francisco, Stockton, and Sacramento.

By the mid-1880s, higher quality coal from the Pacific Northwest and the increasing use of oil spelled disaster for the coal miners here, and the town sites soon were abandoned, their buildings dismantled board by board for use elsewhere. The area had a brief rebirth from the 1920s to 1949 as a source of sand for both glass-making and steel-casting: more than 1.8 million tons of sand were extracted. The East Bay Regional Park District began acquiring land here in the early 1970s and currently oversees some 5985 acres of grassland, foothill woodland, mixed evergreen forest, chaparral, and riparian vegetation. One of the tasks faced by the District to make the preserve safe for public access was to locate potentially hazardous mine-shaft openings; the district even enlisted the help of a specially trained dog to aid its ground search teams. Most openings that were found were securely sealed, but Prospect Tunnel, just off the Stewartville Trail and marked on EBRPD's map, has about half of its 400-foot length open to the public on ranger-led tours.

The Greathouse visitor center, above the picnic area at Somersville town site, has displays of mining history, including artifacts and photographs, in an underground center at the entrance to the Greathouse Portal. The visitor center is open 9 A.M. to 3:30 P.M. on weekends from March to November. In addition to the visitor center and Prospect Tunnel, Black Diamond's attractions include seven other mining sites, also marked on the EBRPD map, and Rose Hill Cemetery, which sits on a hill just west of the Somersville

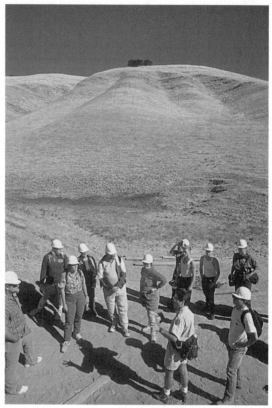

Ranger-led interpretive tours are popular at Black Diamond Mines Regional Preserve.

town site and the preserve's main entrance. The cemetery, containing graves of miners killed in accidents, wives who died in childbirth, and children who died in epidemics of smallpox, typhoid, diphtheria, and scarlet fever, is a fascinating place to visit.

More than 100 species of birds have been recorded in the preserve, including golden eagles, hawks, and falcons. The area is noted for its wildflowers and plants, including a few—Mt. Diablo manzanita, Mt. Diablo sunflower, and Mt. Diablo globe lily—found only here and on Mt. Diablo. The coal miners brought with them nonnative trees, which can still be seen, including black locust, tree of heaven, peppertree, almond, and eucalyptus. Located on the edge of the Central Valley, the area's 34 miles of trails are best enjoyed during fall, winter, and spring.

Park gates open: 8 A.M. to dusk

Visitor center: (925) 757-2620

Camping reservations: (510) 636-1684; Stewartville backpack camp (general public); Star Mine group camp (non-profit groups)

CHAPARRAL LOOP

Length: 2.3 miles

Time: 1 to 2 hours

Rating: Moderate

Regulations: EBRPD; parking fee; hiking only.

Facilities: Picnic tables, water, toilet.

Directions: From Highway 4 in Antioch, take the Somersville Road exit and go south, staying in the left lane as you approach and pass Buchanan Road. At 1.5 miles, follow Somersville Road as it continues straight, while the main road, now called James Donlon Blvd., bends sharply left. At 2.6 miles from Highway 4, you reach the entrance kiosk, park office, and emergency telephone; continue another 0.9 mile to a large parking area, right, with an overflow area, left. The trailhead is at the south end of parking area.

If you have only a few hours to spend in this wonderful preserve, consider this loop as an introduction to some of the attractions that make visiting here worthwhile: beautiful scenery, diverse plant life, and a reminder of the area's not-so-distant past as a thriving coal-mining district. This trip can easily be combined with a visit to historic Rose Hill Cemetery. (Numbers in **boldface** in the route description refer to sites on the EBRPD map and accompanying text.)

From the south end of the parking area, pass a gate and continue uphill on the Nortonville Trail, a paved road, for about 200 feet to a level area and a junction, left, with the Stewartville Trail, a dirt road. Turn left and begin walking uphill on a moderate grade that soon levels, heading southeast through open country. This part of the preserve has native trees common to inland areas of the East Bay—gray pine, blue oak, California buckeye—along with nonnatives brought in by early settlers, including eucalyptus, black locust, tree of heaven, and peppertree, a transplant from Peru with aromatic leaves and pink, peppercorn-like fruit.

A steep, grassy ridge, lush green in winter and early spring, rises left, forming a backdrop for grazing cattle. If you turn around and look west, you can see Rose Hill Cemetery, the last resting place for some of the miners, their wives, and children, who came here in the 1860s hoping to strike it rich on coal—"black diamonds." (The cemetery, well worth a visit, is a short climb from the parking area on the Nortonville Trail.)

Once through a cattle gate, you pass the Railroad Bed Trail, left, which follows part of the old Pittsburg Railroad route, used to haul coal from the Somersville town site, near the parking area, north to Pittsburg Landing, about halfway between present-day Pittsburg and Antioch. Ahead on the right is the Pittsburg Mine Trail. Continue straight on the Stewartville Trail, climbing southeast to an obvious notch in the skyline ridge. (The Stewartville Trail is part of the Mt. Diablo-to-Black Diamond Regional Trail, an 11.6-mile route from Contra Loma Regional Park to the north edge of Mt. Diablo State Park.)

The open grasslands and high ridges that make up this preserve are especially favorable to raptors—birds of prey such as hawks, falcons, and eagles—as well as turkey vultures. As you climb, keep an eye out for dark shapes circling overhead.

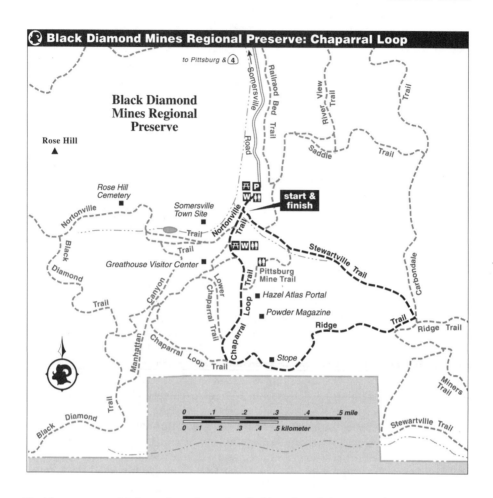

Besides common birds such as the red-tailed hawk and American kestrel, this preserve has been visited by golden eagles, huge brown birds often confused at a distance with large hawks or young bald eagles.

As you crest the ridge, you come to a 4-way junction with the Ridge Trail, right, and the Carbondale Trail, left, just before you reach a barbed-wire fence with a cattle gate. Turn right and follow the Ridge Trail, a dirt road, on a gentle uphill grade through a wooded area of blue oak and California buckeye. Just before a steep section, you pass an unsigned trail, right, and then climb to a dramatic high point with a 360-degree view that takes in much of this preserve, along with landmarks such as Mt. Diablo and the Central Valley.

On the way up, you will see some of the trees and shrubs that give the hot and dry areas of the East Bay their special character, such as gray pine, interior live oak, chamise, yerba santa, and narrow-leaf bush sunflower. Two plants that deserve special mention are Coulter pine, which reaches its northern limit in this preserve, and Mt. Diablo manzanita, found here and on its namesake mountain only. Coulter pine resembles gray pine but has larger cones, denser foliage, and stouter limbs.

Mt. Diablo manzanita has gray, felt-like leaves that attach to the plant's limbs without stems.

Now on the crest of a ridge, you pass two unsigned trails, one on each side of the trail, and begin a moderate descent, with several side trails heading left to viewpoints. The rock here is multicolored, and would not look out of place in the canyons of Utah or Arizona. Growing close to the ground here in small clumps is heath warrior, recognized by its brushy red and green leaves, and magenta flowers that appear in late winter through spring. A relative of paintbrush, heath warrior is a parasite, dependent on manzanita and madrone for its survival: When you see it, the host plants are sure to be nearby.

After a steep drop, the route reaches a four-way junction and the end of the Ridge Trail. To the left, a path dead-ends in a manzanita grove. Ahead and also to your right is the Chaparral Loop Trail. Turn right and descend on the Chaparral Loop Trail, a broad dirt path that crosses more exposed rock in places, through a wonderful area of manzanita, toyon, and Coulter pine. Soon you veer right at a junction with the Lower Chaparral Trail to stay on the Chaparral Loop Trail. At an upcoming fork, stay right again. Nearby rocks offer places to sit and enjoy the views.

A trail post, right, marks paths to the Powder Magazine, **6**, an artificial cave used to store explosives for mining, and to the Stope, **7**, a huge sandstone chamber where miners blasted rock for glass making. Bending left here, the route passes through a rocky area, with a view north to Somersville Road and the preserve entrance, and brings you to the Hazel Atlas Portal, **5**, where sand for glass-making was mined from the 1920s through 1940s. A set of narrow-gauge rail tracks disappears into a gated tunnel just uphill.

The trail now takes you past two junctions with the Pittsburg Mine Trail, right, one leading across a small wooden bridge. The trees lining the road here are called tree of heaven, a hardy nonnative known for its ability to take root under the most adverse conditions. After the tree flowers, it forms clusters of flat, winged fruit that rustle in the breeze.

In about 50 feet you come to a junction: here the Chaparral Loop Trail, a dirt road, turns left, but you continue straight, passing a picnic area, left, and a road heading left to the Greathouse Portal, **3**, another tunnel that was the original entrance for the sand mine and now serves as a visitor center. As the route bends right, you pass a large area of mine tailings and soon meet the Nortonville Trail. Turn right and follow the Nortonville Trail, a partially paved road that soon becomes completely paved, uphill to the junction with the Stewartville Trail, right. Continue straight, retracing your steps to the parking area.

NORTONVILLE LOOP

Length: 5.5 miles, excluding detours to visit Rose Hill Cemetery and mining sites.

Time: 3 to 5 hours

Rating: Moderate

Regulations: EBRPD; parking fee.

Facilities: Picnic tables, water, toilet; horse staging at a parking area, left, just past the entrance kiosk.

Directions: From Highway 4 in Antioch, take the Somersville Road exit and go south, staying in the left lane as you approach and pass Buchanan Road. At 1.5 miles, follow Somersville Road as it continues straight, while the main road, now called James Donlon Blvd., bends sharply left. At 2.6 miles from Highway 4, you reach the entrance kiosk, park office, and emergency telephone; continue another 0.9 mile to a large parking area, right, with an overflow area, left. The trailhead is at the south end of parking area.

This semi-loop, using the Nortonville and Black Diamond trails, takes you through in one of the East Bay's most remote, beautiful, and historic parks. The lands here were part of California's largest coal-mining area, active from the 1860s through the early 1900s. On the edge of the Central Valley, the preserve is best enjoyed during cool weather, but the trails do get very muddy during wet weather. In late winter and spring, wildflowers abound here, and it is during this time, before the trees and shrubs leaf out, that the preserve's numerous birds are easiest to spot. (Numbers in **boldface** in the route description refer to sites on the EBRPD map and accompanying text.)

Starting off on a paved road, the continuation of Somersville Road, you head south and gradually uphill from the parking area, following signs to CEMETERY, MINES, AND NORTONVILLE, all straight ahead. This preserve is characterized by rolling hills, grassland, and blue-oak savanna; other native trees include coast live oak, gray pine, Coulter pine, and California buckeye. There are also prominent stands of nonnative trees, including tree of heaven and black locust, which flowers fragrantly in the spring. A short distance from the parking area, you pass a junction with the Stewartville Trail, left, and continue straight on the Nortonville Trail, part of the Mt. Diablo–to–Black Diamond Regional Trail, an 11.6-mile route between Contra Loma Regional Park and the north side of Mt. Diablo State Park.

Soon the pavement changes to dirt, and when you reach a fork, bear right, continuing gently uphill on the Nortonville Trail toward Rose Hill Cemetery. Along the way, you pass the Manhattan Canyon Trail, left. Black Diamond Mines Regional Preserve, located on the edge of the Central Valley, is very hot in summer, but lovely during the rest of the year. Whether the grassy hills here are lush green after winter rains, or gold-hued in autumn, they appear sharply etched against the typically bright blue sky. Frog croaks and bird calls may be coming from a pond, right, fringed with cattails. This preserve is home to many birds, from huge turkey vultures to tiny hummingbirds, and from aerialists like the American kestrel to ground dwellers such as the golden-crowned sparrow.

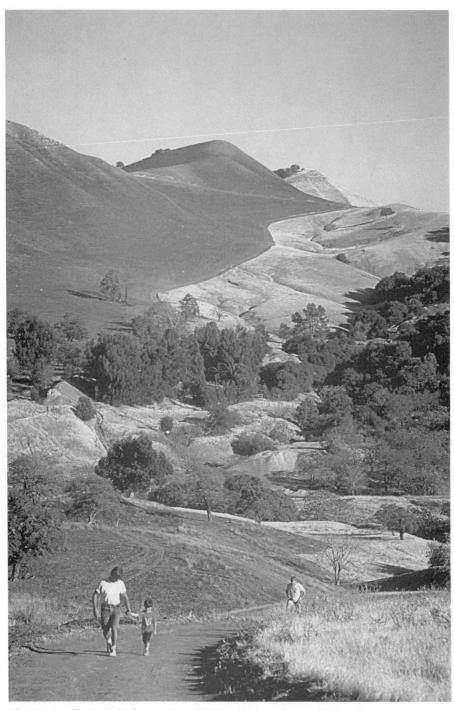

The Nortonville Trail climbs past Rose Hill Cemetery to Nortonville Pass.

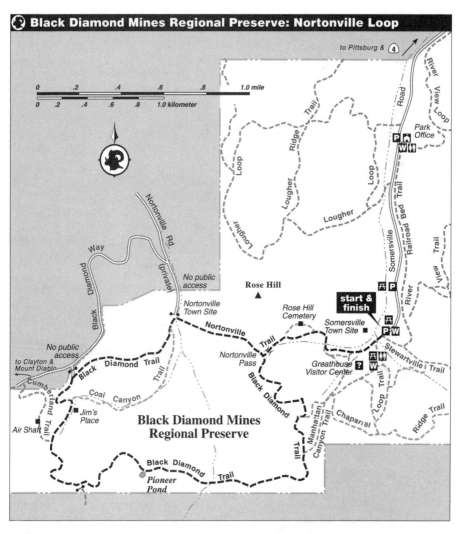

Black Diamond Mines Regional Preserve: Nortonville Loop

Just before the route makes a sweeping right turn, you pass another junction with the Manhattan Canyon Trail, a faint trace leading left. Now climbing on a moderate grade, you begin to get views east, toward the Stewartville section of this preserve, a remote area worth exploring on another day. If you want to visit the Rose Hill Cemetery, turn right at a signed junction and climb a dirt path until you reach a few wooden steps and the cemetery's main entrance, graced by a planting of peppertrees.

Most of the graves in Rose Hill Cemetery are from the mid-to-late 1800s, when this was California's largest coal-mining area. Five mining towns were active nearby—Nortonville, Somersville, Stewartville, West Hartley, and Judsonville. Among those buried here are David Watts, Theophilus Watts, and Thomas D. Jones, three young Welshmen, seeking a better life far from home, killed in an 1876 mine accident. Other graves hold miners' wives and children, victims of disease and the hazards of childbirth. It's hard to imagine, as you walk past the quiet grave sites and look out over the peaceful hills, that this area bustled not long ago with miners wielding pick and shovel, intent on digging nearly four million tons of coal—"black diamonds"—out of the earth.

After walking uphill and west through the cemetery, which has tall Italian cypress and other exotic plants, you take your leave via a gate and a dirt road, which soon joins the Nortonville Trail. Now the route climbs on a moderate grade toward Nortonville Pass, a notch in the western skyline. Just before reaching the pass, you go by a junction with the Black Diamond Trail, left, which you will use later on your return. Red-tailed hawks favor this area, perhaps because they can perch on nearby power-line towers, whereas colorful western bluebirds prefer to sit on the lines themselves. Look here also for lesser goldfinches, the males bright yellow with a black cap, black wings, and greenish backs.

Descending from the pass into a bowl-shaped valley, where Nortonville was located, you pass by mounds of earth, remnants of mining operations, then cross a creek that flows through a culvert, and soon reach a T-junction and the end of the Nortonville Trail. Here the dirt-and-gravel Nortonville Road goes right, but your route, the Black Diamond Trail, heads left. Passing through a cattle gate, you begin an uphill walk on a dirt road, heading south past a marshy area and a junction with the Coal Canyon Trail, left. Veer right and stay on the Black Diamond Trail as it climbs past a grove of black locust, then through a rocky draw to an area dominated by blue oak. On this part of the route you may also see coast live oak and interior live oak, along with California buckeye and gray pine. But the tree to watch for, growing here at the northern limit of its range, is Coulter pine, a stout, long-needled pine with huge cones.

As the route levels and meets Black Diamond Way, a paved road coming sharply from the right, you continue straight on the now-paved Black Diamond Trail, climbing on a gentle grade past a pond, left, and crossing over a culvert. The road makes several S-bends and reaches a clearing: look here for a metal trail post and a wide dirt path leading left a few hundred feet to Jim's Place, **2**, and the Coal Canyon Trail. Guarded by a towering Coulter pine, Jim's place is an underground dwelling of unknown origin, with a square skylight, round stovepipe hole, and shelves cut into the rock. Nearby, on the south edge of the clearing, is a marker for a placer-mining claim.

After visiting Jim's Place, continue uphill on the paved road to a heavily wooded area, stopping to admire a fine stand of manzanita, decorated in winter with white, globe-shaped flowers. A streambed, left, its banks carpeted with leaf litter, may attract woodland birds, such as dark-eyed juncos or perhaps a varied thrush, looking similar to its cousin, the American robin. Beyond the 2-mile point, you reach a junction with the Cumberland Trail/Mt. Diablo-to-Black Diamond Regional Trail, right, which leads past the Air Shaft, **1**, another mining site.

Still on the paved Black Diamond Trail, you wind moderately uphill, through a beautiful blue-oak savanna, switchbacking sharply several times. The sweeping view north from this upland area takes in Pittsburg, Antioch, the hills of Napa and Solano counties, and, on a clear day, Mt. St. Helena. Two dirt roads, one just past the other, head right, while a third, a bit farther on, goes straight and downhill to the preserve boundary. Your route follows pavement and continues to climb, soon revealing San Pablo Ridge, the Berkeley/Oakland hills, and, on the distant horizon, Mt. Tamalpais.

The route continues southeast, following an open ridgetop above steep canyons on either side, and soon reaches a junction with a wide dirt road, left—the continuation of the Black Diamond Trail. Leaving the paved road (marked NO TRESSPASSING), you descend east, enjoying a view that extends to the Antioch Bridge, the west delta, the Central Valley, and, if the day is clear, the snow-capped Sierra. Passing two overgrown dirt roads, left, you continue a gentle descent to a fenced pond, then begin a series of moderate ups and downs through a wooded area, passing over a creek flowing through a culvert. Across a deep valley, left, are the exposed rock cliffs of the Domengine Formation, 52-million-year-old marine sandstone that contains the coal for which this area became known.

Crossing an unnamed pass which offers great views, the route enters a dry, rocky area, then swings north past a pond, and reenters the trees. Just past the 4-mile point, you go through a gate and come to a rest bench under an oak. Here the steep Manhattan Canyon Trail veers right, but you stay on the Black Diamond Trail. A large area of chamise grows nearby, along with bush monkeyflower, black sage, pitcher sage, yerba santa, and manzanita. (The preserve has several types of manzanita, including the highly restricted Mt. Diablo variety, known by its stemless, clasping gray-green leaves and white flowers tinged with pink.)

At the next junction, where a connector to the Manhattan Canyon Trail heads right, you continue straight and begin a moderate climb, with power-line towers just ahead. Passing through a cattle gate and reentering oak woodland, the route makes several changes of direction before leaving the trees and descending in the open to Nortonville Pass. From here, turn right and retrace your route to the parking area.

STEWARTVILLE LOOP

Length: 7.6 miles

Time: 4 to 6 hours

Rating: Difficult

Regulations: EBRPD; parking fee; bicyclists and equestrians can follow a modified version of this loop by staying on the Stewartville and Ridge trails.

Facilities: Picnic tables, water, toilet; horse staging at a parking area, left, just past the entrance kiosk.

Directions: From Highway 4 in Antioch, take the Somersville Road exit and go south, staying in the left lane as you approach and pass Buchanan Road. At 1.5 miles, follow Somersville Road as it continues straight, while the main road, now called James Donlon Blvd., bends sharply left. At 2.6 miles from Highway 4, you reach the entrance kiosk, park office, and emergency telephone; continue another 0.9 mile to a large parking area, right, with an overflow area, left. The trailhead is at the south end of parking area.

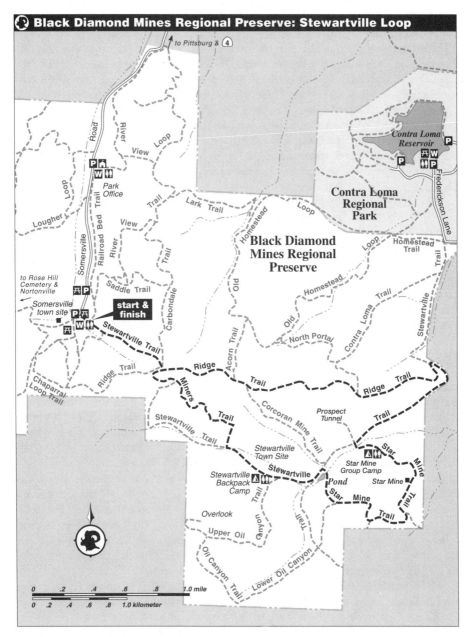

Black Diamond Mines Regional Preserve: Stewartville Loop

Following the Stewartville and Ridge trails past Star Mine and the Stewartville town site is like stepping back in time, when this area echoed with the clang of pick and shovel as eager miners tried to pry coal loose from the surrounding rocks. The Old West is evident here in other ways too, as you walk through grassy valleys dotted with grazing cows or contemplate sweeping vistas from high ridgetops. Parts of this route may be extremely muddy in wet weather. (Numbers in **boldface** in the route description refer to sites on the EBRPD map and accompanying text.)

From the south end of the parking area, pass a gate and continue uphill on the Nortonville Trail, a paved road, for about 200 feet to a level area and a junction, left, with the Stewartville Trail, a dirt road. Turn left and begin walking uphill on a moderate grade that soon levels, heading southeast through open country.

Once through a cattle gate, you pass the Railroad Bed Trail, left, which follows part of the old Pittsburg Railroad route, used to haul coal from the Somersville town site, near the parking area, north to Pittsburg Landing, about halfway between present-day Pittsburg and Antioch. Ahead on the right is the Pittsburg Mine Trail. Continue straight on the Stewartville Trail, climbing southeast to an obvious notch in the skyline ridge.

As you crest the ridge, you come to a 4-way junction with the Ridge Trail, right, and the Carbondale Trail, left, just before you reach a barbed-wire fence with a cattle gate. From here, your route, the Stewartville Trail, joined for a short distance by the Ridge Trail, continues straight through the gate to a T-junction, where the Stewartville Trail heads right and the Ridge Trail turns left. You turn left and head uphill on the moderate, then steep, Ridge Trail, a dirt road, soon arriving at another ridgetop, where your view extends to Antioch and the waterways of the west delta, spanned by the Antioch Bridge and scenic Highway 160. Mt. Diablo's North Peak (3557') looms impressively just west of south.

Late winter and early spring, when the blue oaks here sport mistletoe but no obscuring leaves, is a great time to look for songbirds such as western bluebirds and yellow-rumped warblers, along with jays and nuthatches. As you turn east and follow the narrow ridgetop on a generally level course, you may spot California buttercups in bloom, yellow flowers poking through the grass. Passing a junction, left, with the Acorn Trail, you continue straight and begin to climb; a stock pond here may be overflowing onto your route. Just past the pond you come to a junction, right, with the Corcoran Mine Trail. (One morning here in February I heard coyotes, their yips and yowls shattering the silence.)

Bear left on the Ridge Trail, and as you gain elevation, your view extends east to the Central Valley, and south across a fantastic assortment of ridges and valleys, to the lands of Morgan Territory and Round Valley regional preserves. The route alternates between the north and south sides of a ridge, then runs along its crest, following it moderately downhill. In addition to blue oak, this preserve also contains the East Bay's two other common deciduous oaks, black oak and valley oak, as well as two evergreen oaks, coast live oak and interior live oak.

After leveling, the route climbs gently, staying mostly in the open, then descends to a junction, just past the 2-mile point, with the Contra Loma Trail, left. Continuing straight on the Ridge Trail and making a moderate and then steep descent, you can see Contra Loma Reservoir, the heart of Contra Loma Regional Park, to your left. The Stewartville Trail, which you will rejoin soon, is the gravel road heading south from the park. The steep ridges you passed earlier begin to flatten out ahead, as you walk down the eastern edge of the East Bay hills toward the level Central Valley. Now at the end of the ridge, the road makes an almost 180-degree bend left and soon reaches the Stewartville Trail.

Here you turn right and follow the level Stewartville Trail, a dirt-and-gravel road with sections of broken pavement, as it swings right, turning the end of the ridge you just descended. Now heading southwest, directly for Mt. Diablo's North Peak, you are in open country, with a long valley, perhaps dotted with grazing cattle, stretching back to the east. The coal in these hills lies embedded in rocks called the Domengine Formation, a 52-million-year-old layer of marine sandstone, and there are remnants of mines nearby. After walking almost a mile from the last junction, you pass a creek flowing under the road through a culvert, and come to a four-way junction, marked by a trail post, left. Here the Stewartville Trail continues straight; the trail to Prospect Tunnel, 8, which can be explored on ranger-led tours, heads right; and the Star Mine Trail goes left through a cattle gate.

Turn left onto the Star Mine Trail, here a dirt-and-gravel road with paved sections, and follow it through a cattle gate, across another culvert, and past Star Mine Group Camp (picnic tables, toilet), where the trail begins to climb on a gentle and then moderate grade. (Bicyclists and equestrians wishing to visit the Star Mine should follow the Star Mine Trail, but will have to backtrack to the four-way junction and use the Stewartville Trail to complete a loop back to the parking area.)

Once past the campground, the road turns to dirt, and along its embankment you may see miner's lettuce, appropriately, and shooting stars. Hummingbirds, western bluebirds, and dark-eyed juncos add color and song as you climb to a low point on the skyline ridge ahead. Once across the ridge, you descend to a beautiful area of open hillsides dotted with oak, buckeye, and pine. At about the 4.3-mile point, approximately 50 feet to the right of the road, you can see the gated tunnel of Star Mine, 9, one of the last coal mines in the area to shut down. Nearby piles of dirt—mine tailings—are mute testimony to the miners' Herculean efforts.

The route turns southwest here, climbs through a rocky canyon where shrubs such as toyon and yerba santa flourish, and levels in a pine forest. Here you bear right at a fork, staying on the Star Mine Trail. Soon you reach one of the star attractions of this route, in addition to the mines—a

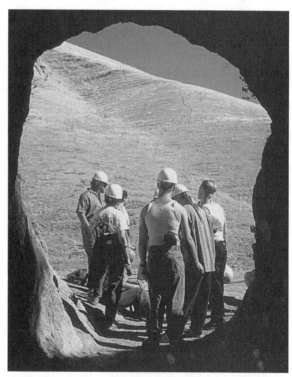

Prospect Tunnel, a coal-mine shaft, is near the junction of the Stewartville and Star Mine Shafts.

manzanita forest. You may notice two kinds of manzanita growing here: one of them, Mt. Diablo, is restricted to its namesake mountain and this preserve; the other, common manzanita, is found on Mt. Diablo and in Morgan Territory Regional Preserve.

The difference between these two species can best be studied where they grow side by side. Mt. Diablo manzanita has gray, felt-like leaves that clasp the branch and attach without a stem; there is an indentation in the leaf where it attaches to the branch. Common manzanita, on the other hand, has leaves that are green, shiny, and smooth, and attach to the branch with stems. Manzanitas flower in winter or early spring, bedecking themselves with masses of white or white-and-pink blossoms. Also growing here is chamise, one of the most common chaparral plants, perfectly adapted to dry, rocky soils.

The climbing is steep here, but beautiful views of angled ridges and oak woodlands reward your efforts. Mt. Diablo, the Central Valley, and the long east–west ridge you explored earlier on the Ridge Trail, are points of orientation. A nearby rest bench gives you a place to relax and enjoy the view. At about the 5-mile point, just past the rest bench, your route leaves the road, turns right, and descends on a single track, closed to bicycles and horses. Losing elevation as you switchback down a grassy hillside, past pine, oak, and buckeye, you reach a beautiful broad valley located east of the Stewartville town site. Here you pass through a wooden gate in a barbed-wire fence, and in about 75 feet reach a fork in the route. The left fork, a path through the grass, connects to the Lower Oil Canyon Trail. The right fork, your route, leads to a junction with the Stewartville Trail. Once around the corner of a ridge, you can see a cattle pen, located in the center of a Y-shaped valley that opens to the north.

The route circles a wet area, climbs an embankment, and meets the Stewartville Trail, a dirt road. Turning left, you walk toward the cattle pen, and, once past it, stay to the right as the road briefly splits in two. Just after the segments rejoin, you pass a junction, left, with the Lower Oil Canyon Trail. Continue straight and level, walking by grassland where cows may be grazing, following a creek on your right. Soon you come to the next junction, where the Upper Oil Canyon Trail heads left. (The Oil Canyon trails are worth exploring if you have time, or perhaps on another day.)

Again continue straight, passing the Stewartville backpack camp, left, where a toilet and three shaded picnic tables are available; then walk through a grazing area, which may be flooded, to a junction marked by a trail post, right. Nearby is the site of Stewartville, one of five mining towns that thrived in this area between the 1860s and the turn of the century.

Now you turn sharply right on the Miners Trail, a single track closed to bicycles and horses, and begin a gentle climb, soon finding another trail post, left. An old dirt road runs east–west here, across your route, but you continue uphill, steeply now, on the single track, past mine tailings and the remnants of a wooden structure. Tall gray pines are joined here by black locust, perhaps planted for shade. You will also encounter on this part of the route interior live oak, manzanita, toyon, chamise, black sage, and California sagebrush. As you climb higher, now on a narrow track cut from the hillside, you can see the Stewartville Trail, downhill and left. The drop-off is extreme, so use caution on this rocky and eroded trail.

The grade eases to moderate as the trail follows the indentations of the east–west ridge that is topped by the Ridge Trail. After crossing a possibly wet area on a small wooden bridge, you join the Stewartville Trail at the elbow of a sharp switchback, about the 7-mile point, where you bear right and continue to climb on a moderate grade. (If wet, this is the muddiest section of the hike.) After making a switchback to the right, you pass a rest bench and reach a flat area where the Stewartville and Ridge trails meet. Turn left, go through the gate, and retrace your route to the parking area.

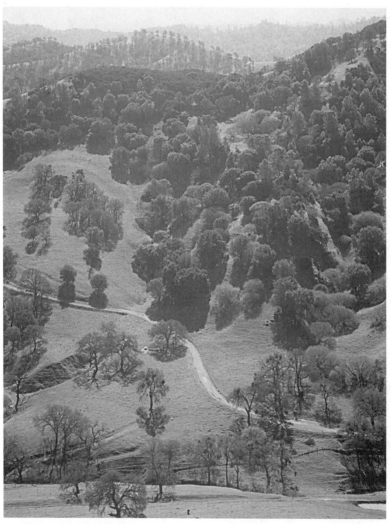

The Ridge Trail affords views of the preserve's characteristic oak woodlands and rolling hills.

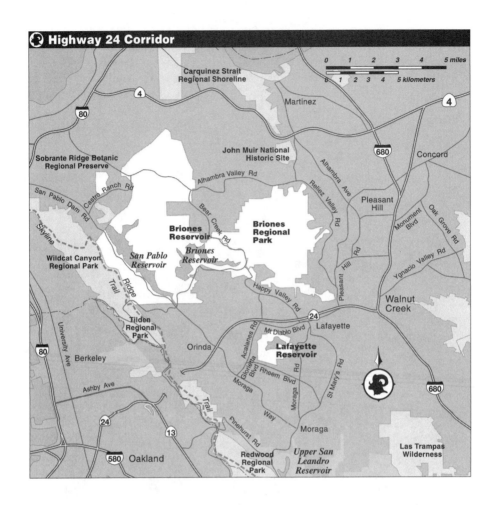

♦ Highway 24 Corridor ♦

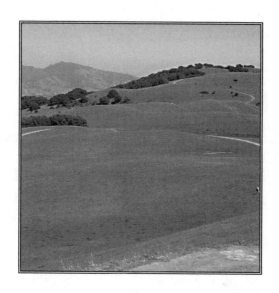

◆Briones Reservoir ◆

BEAR CREEK TRAIL

Length: 8 miles round-trip; 4 miles with car shuttle.

Time: 3 to 4 hours; half that with car shuttle

Rating: Moderate; easy with car shuttle

Regulations: EBMUD; trail use permit required; no bicycles, no dogs.

Facilities: Toilet; horse staging.

Directions: From Highway 24 in Orinda, take the Orinda exit and go 2.2 miles northwest on Camino Pablo to a junction with Bear Creek Road. Turn right and go 4.2 miles to EBMUD's Bear Creek staging area, left, just past the junction with Happy Valley Road. The trailhead is at the southwest corner of parking lot.

(If you are doing this as a shuttle trip, leave a car at the EBMUD Briones Overlook staging area, 1.4 miles northeast of Camino Pablo on Bear Creek Road. Then continue, as above, to the Bear Creek staging area.)

This pleasant out-and-back walk on EBMUD land, using the Bear Creek Trail, skirts the south and east shores of Briones Reservoir and ends near Briones Overlook staging area. A wide variety of trees, shrubs and flowers makes this an ideal nature-study trip.

Just beyond the gate at the trailhead are an EBMUD register and a sign for the Bear Creek Trail. After signing the register, turn left and descend the Bear Creek Trail, here a gravel path, to a clearing where Bear Creek flows in from the left. All the elements that make this a wonderful hike are present at the start—a wide variety of trees and shrubs, and the proximity of water. Trees here include California bay, coast live oak, and willow. Coyote brush, snowberry, and poison hemlock are also here, along with ferns.

After crossing the creek—this may be tricky during periods of high water—climb steeply on an eroded dirt path and, in about 200 feet, reach a trail post indicating the Bear Creek Trail and the Overlook staging area, 4 miles distant. Also on the trail post is an emblem for the Mokelumne Coast to Crest Trail. This 300-mile recreational trail, still in the early stage of development, will one day link the Bay Area to the Sierra Nevada. More than a dozen public and private organizations, including EBMUD, EBRPD, the U.S. Forest Service, and the National Park Service, are working together to complete this ambitious project (for more information, visit www.mc2ct.org).

About 75 feet uphill from the trail post you reach a gate; go through it and immediately come to a junction with an old paved road, shown on the Olmsted map as Shuetman Road. Turn right at this T-junction—you are still following the Bear Creek Trail—and walk west on a level grade through grasslands bordered with colorful wild radish and blue elderberry. Look for western meadowlarks and red-winged blackbirds in the shrubs, and turkey vultures gliding overhead.

Soon you get your first glimpse of Briones Reservoir ahead. To your left is a heavily forested area, but across the water are rolling, grassy hills dotted with oaks. At about the 0.5-mile point, you pass through a gate, and in 125 feet or so reach a fork. Here the pavement continues to the water's edge, where you might spy frogs and tadpoles. Your route, the Bear Creek Trail, now a wide dirt road, veers left into dense woodland.

Shady and level, this part of the route stays near but not beside the water. Take a moment to stop, look, and listen for birds, from small— chickadees—to large— Canada geese. Trees here include bigleaf maple, bay, California buckeye, black oak, and madrone. Snowberry, coffeeberry, and toyon grow nearby, as do spring wildflowers such as Ithuriel's spear, milkmaids, and California buttercup.

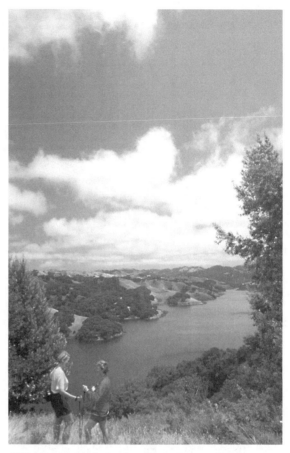

Hikers pause to admire the view east across Briones Reservoir from about the 2-mile point on the Bear Creek Trail.

Around the 1-mile point, you pass a rest bench at an overlook, then begin an easy climb. Opposite an upcoming trail post, look left into the trees for a glimpse of the foundation and stone stairway of an old house. Several tall walnut trees stand proudly beside the trail, which soon enters an overgrown area where ferns and mosses give a rain-forest feel. You may see a large bird box or two nailed high on a tree. These are for wood ducks, highly colorful birds which nest locally. This is also a good area for sighting northern flickers and spotted towhees.

The trail narrows to single-track width as it rises gently across a steep hillside, where a few clearings, right, offer views of the reservoir and the hills beyond. Sunlight filters through the trees here, giving a dappled effect. At one point the trail comes out of the forest and passes within 50 feet of Bear Creek Road; look here for owl's clover growing low to the ground. After crossing over two drainage ditches you reenter the forest, where you can add to today's list of trees and shrubs canyon

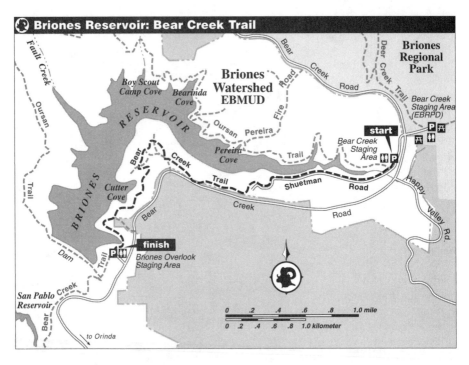

live oak, hazelnut, madrone, manzanita, and bush monkeyflower. Listen for the western scrub-jay's loud screech and the wrentit's repetitive one-note stutter.

After about 2 miles of easy walking, you enter a clearing and almost join a dirt fire road, closed to the public, running at right angles to your route. But just before reaching the road, a trail post directs you to follow the Bear Creek Trail as it veers right and starts uphill, passing a meadow full of thistle and poison hemlock. Now you climb steeply into an area of coastal scrub, including coyote brush, California sagebrush, bush monkeyflower, and blue bush lupine. The route is perched on the side of a steep hill with southern exposure in an area loaded with poison oak. From this vantage, you have a good look at the reservoir and the dam at its southwestern edge. Soon you come to a grassy area with a couple of inviting rest benches. Watch for hillside gooseberry along this part of the route, its thorny fruit looking like a medieval weapon.

The trail, now swinging around Cutter Point and bending southwest, crosses the fire road you met earlier, and soon comes to an open hillside dotted with blow wives, lupine, Ithuriel's spear, and blue-eyed grass. A large power-line tower here is the only intrusion on an otherwise lovely scene. The route now crosses another branch of the fire road and descends slightly, soon reaching a dense forest of bay and coast live oak. A large grove of madrone trees grows here on a north-facing hillside overlooking the reservoir.

At about the 3-mile point, you break out into a clearing and walk under a set of power lines. Here are chaparral plants, including manzanita, bush poppy and chamise, both of which bloom in late spring. The trail passes through a grove of pines, then moves into the open. The reservoir is on your right, and your destination, the Briones Overlook staging area, is straight ahead. From here you descend slightly to water level, with willow, madrone, bush monkeyflower, lupine, and California poppy growing beside the trail.

Just a bit farther and uphill is an unsigned fork in the trail. If you are doing this hike with a car shuttle, bear left and continue uphill to the staging area (there is a toilet there). If not, turn around and retrace your route to the Bear Creek staging area.

RESERVOIR LOOP

Length: 14 miles

Time: 6 to 8 hours

Rating: Very difficult

Regulations: EBMUD; trail use permit required; no bicycles, no dogs.
Facilities: Toilet; horse staging.
Directions: From Highway 24 in Orinda, take the Orinda exit and go 2.2 miles northwest on Camino Pablo to a junction with Bear Creek Road. Turn right and go 4.2 miles to EBMUD's Bear Creek staging area, left, just past the junction with Happy Valley Road. The trailhead is on the west side of Bear Creek staging area.

This loop, combining the Bear Creek and Oursan trails, is one of the longest in this book, taking you completely around Briones Reservoir. The route passes through a variety of terrain, from dense oak and bay forest near the reservoir's shore to open grassland high atop Sobrante Ridge. Along the way you will encounter grand vistas, an assortment of trees and shrubs, spring wildflowers, and birds by the dozen. Except for about 3 miles of the Bear Creek Trail, the entire trip is on well-graded dirt roads. (Be alert for vehicles, which use the roads.)

Just beyond the gate at the trailhead are an EBMUD register and a sign for the Bear Creek Trail. After signing the register, turn left, and descend the Bear Creek Trail, here a gravel path, to a clearing where Bear Creek flows in from the left. After crossing the creek—this may be tricky during periods of high water—climb steeply on an eroded dirt path and, in about 200 feet, reach a trail post indicating the Bear Creek Trail and the Overlook staging area, 4 miles distant.

About 75 feet uphill from the trail post you reach a gate; go through it and immediately come to a junction with an old paved road, shown on the Olmsted map as Shuetman Road. Turn right at this T-junction—you are still following the Bear Creek Trail—and walk west on a level grade. Soon you get your first glimpse of Briones Reservoir ahead. To your left is a heavily forested area, but across the water are rolling, grassy hills dotted with oaks. At about the 0.5-mile point, you pass through a gate, and in 125 feet or so reach a fork. Your route, the Bear Creek Trail, now a wide dirt road, veers left into dense woodland.

Around the 1-mile point, you pass a rest bench at an overlook, then begin an easy climb. The trail narrows to single-track width as it rises gently across a steep hillside, where a few clearings, right, offer views of the reservoir and the hills beyond. Soon you enter a clearing and almost join a dirt fire road, closed to the

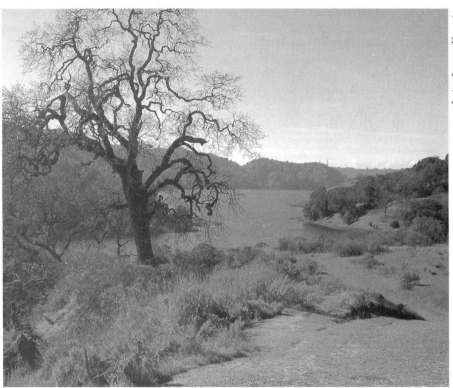

Briones Reservoir from the Oursan Trail.

public, running at right angles to your route. But just before reaching the road, a trail post directs you to follow the Bear Creek Trail as it veers right and starts uphill.

Now you climb steeply into an area of coastal scrub. The route is perched on the side of a steep hill with southern exposure in an area loaded with poison oak. From this vantage, you have a good look at the reservoir and the dam at its southwestern edge. Ahead is a grassy area with a couple of inviting rest benches. The trail, now swinging around Cutter Point and bending southwest, crosses the fire road you met earlier, and soon comes to an open hillside. The route now crosses another branch of the fire road and descends slightly, soon reaching a dense forest of bay and coast live oak.

At about the 3-mile point, you reach an area of chaparral. Next comes a grove of pines, and then open ground. With the reservoir on your right, you descend slightly to water level, with willows and madrones growing beside the trail. Just a bit farther and uphill is an unsigned fork, just below EBMUD's Briones Overlook staging area.

When you reach the fork, at about the 4-mile point, continue straight on a level grade, passing through an area of coast live oak, madrone, and pine. Soon another connector to the staging area merges on the left, and a paved road appears on your right, running parallel to the trail. After a short distance, the trail joins this road, and a few paces farther you come to a T-junction with another paved road, one that comes from Bear Creek Road and heads northwest across the dam that impounds Briones Reservoir. At this point you leave the Bear Creek Trail, turning right to cross the dam. (Use caution, as this road is traveled by trucks.)

Out in the open now, you have a wonderful view of the reservoir, which is surrounded by rolling hills. Overhead you may see vultures circling, while closer at hand, if it's spring, western bluebirds and swallows dart through the air hunting insects. (If you see bird boxes with small holes, they are probably for the bluebirds. Large-holed boxes are generally for wood ducks.)

As you cross a bridge over the spillway and get on the dam, you have a deep valley on your left, where San Pablo Dam Road skirts the southwest edge of San Pablo Reservoir, several hundred feet below. The dam also affords you a fine view, southwest, of San Pablo Ridge and the Berkeley Hills.

On the other side of the dam, the paved road changes to dirt and gravel, bends right, and passes an unsigned junction with a gated dirt road, left. Ahead are several boat houses near the reservoir's shore. (This poorly signed and not particularly attractive section of the route is near a dumping area for clean fill.) Follow the road as it turns left and climbs uphill, past the boat houses. You will notice several unofficial trails and side roads as you walk northwest, away from the reservoir: ignore them all. Keep the dumping area to your right as the road levels and begins to descend. Soon the road splits at a fork; here you bear right, and in about 200 feet pass a connector to the left-hand road.

You are now on the Oursan Trail, which you follow as it climbs more and more steeply toward a set of large power-line towers. The terrain is mostly open and rolling, with some groves of California bay and coast live oak. Passing through a gate, you continue to gain elevation, now on a gentle grade, giving you an opportunity to pick out landmarks such as Inspiration Point (southwest), Vollmer Peak (south), and Round Top (just east of south). The Briones Overlook staging area is just across the reservoir to the southeast. The route now turns northeast and begins to climb Sobrante Ridge, passing an unsigned junction with a road climbing steeply left. A wonderful display of spring wildflowers—California poppies and bluedicks—decorates a rocky road cut, and clumps of California sagebrush claim footholds on the open hillside.

At about the 6-mile point, the route swings north, away from the reservoir, to run along the crest of Sobrante Ridge. Coffeeberry and hillside gooseberry are here, along with soap plant and shooting stars. As the route levels, you pass a restricted-access road, right, and then begin to climb again, getting a glimpse of Mt. Tamalpais, west, peeking over San Pablo Ridge. Below and left is Sather Canyon, a deep gash in the landscape with a creek at the bottom that drains into San Pablo Reservoir. Almost due east is Mt. Diablo, and to the southeast rise Las Trampas and Rocky ridges, the latter topped by a single antenna, forming the parallel walls of Bollinger Canyon.

Spring wildflowers put on a beautiful display here, as California poppy, California buttercup, and blue-eyed grass color the grassy slopes with dabs of orange, yellow, and blue, sharing the limelight with blue bush lupine. Once atop the ridge, the route is mostly level, but it drops slightly to pass through a shady tunnel of bay and coast live oak. The far end of this tunnel frames a lovely view

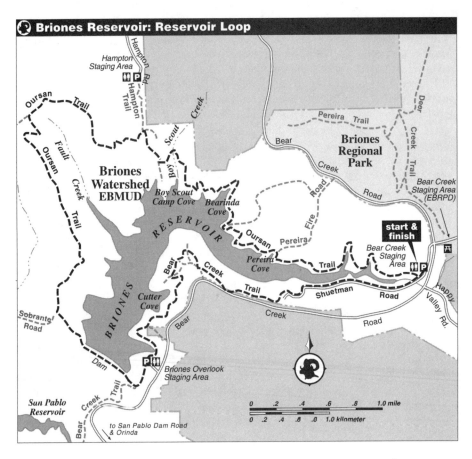

north toward the Carquinez Strait and Suisun Bay, across an area of open space checkered with densely packed housing developments. In the far distance rises Mt. St. Helena, visible on a clear day.

Now the route makes a 180-degree bend right and begins to work southeast toward Briones Reservoir across open terrain, some of it prone to landslides. Fault Creek flows into the reservoir through a deep valley to your right. As the route turns east and heads directly toward Mt. Diablo, you pass a junction, marked by a trail post, with a road that heads south. In 100 yards or so, you pass another road, this one restricted access. You are descending on a gentle grade, and soon pass a wooded area, right, on your way to a T-junction with a paved road, the Hampton Trail. Just before reaching the junction, at about the 8.5-mile point, you pass through a gate, directly under a set of power-line towers.

From here, the Hampton Trail heads north, and in about 0.5 mile becomes Hampton Road. Your route, the Oursan Trail, turns right and follows broken pavement downhill on a gentle grade, soon reaching a fork, where you bear left, pass through a gate, and begin to climb on a dirt road. A narrow path, right, leads to a corral and an inviting grove of trees, a good spot for a picnic. From here back to the Bear Creek staging area, your route follows the ins and outs of the reservoir's shoreline, often rising to cross a small ridge, then descending to a little gully, where a creek may flow through a culvert under the road and into the reservoir. At the first of these gullies, where Scout Creek flows into Boy Scout Camp Cove, you pass another restricted-access road, left, and then cross the creek. Near the creek, willows grow in a wet area, downhill and right, and California poppies decorate a hillside, left. You may see a wedge of Canada geese flying across the reservoir, keeping a tight formation and honking to each other.

A moderate climb takes you through a little notch and over a shoulder, and then you descend in the shade of coast live oaks to another creek, where bay and California buckeye flourish in the moist soil. Leaving the trees, you start climbing again, away from the reservoir and over a rise, where a gate lets you pass through a fence that crosses the road. Now the route descends, then levels and again follows the shape of shoreline. If the water level is low, you may see large marshy areas with dried-out bulrushes.

At about the 10-mile point, your route leads into Bearinda Cove, past a junction, left, with a restricted-access road. After crossing a creek, you veer right as the route heads back toward the reservoir, passing a hillside overgrown with blackberry vines and snowberry, and shaded by bay and buckeye. These occasional shady areas, interspersed with long stretches of open terrain, are welcome on a warm day.

Your course is now generally east, along the north shore of the slender eastern arm of the reservoir. Here you leave behind the sweeping, rolling hills and begin to enjoy the shade of trees and the sight of many birds enjoying the wetlands. At Pereira Cove, you pass a path heading uphill and left, closed to hikers and horses, as the route swings right, toward the water. In the open parts of the route, you may see red-tailed hawks, red-shouldered hawks, or turkey vultures circling above, but in wooded areas, be on the lookout for the varied thrush, which resembles its cousin, the American robin. Just past Pereira Cove, in an open area, you pass a path going left and uphill; bear right and enter an oak woodland where you may be greeted by raucous western scrub-jays.

Climbing for the first time in a while, the route veers north into the first of two narrow, north-pointing ravines, with a finger of the reservoir below and right. After a short, steep climb, you descend moderately to a creek, passing a hillside covered with long strands of vine honeysuckle and low-growing periwinkle. As the route levels after climbing from the creek, you pass a restricted-access road, left; here you bear right and begin a gentle descent in the open, toward the reservoir. This process is repeated at the second of the two ravines. Along the way, you may be startled by the loud flapping of wings as a flock of band-tailed pigeons departs from the nearby oaks. These are closely related to rock doves, our common urban pigeons, but are a few inches larger, uniformly patterned, and much more elegant.

Now out in the open, the route crosses an area that may be flooded in wet weather, then climbs over a shoulder on a moderate grade near the east end of the reservoir. Here the terrain drops steeply toward the reservoir's shoreline, right, at the inflow of Bear Creek. After a few more ups and down, you reach a junction with the Bear Creek Trail, just before the Bear Creek staging area. Turn right and pass through a gate to the parking area.

✦Briones Regional Park ✦

BRIONES CREST

Length: 6.8 miles

Time: 4 to 6 hours

Rating: Moderate

Regulations: EBRPD; fees for parking and dogs.

Facilities: None at the trailhead; picnic tables, water, and toilets are located at other parking areas near the trailhead; horse staging.

Directions: From Highway 24 in Orinda, take the Orinda Exit and go northwest 2.2 miles on Camino Pablo to Bear Creek Road. Turn right and go 4.5 miles to the park's Bear Creek Valley entrance, which is just beyond Happy Valley Road. Turn right, and after 0.3 mile reach the entrance kiosk; continue 0.1 mile to the last parking area. The trailhead is at the end of the park entrance road, just past the last parking area.

This rambling loop, which includes parts of the Homestead Valley, Briones Crest, Table Top, Mott Peak, and Black Oak trails, offers a great introduction to the south half of this expansive, 6117-acre park, an area of rolling hills, high ridges, and forested canyons. The rewards for climbing along the Briones Crest include spring wildflowers and 360-degree views.

Part of this scenic loop follows a route named for Ivan Dickson, a dedicated member of the Berkeley Hiking Club and park enthusiast who, upon his death in 1993 at age 95, left a surprise bequest of $500,000 to the regional park district. The yearly interest on this account is used for trail maintenance programs involving groups, organizations, and individuals.

Passing a trail post with the Ivan Dickson Memorial Loop emblem, you go through a gate and follow a paved road—the continuation of the park entrance road—east through a brushy area, soon reaching a fork and the end of pavement. Here the Old Briones Road Trail, once the main route between Orinda and Martinez, heads left, and the Homestead Valley Trail, your route, goes right. Bearing right and descending on a wide dirt road, you cross Bear Creek, its banks lined with coast live oak, California bay, willow, madrone, and bigleaf maple.

Much of your route is in the open, climbing high atop the rolling hills that characterize this regional park, so enjoy while you can the shady canyon that holds Bear Creek and the wide variety of trees that grow here. Birds appreciate this oasis too, and you may hear the sharp cry of a northern flicker or the call of a California quail as you climb out of the canyon, through a cattle gate, and into the open. Reaching a junction with the Crescent Ridge Trail, which goes straight, you turn right and continue on the Homestead Valley Trail, and in about 100 yards pass a junction with the Bear Creek Trail, right. A nearby swampy area is home to noisy flocks of red-winged blackbirds.

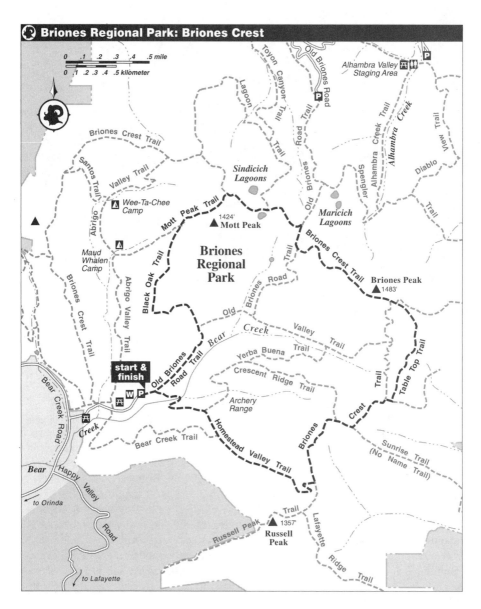

With a tributary of Bear Creek on your right, the route passes a few venerable coast live oaks, their many branches spreading from twisted trunks, and several California buckeyes, flowering beautifully in late spring. As the route begins to climb on a moderate grade, through a forest of oak and bay, you may notice other spring bloomers, such as blue bush lupine and bush monkeyflower. This woodland habitat is ideal for two common towhees, California and spotted, which love to scrape through leaf litter for food. Turkey vultures and red-tailed hawks may be

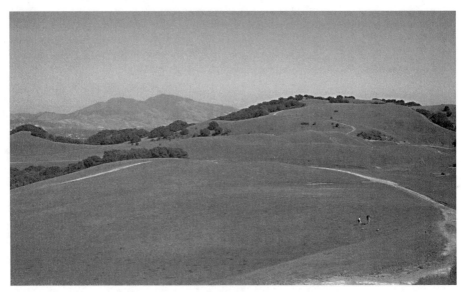

View from the Black Oak Trail extends east to Mt. Diablo State Park.

circling overhead, and western scrub-jays, if here, will probably announce your presence.

Breaking into the open and sweeping uphill on several sharp bends, the route passes through a gate and reaches the Briones Crest Trail. Turning left, you now follow the rolling ridgecrest through a wooded area, where dark-eyed juncos flit from tree to tree, and spring wildflowers such as California poppy, Ithuriel's spear, and winecup clarkia emerge from the grass, dappled by sunlight. The view east is of Walnut Creek and Mt. Diablo, beautifully set off by a foreground of rolling hills.

At about the 2.3-mile point, you pass a junction, left, with the Crescent Ridge Trail. Heading straight and east, toward Mt. Diablo, the Briones Crest Trail stays in the open, on top of the world. When you reach a fork with the Sunrise Trail, right, bear left and descend past several cattle gates through a lush wildflower meadow sprinkled with blue-eyed grass, owl's clover, bluedicks, and paintbrush. At the next junction, leave the Briones Crest Trail as it veers left; continue straight on the Ivan Dickson Memorial Loop to the Table Top and Spengler trails. Where the Spengler Trail makes a hard right, you continue straight on the Table Top Trail, past an area of chamise and California sagebrush, heading toward the high ground around Briones Peak (1483').

A short, steep climb rewards you with views, west, to the Berkeley Hills, while directly ahead you can see a large cable-television facility. As you continue climbing along the crest of a ridge, more of the East Bay becomes visible to the north, including Martinez, Benicia, the Carquinez Strait, and Suisun Bay, home to the mothball fleet of World War II ships. When you come to a cattle gate, you have reached the next junction. Here, the Table Top Trail bends sharply right and downhill, but you continue straight through the gate, and in a few feet rejoin the Briones Crest Trail, merging from the left.

Three birds whose names are similar—horned lark, western meadowlark, and lark sparrow—may be present nearby. Unrelated, but sharing the same habitat—open fields and grassland—each of these songbirds has distinctive markings. The lark sparrow, smallest of the three, shows a rust-and-white face pattern and a dark spot on its light gray breast. The horned lark, slightly larger, sports black tufts on its forehead, a black stripe under its eye, and a black bib under its throat. The western meadowlark, almost robin-sized, has white head stripes and a wide black bib on a yellow breast. Each bird flashes white tail feathers in flight.

After climbing to and passing through a small grove of oaks, just before the route begins to descend, you come upon two unsigned paths, one left, the other right. The right-hand path leads up to the summit of Briones Peak, where a rest bench and terrific views await you. After a well-deserved break, return to the main route, turn right, and continue northwest over rolling terrain, mostly descending, to a fork with the Old Briones Road Trail. At this point, about 4.3 miles, the Briones Crest Trail, your route, turns right and follows the same downhill route as the Old Briones Road Trail, leaving it in about 0.1 mile at a junction, where you turn left.

With one of the two Sindicich Lagoons on your left, you pass the Lagoon Trail, right, and a narrow path, left. Continue straight and uphill, looking back from time to time to admire an unobstructed view of Mt. Diablo, east, and the other, larger lagoon, north. The lagoons are the breeding grounds for thousands of California newts, which migrate here in early spring from hiding places in nearby forests.

Soon you come to a junction with the Mott Peak Trail, a wide dirt road, where you turn left and climb toward a saddle just north of Mott Peak (1424'). Mott Peak was named for William Penn Mott Jr., general manager of EBRPD from 1962 to 1967, who led an expansion drive that incorporated Briones, among others, into the regional park system. Mott left EBRPD to become director of California's Department of Parks and Recreation, and was later named head of the National Park Service.

Once across the saddle, you descend to a cattle gate and continue downhill on a moderate grade, with a view west to the Oakland and Berkeley hills, anchored by Round Top and Vollmer Peak, and beyond to Mt. Tamalpais. At the next junction, leave the Mott Peak Trail, which heads right, and continue straight on the Black Oak Trail. This stretch is level for a short distance, but then drops past a connector, right, to the Mott Peak Trail. A short, steep uphill section leads you to the top of a rise, where a nearby rest bench beckons. Now the route heads downhill on a gentle and then moderate grade, following the crest of a narrow ridge. At the next rest bench the route turns left and makes a steep descent on loose dirt, past the grove of black oaks that gives this trail its name, to the valley floor.

Buckeye, blue elderberry, bay, and willow grace this grassy area, and you soon reach a T-junction with the Old Briones Road Trail, just past the 6-mile point. Here you turn right, crossing a tributary of Bear Creek flowing under the road via a culvert, and meander through a level, shady area that soon gives way to open grassland. Continue on a pleasant, level course for about 0.5 mile, at the end of which is a cattle gate. After passing through the gate, you arrive, in about 250 feet, at the junction with the Homestead Valley Trail to close the loop. Bear right, now on pavement, and retrace your route to the parking area.

✦Lafayette Reservoir✦

RIM TRAIL

Length: 4.7 miles

Time: 2 to 3 hours

Rating: Moderate

Regulations: EBMUD; parking fee; Trail Use Permit not required; no horses or dogs, no skateboarding. Bikes and roller skates are allowed Tuesdays and Thursdays, 12 P.M. to closing; Sunday mornings, opening to 11 A.M.

Facilities: Visitor center/boat house, picnic tables, children's play area, restrooms, toilet, phone, water.

Directions: From Highway 24 eastbound in Lafayette, take the Acalanes Road/Mt. Diablo Blvd. exit and go east 0.8 mile on Mt. Diablo Blvd. to the entrance to EBMUD's Lafayette Reservoir Recreation Area. Turn right and go 0.2 mile uphill on the one-way entrance road, then turn left for the main entrance, or right for the annual-pass entrance. The trailhead is at the foot of the concrete staircase at the west end of parking area.

From Highway 24 westbound, take the Acalanes/Upper Happy Valley Road exit, go south under the highway, turn left (east) on Mt. Diablo Blvd., and then follow the directions above.

Parking is on top of the dam. There are meters for up to 2 hours; the meters take only quarters, and no change is available (25 cents per 15 minutes). Parking regulations are strictly enforced, as are closing times, which vary seasonally. Alternatively, you can buy an all-day pass at the entrance station, $6 for cars and motorcycles, $15 for vans. If the entrance station is closed, you can buy an all-day parking pass at a machine that accepts only $1 and $5 bills, or at the visitor center, 0.25 mile west around the reservoir. (An EBMUD Trail Use Permit, not needed here but required for trips to Briones and Upper San Leandro reservoirs, is also available at the visitor center.)

This loop around Lafayette Reservoir on the Rim Trail, with great bird-watching opportunities and several high points affording 360-degree views, is a great introduction to the parklands administered by EBMUD. (Note: the route is almost impassible during wet weather due to mud.)

From the trailhead, walk up the concrete stairs and continue straight on a wide dirt path through a picnic and children's play area. Below and left is the Shore Trail, a paved road that circles the reservoir—another fine hike. After leaving the picnic area, you join a dirt road, right, and pass another, left, as you continue uphill on a moderate grade.

Open grasslands with valley oaks appear as you near a ridgecrest, while overhead a red-tailed hawk may be gliding on the wind. The route turns west and heads for a flat spot on the ridge ahead; turn around here and enjoy a great view of Mt. Diablo, with the reservoir in the foreground, its waters perhaps shimmering

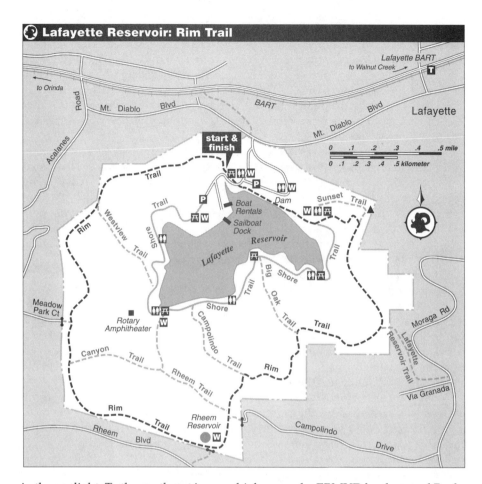

Lafayette Reservoir: Rim Trail

in the sunlight. To the southeast is more high ground—EBMUD land around Rocky Ridge, and Las Trampas Wilderness. To the north is busy Highway 24, and beyond, the hills of Briones Regional Park. At several points along the way, trails connecting with the reservoir's Shore Trail drop from the rim.

Birds are plentiful around Lafayette Reservoir. Double-crested cormorants roost on the intake tower, great blue herons stalk the shallows near shore, hummingbirds buzz and dart among the shrubs, warblers flit through the Monterey pines and coast live oaks, and California towhees scratch through leaf litter for food. California quails and wild turkeys are common, and bald eagles have been known to nest here.

Easy walking brings you, at about the 0.8-mile point, to the first junction, where the Westview Trail heads left. Now climbing on a moderate grade, you pass a grove of California bay on your way to the next high point, near a residential area at the park's western boundary. Here the route levels, descends into a forested area, and then climbs steeply as it swings south, alternating between sun and shade. Another descent takes you to a rolling section around the 1-mile point, where the trees give way to grass and coyote brush.

Lafayette is the smallest of five EBMUD reservoirs in the East Bay that have public trails along their shores. Built in the mid-1920s and designed as a much larger facility to hold water from the Sierra, its size was reduced when, during construction, the dam settled and cracked. For safety's sake the dam was widened and the size of the reservoir reduced. The intake tower, which stands high and dry above the water near the dam, was built before problems arose; its height shows the planned depth of the reservoir. Today the reservoir, with 126 acres of surface area, is a recreation area and emergency water supply.

A moderate climb, followed by a moderate descent, brings you to a junction with a path that heads left to a viewpoint. Passing that, you soon reach a low point and a path, right, leading to Meadow Park Court, off Glorietta Blvd. Continuing straight through a possibly muddy area, where animal tracks, especially those of deer, may be evident, you begin a very steep climb, with the reservoir now obscured by a ridge, left. As you walk past groves of pine and coast live oak, the route levels briefly but then plunges steeply to another low spot, with a residential area, right, and a junction with the Canyon Trail, left.

More up-and-down travel brings you to the summit of a high ridge where the grade eases off, and now you pass fine stands of coast live oak, pine, eucalyptus, and California buckeye. Listen carefully and you may hear the sharp cry of a northern flicker as it moves from tree to tree, probing for insects. Southwest from here is Round Top, an extinct volcano in the Sibley Volcanic Regional Preserve, its forested summit topped with communication towers. Mt. Diablo, which resembles a volcano but is actually made from uplifted layers of rock that were originally underwater, still dominates the eastern skyline.

When you reach a large water tank, follow a paved path around it to the right, and pass a paved road heading right and downhill. Continue around the tank, where drinking water is available for you and your pet, and climb on pavement through a pine grove. Now the pavement ends and you are back on a dirt road, walking east through a treeless area of grasses and shrubs. Climbing steeply, you soon reach the route's high point (1038'), and the road divides to go around it. If you spot a small gray hawk, it is probably a white-tailed kite, one of the few birds that can truly hover. This raptor, which feeds on rodents and insects, is expanding its range and increasing in numbers.

This high point affords you 360-degree views: from the Oakland and Berkeley hills to Walnut Creek, Alamo, and Mt. Diablo; from Orinda, Moraga, and Rheem Valley to Briones Regional Park. After enjoying your time on the summit, continue east and immediately begin a steep drop on a dirt fire break, which may be muddy and eroded. Pick your way carefully down this short, steep section, and as the route swings north look for blue bush lupine on your left, and some beautiful oaks. As the grade eases you reach a junction: to your left is a dirt road, shown on the EBMUD map as the Rheem Trail; to your right is a path leading to a gate at the end of Campolindo Dr., off Moraga Road. As you continue straight the route climbs in the open, reaches a high point, turns northeast, and descends to a junction with the Campolindo Trail, a dirt road heading left.

Here you may spot another hovering bird, the American kestrel, the smallest North American falcon. Compare the hovering birds you may have seen so far with the ever-present turkey vulture, a large black raptor that glides and soars on air currents, tipping from side to side, its wings held in a V-position. While some birds hunt from the air, many feed on the ground. Ground feeders that prefer open sites, such as gold-crowned sparrows, flock together for safety, whereas birds that feed in dense cover, such as spotted and California towhees, can afford to do so singly or in pairs. Check both kinds of habitat here for these birds and others like them.

The route now bends right and climbs, giving you good views of the reservoir, the dam, and Highway 24. As you walk east over level ground, western scrub-jays may herald your arrival with their raucous calls. Turning north and descending gently, you pass a residential area, right, and enjoy a pleasant respite from the constant roller-coaster terrain. Just past the 3-mile point, you come to a junction with the Big Oak Trail, left. Your route veers right and continues over open, level ground, past stands of pine and eucalyptus. The next junction is with the Lafayette Reservoir Trail to Moraga Road, which goes right and uphill.

A short, moderate climb brings you to another high point with 360-degree views, increasing significantly the "scenery per mile" quotient of this hike. As you descend, you reach a junction with the Sunset Trail, heading straight, but your route turns left and continues downhill on a moderate grade, meandering past oaks loaded with mistletoe. At about the 4.3-mile point, you come to a junction with the Shore Trail, the paved path that circles the reservoir. Turn right and walk through a picnic area toward the dam, descending gently before reaching the parking area.

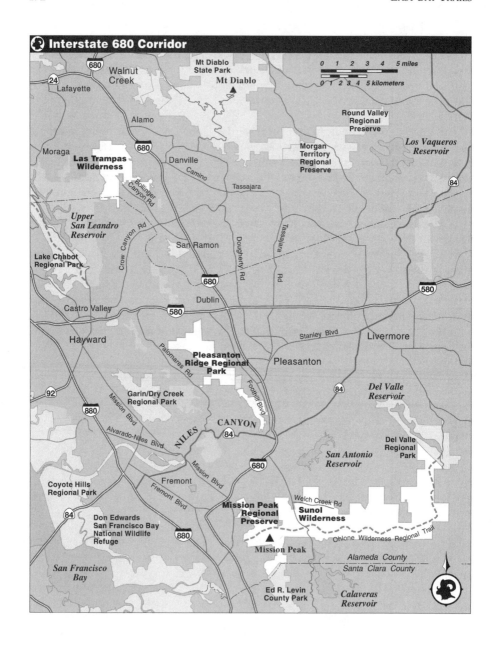

Interstate 680 Corridor

◆ Interstate 680 Corridor ◆

✦Las Trampas Wilderness ✦

Las Trampas Wilderness, 4811 acres of convoluted, oak-studded hills and wind-swept, chaparral-cloaked ridges, is one of the great undeveloped parks in the EBRPD system. The park is dominated by two high ramparts, Las Trampas Ridge and Rocky Ridge, guarding the deep slash of northwest–southeast trending Bollinger Canyon. The high point on Las Trampas Ridge, Las Trampas Peak, is 1827 feet in elevation. The top of Rocky Ridge, a little more than a mile south, stands at 2024 feet. Rocky Ridge, once used as a Nike missile site, now sports a communication tower on its summit. Fine views of Mt. Diablo can be had from the top of Las Trampas Peak or along the "Corduroy Hills" route. From the top of Rocky Ridge, the vista extends southwest across EBMUD lands to Upper San Leandro Reservoir. The twin walls of Rocky and Las Trampas ridges, rising between the Oakland and Berkeley hills and Mt. Diablo, are landmarks easily seen from many vantage points in the East Bay.

Las Trampas in Spanish means "The Traps," perhaps a reference to the Ohlone Indian practice of trapping deer and elk by driving them into the area's steep box canyons, or perhaps, as Erwin G. Gudde writes in *California Place Names*, a reference to traps set in chaparral to catch elk. Like many other East Bay parks, Las Trampas was at one time a large rancho, but after California became a state, its lands fell into American hands. The names of nearby valleys and canyons— Bollinger, Cull, Hunsaker, Stone, and Tice—commemorate the early settlers who benefited from the misfortunes of the rancho's original owners, the Romero brothers. The East Bay Regional Park District purchased the parklands in the 1960s, using state bond money and federal grants.

Las Trampas is one of the finest places in the East Bay to study chaparral, and it is one of the few places to see scrub oak, the plant whose Spanish name, *chaparro*,

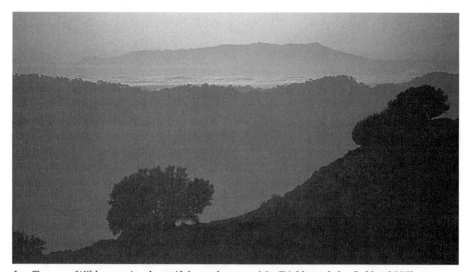

Las Trampas Wilderness is a beautiful area between Mt. Diablo and the Oakland Hills.

gives us the word for this hardy plant community. The park, which contains the Las Trampas and Bollinger faults, is also of great interest to geologists and paleontologists: its high ridges were at one time part of the ocean floor, and the sandstone outcrops and cliffs of Rocky Ridge and Las Trampas Ridge contain shells and fossils of animals long extinct, such as primitive camels, a three-toed horse, and a four-tusked elephant-like animal. Present-day mammals that may be seen in the park, according to the EBRPD brochure, include raccoons, foxes, opossums, bobcats, skunks, squirrels, and deer. Sightings of mountain lions have been reported in recent years.

Las Trampas is best enjoyed during cool weather, but mud can be a problem after rainy periods. Parking-area gates close at dusk: be careful not to get locked in, especially if you are doing the long "Corduroy Hills" trip.

CORDUROY HILLS

Length: 6.1 miles

Time: 4 to 6 hours

Rating: Very difficult

Regulations: EBRPD; no bicycles or horses.

Facilities: Picnic tables, toilet, water (may not be available year-round).

Directions: From Interstate 680 in San Ramon, take the Crow Canyon Road/San Ramon exit and go west 1.1 miles on Crow Canyon Road to Bollinger Canyon Road. Turn right and go 4.5 miles to the end of the road, past the first Las Trampas Wilderness entrance, and turn left into the parking area. The trailhead is at the parking area entrance on Bollinger Canyon Road.

From Interstate 580 eastbound in Castro Valley, take the Center St./Crow Canyon Road exit, go left over the freeway, then right on Castro Valley Blvd., which soon becomes E. Castro Valley Blvd., 0.7 mile to Crow Canyon Road. Turn left and go 7.5 miles to Bollinger Canyon Road, then follow the directions above.

From Interstate 580 westbound in Castro Valley, take the Castro Valley exit, turn left onto E. Castro Valley Blvd. and go 0.1 mile to Crow Canyon Road. Turn right and follow the directions above.

This rugged loop joins all or parts of the Chamise, Las Trampas Ridge, Corduroy Hills, Madrone, Virgil Williams, Del Amigo, Sulphur Springs, Trapline, and Mahogany trails, leading you through an amazing variety of terrain, from sun-baked chaparral to shady forest. Some of the best views in the East Bay of Mt. Diablo are to be found on this loop, which passes through a stunted forest of scrub oak and other interesting plant communities. Wet weather may bring mud and even landslide activity to parts of this route. Bring plenty of water and start early; the parking area gate may be locked at 5 P.M.

Turn right on Bollinger Canyon Road and walk 500 feet to a turnout, left. Go through a gate and follow the single-track Chamise Trail as it climbs southeast across an open hillside to a junction with the Bollinger Canyon Trail. Stay on the Chamise Trail by veering left and ascending a series of well-graded switchbacks.

Across Bollinger Canyon rises the southern segment of Las Trampas Wilderness, dominated by the steep escarpment of Rocky Ridge, worth exploring on another day. As you gain elevation you may see turkey vultures circling overhead, or hear the sharp cry of a northern flicker.

The Chamise Trail takes its name from a hardy, widespread shrub, also known as greasewood, which grows here in the company of two other chaparral plants, buckbrush and black sage. Looking like a small evergreen tree, chamise sports white flowers in late spring, then turns brown when its rust-colored fruit appears. As the trail bends left, you pass a junction with the Mahogany Trail, part of your return route, heading straight and steeply downhill. To the northeast is Las Trampas Ridge, a rugged, chaparral-covered barrier you will cross later. Continuing to climb moderately along the crest of a narrow north–south ridge, you pass through a corridor of chaparral—a great place to study the plants up close—and, in a grove of coast live oak, reach the other end of the Mahogany Trail, right.

Now in the open, the route climbs a grassy hill and approaches the north-west–southeast spine of Las Trampas Ridge, right, guarded by massive rock cliffs. In addition to the chaparral plants, another shrub to admire here is a thorny relative of the flowering currants, hillside gooseberry, whose delicate white-and-purple flowers appear in late winter. A flat area and a T-junction mark the point where the ridge you are on intersects Las Trampas Ridge. The Chamise Trail ends here, and you bear left on the Las Trampas Ridge Trail, enjoying views of Mt. Diablo, northeast, and Rocky Ridge, sporting a lone communication tower, southwest.

Just past the junction, you encounter a large grove of scrub oak, right, a low-growing shrub with light bark and small, pointed leaves. The Spanish word for scrub oak, *chaparro*, gives us "chaparral," but chaparral in the East Bay almost always contains a wide variety of shrubs adapted to dry conditions. One of these, also found here, is spiny redberry, whose round, prickly leaves make it resemble a small live oak.

Passing through a fence, you descend a steep, narrow track, muddy at times, past more scrub oak, soon reaching a clearing where the route levels. Back in chaparral, with occasional pockets of shade offered by oak and California bay, the trail follows a rolling course on the edge of a steep canyon, right. The designation of this area as an EBRPD "wilderness" is appropriate: except for the trail, human intervention is nowhere to be seen. In one of the shady areas, just east of Vail Peak (1787'), you reach a fence, right, and a junction with the Corduroy Hills Trail. Here your route, a single track, turns right and steeply downhill, following at first some wooden steps, then switchbacks, to an open, grassy hillside. A small divide, which you cross, separates two canyons, the left one formed by two ridges, Las Trampas and Nordstrom. Just ahead is Eagle Peak (1720'), a high point on the southeast end of Nordstrom Ridge.

A steep ascent, in places a scramble over rocky ground and boulders, puts you atop a cliff with a tall rock outcrop just west of Eagle Peak, a nice rest stop. The view from here is spectacular, taking in Walnut Creek, Concord, Suisun Bay, and the west delta. Once on level ground, you reach a trail junction where the Corduroy Hills Trail continues left and downhill, via wooden steps, and a spur trail to Eagle Peak heads right and uphill. After turning left and descending the steps, you traverse the north side of Eagle Peak on a trail carved in a steep cliff, enjoying

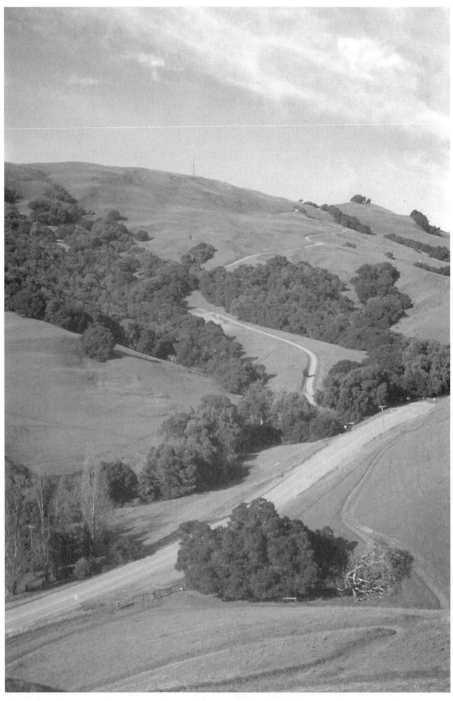

View west from the Chamise Trail across Bollinger Canyon Road to Rocky Ridge.

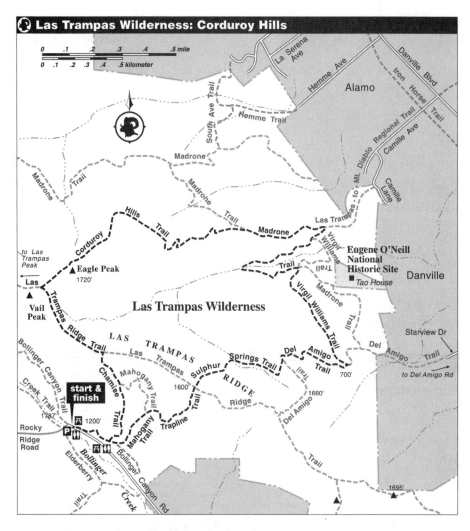

Las Trampas Wilderness: Corduroy Hills

a terrific view of Mt. Diablo. Soon you begin to descend steeply on more wooden steps, then less so, through a wooded area along the crest of a ridge.

In a grassy meadow the route levels, bends right, and begins to climb. This dramatic part of Las Trampas Wilderness, the Corduroy Hills, is characterized by deeply convoluted canyons and ridges. Black oak makes an appearance here, favoring warmer, drier slopes. Now beginning a long, moderate descent, you break out of the trees and wind down through open grassland to a T-junction, just after some switchbacks, with a wide dirt road. Turn left—the arrow pointing straight on a trail post here is confusing—and continue your descent, following the road as it heads first toward Mt. Diablo, then zigzags down a ridge, soon joining a road coming from the right-hand branch of the previous junction.

At about the 2.5-mile point, the Corduroy Hills Trail ends, and you merge with the Madrone Trail, coming from the left. Here you go straight, passing an area that may be quite muddy in wet weather, and continue to descend. As the road makes an almost 180-degree bend right, you pass the Las Trampas–to–Mt. Diablo Regional Trail, which departs left. Stay on the Madrone Trail, descending past the single-track Virgil Williams Trail, which also goes left.

Just ahead, you reach a dense forest with a creek on your left, and now the route begins to climb southwest on a moderate grade that soon eases. This area too may be muddy or even flooded in wet weather. Trees thriving here in the cool, moist soil include California buckeye, bigleaf maple, and white alder, along with the usual bay and coast live oak. With trees that lose their leaves in winter, it is sometimes easier to identify them by looking down at the leaf litter, instead of up at their bare branches.

The road bends left and crosses the creek, which flows through two large culverts, and continues to climb, soon reaching a four-way junction with the Virgil Williams Trail. Here you turn right, go through a gate, and climb through dense forest on moderate and occasionally steep grades. Left through the trees is Tao House, the one-time home of playwright Eugene O'Neill, preserved by the National Park Service as a National Historic Site. It was in Tao House, where he lived from 1937 to 1944, that O'Neill wrote *The Iceman Cometh* and *A Long Day's Journey Into Night*, two of his best-known dramas. Arrangements to visit Tao House can be made by calling (925) 838-7546.

As the route levels, you pass through an area of chaparral, then make another steep climb, go through a gate, and descend to a junction with the Del Amigo Trail, a wide dirt road. Turning right, you come to the steepest part of the route, a climb that helps earn for this hike its "difficult" rating, and putting it in company with "Ramage Peak," the "Grand Loop" on Mt. Diablo, and a few others as among the most challenging in this book. Speaking of Mt. Diablo, it is worth turning around from time to time as you grunt and sweat your way uphill to view its hulking form across the Interstate 680 corridor.

On your way up the steep slope, you may encounter shrubs such as coffeeberry, bush monkeyflower, California sagebrush, and blue bush lupine, growing here in the company of black oak and bigleaf maple. As the grade eases, the Del Amigo Trail enters a lovely clearing, bends sharply left, and reaches a junction on level ground with the Sulphur Springs Trail, where you turn right. (The arrows on the signs are potentially confusing here, and the trail going straight, signed SUMMIT TRAIL, is the continuation of the Del Amigo Trail on the park map).

As you begin to descend the Sulphur Springs Trail, a steep dirt road, note a narrow path on the right, about 150 feet from the junction, leading through the grass to a group of boulders, shaded in the afternoon and conveniently sized for sitting. This area makes a good rest stop. After you are again underway, descend into a beautiful, shady canyon, then follow a creek, which may be flowing across the road in more than one spot, downstream to several horse watering troughs in a grove of coast live oak. Here your route, the Sulphur Springs Trail, turns left, crosses the creek at a trail post, and, as an eroded single track, begins climbing uphill on a moderate grade.

A pleasant climb through oak woodland and past a meadow, possibly flooded, wins back some of the elevation you recently lost and soon brings you to a four-way junction in a meadow and the end of the Sulphur Springs Trail. Here the Las

Trampas Ridge Trail crosses left to right, and your route, the Trapline Trail, goes straight. In about 100 feet you reach a saddle on the crest of Las Trampas Ridge, where an opening in a barbed-wire fence allows you to pass through. Directly ahead, about 0.5 mile away, is Bollinger Canyon, with Rocky Ridge rising up behind, a sure sign you are nearing the finish. Now you follow the Trapline Trail, here a rock-and-dirt path, down through a corridor of chaparral, where you may find mountain mahogany, a large shrub with silver-gray bark and small, translucent green leaves, serrated at the ends.

Soon chaparral gives way to open grassland, then forest, as you lose hard-won elevation, finally reaching the end of the Trapline Trail. Here you join the Mahogany Trail, a single track, by angling left, and continue to descend beside a creek in a steep ravine, right. What a contrast with the dry chaparral of a few minutes ago! Here everything is cool and lush, and you are surrounded by the soothing sound of running water. Most of the East Bay's common oaks—blue, black, canyon live, coast live—are represented in Las Trampas Wilderness, along with one that is rare in our area, Oregon oak. This commercially valuable tree, growing from Central California to British Columbia, resembles valley oak, but its trunk is straighter, and its leaves are slightly larger and have fewer lobes.

After a steep descent, in places on wooden steps, you reach a bridge over the creek near a small waterfall. Once across, you begin to climb a narrow path through an area where bay and toyon, normally a shrub but here a small tree, compete for sunlight. An unusual plant growing in this wooded area is California pipevine, whose flowers, appearing in late winter, resemble miniature saxophones. A steady climb brings you to a fence, and just beyond, a junction with the Chamise Trail, where you turn left and retrace your steps to the parking area.

LAS TRAMPAS PEAK

Length: 3.8 miles

Time: 2 to 4 hours

Rating: Moderate

Regulations: EBRPD; no bicycles on the Chamise Trail or single-track segment of the Las Trampas Ridge Trail. (Bicyclists wishing to ride to Las Trampas Peak must follow the Bollinger Canyon Trail uphill to the multi-use part of the Las Trampas Ridge Trail.)

Facilities: Picnic tables, toilet, water (may not be available year-round).

Directions: From Interstate 680 in San Ramon, take the Crow Canyon Road/San Ramon exit and go west 1.1 miles on Crow Canyon Road to Bollinger Canyon Road. Turn right and go 4.5 miles to the end of the road, past the first Las Trampas Wilderness entrance, and turn left into the parking area. The trailhead is at the parking area entrance on Bollinger Canyon Road.

From Interstate 580 eastbound in Castro Valley, take the Center St./Crow Canyon Road exit, go left over the freeway, then right on Castro Valley Blvd., which soon becomes E. Castro Valley Blvd., 0.7 mile to Crow Canyon Road. Turn left and go 7.5 miles to Bollinger Canyon Road, then follow the directions above.

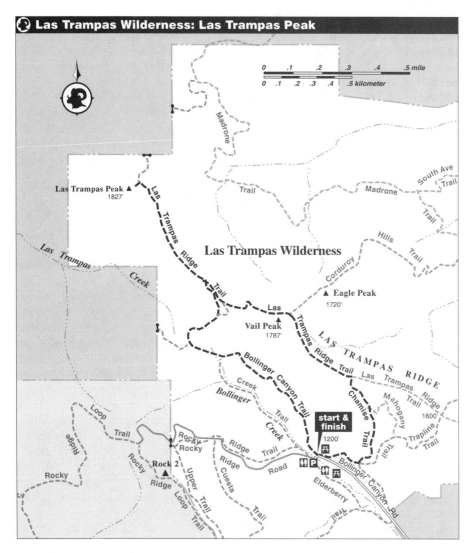

Las Trampas Wilderness: Las Trampas Peak

From Interstate 580 westbound in Castro Valley, take the Castro Valley exit, turn left onto E. Castro Valley Blvd. and go 0.1 mile to Crow Canyon Road. Turn right and follow the directions above.

Exploring Las Trampas Peak via the Chamise, Las Trampas Ridge, and Bollinger Canyon trails is the goal of this semi-loop trip, which passes through oak and bay forest, chaparral, and grassland, on its way to high grounds with great views.

Turn right on Bollinger Canyon Road and walk 500 feet to turnout, left. Go through a gate and follow the single-track Chamise Trail as it climbs southeast across an open hillside to a junction with the Bollinger Canyon Trail. Stay on the Chamise Trail by veering left and ascending a series of well-graded switchbacks.

As the trail bends left, you pass the Mahogany Trail, which goes straight and steeply downhill. Continuing to climb moderately along the crest of a narrow north–south ridge, you pass through a corridor of chaparral—a great place to study the plants up close—and, in a grove of coast live oak, reach the other end of the Mahogany Trail, right.

Now in the open, the route climbs a grassy hill and approaches the northwest–southeast spine of Las Trampas Ridge, right, guarded by massive rock cliffs. A flat area and a T-junction mark the point where the ridge you are on intersects Las Trampas Ridge. The Chamise Trail ends here, and you bear left on the Las Trampas Ridge Trail, enjoying views of Mt. Diablo, northeast, and Rocky Ridge, sporting a lone communication tower, southwest. Passing through a fence, you descend a steep, narrow track, muddy at times, soon reaching a clearing where the route levels. In a shady area, just east of Vail Peak (1787′), you reach a fence, right, and a junction with the Corduroy Hills Trail.

From here you follow the Las Trampas Ridge Trail as it bends left and climbs through a dense forest of trees and shrubs, including coast live oak, canyon live oak, California bay, toyon, and hillside gooseberry, a thorny bush with lovely white-and-purple flowers. Farther up the trail, you may see gooseberry's relative— pinkflower currant, a shrub with pink flowers and no thorns. With a deep canyon on your right, follow the trail as it tops a small rise and begins to descend around the north side of Vail Peak. Big, beautiful madrone trees with reddish bark stand at the edge of an area of chaparral, mostly chamise and buckbrush. Through the trees, right, Mt. Diablo rises behind Alamo, Danville, and the Interstate 680 corridor. In a clearing, lupine and bush monkeyflower soak up the morning sun.

As you come to a clearing at about the 1.4-mile point, a connector to the Bollinger Canyon Trail heads left. (To shorten the trip, turn left and descend about 0.2 mile to the Bollinger Canyon Trail, then follow that trail for about 1 mile to the parking area.) Continue straight, walking northwest, with spectacular views ahead across Moraga Valley to the Oakland and Berkeley hills, topped by Round Top and Vollmer Peak, and behind them in the distance, Mt. Tamalpais. Now passing through a corridor of chaparral, the route begins to climb an ever-narrowing ridge with steep drops on both sides. Nordstrom Ridge rises from a deep, forested valley, right, and behind it looms the hulking form of Mt. Diablo.

After reaching a high point, the route descends to meet the Bollinger Canyon Trail, a dirt road, left. Your route, the Las Trampas Ridge Trail, now also a dirt road, continues straight, with the summit of Las Trampas Peak (1827′) about 0.5 mile ahead. (To shorten the trip, turn left on the Bollinger Canyon Trail and go about 1.2 miles to the parking area.) Stands of madrone, manzanita, and coast silk tassel line the road. After descending to a saddle, the route makes a final push steeply uphill to surmount Las Trampas Peak.

At about the 2-mile point, you reach a junction with a road heading left to the peak's summit. The road you have been on bends right and drops over the edge of a grassy plateau on its way to the park boundary. Before climbing to the summit, walk to the edge of this plateau to enjoy a fine view, which extends north toward Walnut Creek, Concord, Mt. Diablo, Suisun Bay, and the west delta. Now turning back toward Las Trampas Peak, you climb on a moderate grade to its summit for another vista, this one south along Las Trampas Ridge to Pleasanton and beyond.

From the summit, retrace your steps to the junction of the Las Trampas Ridge and Bollinger Canyon trails. Bear right and follow the Bollinger Canyon Trail, a dirt road, downhill on a moderate grade through chaparral—manzanita, chamise, toyon, black sage, and buckbrush. As the route steepens and bends right, you pass the connector to the Las Trampas Ridge Trail, left. Soon you come to an unsigned fork: bear right and continue the descent into Bollinger Canyon. Western scrub-jays and California towhees are two of the most common birds you may see here. The former is one of three species of scrub-jays found in North America; the latter is one of five species of towhees. Ornithologists are constantly learning more about the birds they study, and sometimes this results in birds being renamed or reclassified. Not too long ago, scrub-jays all belonged to a single species, and the California towhee was called brown towhee.

At about the 3-mile point, you pass an unsigned road, right, and continue to descend on the Bollinger Canyon Trail through open areas that may be flooded, muddy, eroded, or all three. Bollinger Creek, bordered by trees, is on your right, and soon you come to a junction with the Creek Trail, right, also very muddy at times. Continuing straight on the Bollinger Canyon Trail, you come after about 0.5 mile to a fence at the end of Bollinger Canyon Road and the entrance to the parking area.

ROCKY RIDGE

Length: 3.8 miles

Time: 2 to 3 hours

Rating: Moderate

Regulations: EBRPD; no bicycles; trails may be closed to horses when wet and muddy.

Facilities: Picnic tables, toilet, water (may not be available year-round).

Directions: From Interstate 680 in San Ramon, take the Crow Canyon Road/San Ramon exit and go west 1.1 miles on Crow Canyon Road to Bollinger Canyon Road. Turn right and go 4.5 miles to the end of the road, past the first Las Trampas Wilderness entrance, and turn left into the parking area. The trailhead is at the northwest corner of parking area, at the green cattle gate.

From Interstate 580 eastbound in Castro Valley, take the Center St./Crow Canyon Road exit, go left over the freeway, then right on Castro Valley Blvd., which soon becomes E. Castro Valley Blvd., 0.7 mile to Crow Canyon Road. Turn left and go 7.5 miles to Bollinger Canyon Road, then follow the directions above.

From Interstate 580 westbound in Castro Valley, take the Castro Valley exit, turn left onto E. Castro Valley Blvd. and go 0.1 mile to Crow Canyon Road. Turn right and follow the directions above.

This short but scenic semi-loop trip, via Rocky Ridge Road and the Cuesta and Upper trails, takes you atop 2000-foot Rocky Ridge, the border between Las Trampas Wilderness and EBMUD lands of the Upper San Leandro Reservoir watershed. Rocky Ridge, a Nike missile site during the Cold War, rises midway

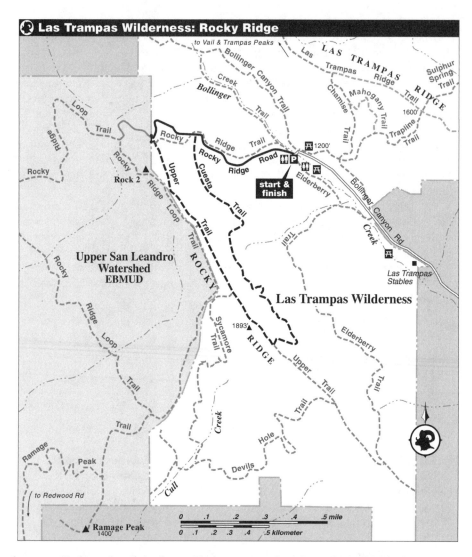

between Redwood and Anthony Chabot regional parks and Mt. Diablo State Park, making it a commanding vantage point with great views.

After passing through the cattle gate, you begin a steep uphill walk on paved Rocky Ridge Road. After a short while the grade eases somewhat, but more climbing is just ahead, past stands of coast live oak and California bay. In wet weather, water may be running here in channels on both sides of the road. If you are here late in the day, listen for the "hoo, hoo, hoo-hoo" of a great-horned owl, but don't be fooled by a mourning dove's plaintive cooing. After climbing for about 0.5-mile, you round a bend and reach a junction with a single-track trail heading left and steeply uphill. Turn left, and immediately come to a fork with a trail post in the middle. Here the Rocky Ridge Trail heads right and the Cuesta Trail, your route, goes left.

Turn left and climb south and then southeast across an open hillside, enjoying views of Bollinger Canyon, Mt. Diablo, and your goal, Rocky Ridge, right. The trail, climbing on a gentle grade, may be muddy and damaged by cows. Along the way uphill you pass many paths joining your route: ignore these and stay on the Cuesta Trail, a well-defined path. Watch for red-tailed hawks soaring overhead and dark-eyed juncos darting from tree to tree. Bigleaf maples join bays and oaks to offer some occasional shade, but the route stays mostly in the open.

Now the route bends sharply right, heads toward Rocky Ridge, and starts to climb across hillside dotted with boulders and clumps of blue bush lupine. Soon you turn left and descend over rough and eroded ground to a fence. Here the grade levels and then begins to climb again. The hillside sweeping up to your right is getting steeper, and across Bollinger Canyon, left, Mt. Diablo rises majestically behind Las Trampas Ridge. The route finally begins a steep climb, via switchbacks, to Rocky Ridge, and now you can see a communication tower on the ridge's high point (2024'). Across Bollinger Canyon in the distance, just right of the antenna, is Las Trampas Peak (1827'), a great destination for another day.

Just before the 2-mile point, after the final switchback, you reach a T- junction with the Upper Trail, a dirt road running southeast to northwest. Turn right and follow the Upper Trail as it climbs in the open over several high points, each with terrific views, especially southwest to EBMUD lands around Upper San Leandro Reservoir. Ramage Peak (1401') stands watch in front of the reservoir, and left of the peak you can see Hideaway Ranch, on private lands at the end of Cull Canyon Road. Descending briefly from these heights, you reach a flat spot and a junction with the Sycamore Trail, a faint trace heading left across the grass.

Staying straight along the ridgecrest, you come to a fence, left, guarding EBMUD's watershed. Here the road goes through a locked gate and becomes part of EBMUD's Rocky Ridge Loop Trail (Trail Use Permit required), but your route, the Upper Trail, continues as a single-track trail on the right side of the fence. Heading northwest, you now have views extending north past Walnut Creek and Concord to Suisun Bay and the west delta. You can also see the parking area where you started this hike, right and downhill.

At about the 2.8-mile point, you reach a gate in the fence, left, marking a junction with EBMUD's Rocky Ridge Loop Trail. As you continue straight, still on the Upper Trail, you cross a steep hillside that drops right. After a moderate descent on rough, eroded trail, you pass the steep Rocky Ridge Trail, right, leading down to the Cuesta Trail. Continue straight, and in a few feet you come to Rocky Ridge Road, gated uphill to your left, with another EBMUD access point on the other side of the road. Turn right and begin a moderate descent on the paved road. At about the 3.3-mile point, you close the loop at the junction with the Cuesta Trail, right. From here, retrace your route downhill to the parking area.

✦Pleasanton Ridge Regional Park ✦

PLEASANTON RIDGE

Length: 12.3 miles

Time: 6 to 8 hours

Rating: Very difficult

Regulations: EBRPD.
Facilities: Picnic tables, water, toilet, horse staging.
Directions: From Interstate 680 in Pleasanton, take the Sunol Blvd./Castlewood Dr. exit and take the first right onto Castlewood Dr., staying straight where Pleasanton–Sunol Road bends left. After 0.3 mile, you reach Foothill Road; turn left and go south 1.6 miles on Foothill Road to the Oak Tree staging area, right. The trailhead is at the west side of first parking area, just beyond the water fountain and information board.

The semi-loop trip along Pleasanton Ridge, combining the Oak Tree, Ridgeline, Bay Leaf, Sinbad Creek, Thermalito, and Olive Grove trails, while one of the longest and most challenging in this guide, is also one of the most rewarding. The views are outstanding, extending from Pleasanton, San Ramon, and Mt. Diablo to Sunol Valley, the Sunol/Ohlone Wilderness, and Mission Peak. The terrain is varied: the route passes through dense woodland, open grassland, and even a restored olive orchard. Bird and plant life flourish in this relatively undeveloped, 4743-acre park. (Numbers in parentheses in the route description below refer to numbered junctions on the park map. These numbers can be found on trail posts along the trail.)

After walking a short distance west from the parking area on a dirt road, you come to a cattle gate; once through, bear left and begin climbing the Oak Tree Trail, also a dirt road. The grade is moderate at first, and the route passes through alternating areas of open grassland and oak woodland—mostly valley oak and coast live oak—on its way up Pleasanton Ridge. Where there are oaks in the East Bay you are likely to find woodpeckers, two of the most common being acorn woodpecker and northern flicker. Acorn woodpecker is a dark bird, slightly smaller than a robin, with a black-and-white face, red crown, white rump, and white wing patches. As its name implies, this woodpecker gathers acorns in the winter—it dines on insects in the summer—and often stores them in holes it drills in oak trees. The northern flicker is a larger bird, brown overall, with a white rump, spotted breast, and horizontally striped back. The male of the "red-shafted" form, found west of the Rocky Mountains, sports a red mustache.

Several hundred yards past the trailhead, you come to a bend in the road and a junction (2) with the Woodland Trail, a single track heading left and uphill. (This trail, closed to bicycles, is an alternate way to reach the ridgecrest, and although it switchbacks steeply at first, most of the climbing is in the shade.) Following the Oak Tree Trail as it climbs on a winding, open course, generally northwest, you begin to see the busy Interstate 680 corridor below and right, and in the distance, the twin summits of Mt. Diablo. Joining oaks as one of the earliest trees to leaf out is California buckeye, with its distinctive fan of five bright green leaflets. Buckeyes adapt to hot weather by shedding their leaves early, sometimes in midsummer. You can identify the leafless tree by its rounded crown and angled branches, which are often colored orange by lichens.

The route continues its gentle and then moderate ascent, crossing a stream that runs under the road through a culvert. Venerable oaks—coast live and valley—give you occasional shade, but most of the time you are in open grassland. As the route turns west, you pass a junction, right, with the Sycamore Grove Trail (3), and you can see some of the large, light-barked trees that give this trail its name. There is a constant hum here from the freeway, but that will soon diminish, to be replaced by the breezy rustling of oak leaves. The route completes a 180-degree bend and now heads south, passing a junction with a grass-covered road, left, that is closed to bicycles. Toyon, blue elderberry, and poison oak grow here beside the road.

At about the 1.3-mile point, you emerge from a wooded area and reach a four-way junction near a barbed-wire fence. The trail merging from your left is the Woodland Trail. Straight ahead, and staying left of the fence, is an unsigned dirt road. Your route, the Oak Tree Trail, turns right and goes through an opening in the fence. About 30 feet beyond the fence is a trail post (5), and a choice of three dirt paths. The left-hand path is the continuation of the Oak Tree Trail. The right-hand path, a rutted single track, is an unfortunate shortcut that has scarred a grassy hillside; a restoration project is underway. The center path, your route, is the Ridgeline Trail.

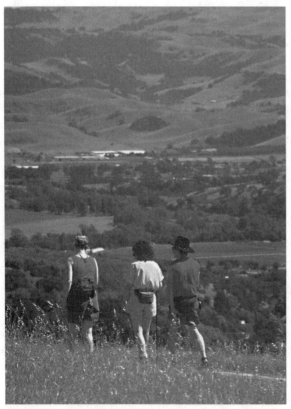

Hikers on Pleasanton Ridge enjoy sweeping vistas from the mostly open ridgetop grasslands.

The view from here is wonderful, taking in Mission Peak to the south, San Antonio Reservoir to the southeast, and behind it, the Sunol/Ohlone Wilderness. Skirting the north side of Mission Peak is Interstate 680, carrying its heavy load of traffic between Fremont and Pleasanton. To the west, heavily forested Sunol Ridge, topped by a single communication tower, rises above Kilkare Canyon and Sinbad Creek, reaching an elevation of just over 2000 feet. The Ridgeline Trail makes a 180-degree bend to gain the ridgetop, passing an unsigned path, right. Bending left, the route reaches a fork marked by a trail post (10). The left-hand fork is a short connector to the Olive Grove Trail; the right-hand fork is the Ridgeline Trail, your route.

The large olive grove ahead is one of several planted here between about 1890 and the 1920s. No record exists of who planted the trees, which are currently being restored by the park district and a private concessionaire. About 125 feet past the fork, you pass a junction, right, with a rough dirt road that runs along a barbed-wire fence. The Ridgeline Trail now parallels this fence, heading generally north-west and climbing past the olive grove on a moderate grade. Just beyond the grove is a water fountain, a watering trough for animals, and another fork, where you continue straight.

Rising steeply over rocky ground, your route, shared by hikers, bicyclists, equestrians, joggers, and dog walkers, passes more olive trees, their leaves quak-ing in the breeze. At the end of the olive orchard, the route levels and comes into the open, with views extending north to Mt. Diablo and south to Mission Peak. The northeast face of Pleasanton Ridge drops steeply to Interstate 680, right and now far below. Just shy of the 2-mile point, you pass a junction (14) with the Olive Grove Trail merging sharply from the left. On its way along the ridgetop, the route climbs over several high points, the first of which is just ahead. (There are two picnic tables atop one of these rounded summits.)

Soon you descend to a flat spot and a four-way junction. Here, on the left, is a short connector (16) to the Thermalito Trail, a route running generally parallel to and southwest of the Ridgeline Trail. The Thermalito Trail takes its name from the Thermal Fruit Company, which was active nearby from 1904 until the 1930s. On the right, an unsigned path climbs to a cattle gate. Your route continues straight,

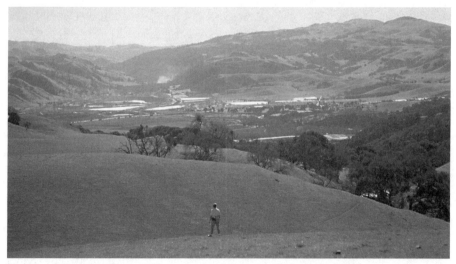

Views south from Pleasanton Ridge extend to Mission and Monument Peaks.

then bends right and climbs steeply to the summit of a grassy hill. Ahead the ridge continues to rise, and on your right is a boundary with the Castlewood Country Club, private property. Twisted and gnarled valley oaks line the route in places. Now you reach a junction, left, with another connector to the Thermalito Trail (18).

Continuing on the Ridgeline Trail, you climb steeply over several more hills, with steep drops in between. On the left you'll find a well-shaded picnic table, bench, and horse-hitching post. Finally, the route leaves the ridgetop, veering right and downhill through a cattle gate (19), then descends on a rutted and rocky road via two switchbacks to a forest of California bay, coast live oak, black oak, and bigleaf maple, with toyon, bush monkeyflower, and vine honeysuckle adding variety to the scene, so different from the ridgetop. At the second switchback, you pass a path that heads right to a gate and the country club, a restricted area. The route resumes its northwest course on a level grade, soon entering the City of Pleasanton's Augustin Bernal Park.

Now out of dense forest, you drop to a flat spot, which may be muddy, and a junction with the Thermalito Trail, a dirt road, left. A beautiful clearing here makes a fine rest spot, and a fallen tree limb may provide you with a comfortable seat. There is drinking water and a trough for animals a short distance down the Thermalito Trail. The valley oaks surrounding this clearing are loaded with mistletoe, especially evident when their limbs are bare. (To shorten your hike, take the Thermalito Trail southwest and follow the route description from about the 8.5-mile point for the return part of this trip.) Leaving the clearing and still on the Ridgeline Trail, you begin a moderate ascent, passing near some stands of blue oak. Flocks of dark-eyed juncos may move from tree to tree just ahead of you, or you may hear the call of a red-tailed hawk and see it circling high above.

Soon the Valley View Trail, a dirt road, appears on your right; it will merge with the Ridgeline Trail at an upcoming junction. Before the junction, a short connector road, right, leads to the Valley View Trail. About 50 feet past the connector road is the single-track Equestrian Trail, left, for horses only. Continuing straight, you pass these junctions and a pond, left. There is a water fountain here. This part of the hike is in the open, but sheltered from the wind, so it may be hot. The route rises to a little saddle and passes a junction, left, with the other end of the Equestrian Trail. Ahead is a gate, the boundary between the city and regional parks.

Once through the gate you arrive at a junction (21). Here a dirt road continues straight, but your route turns right and leads you through a beautiful oak savanna, with a fence marking the park boundary on your right. After a mostly level walk you merge with the road that went straight just after the gate and begin to gain elevation. As the route breaks into the open, you pass a pond, left, which may be full of tadpoles, frogs, or both. A large coast live oak at the water's edge provides shelter for songbirds. There is a junction here with the Sinbad Creek Trail, left, part of your return route (22). Continue straight, passing another small pond and a hill, right, with a bench. Now you enter a wonderful area of rolling hills punctuated by groves of oak. You may see ground squirrels standing at attention in front of their burrows or scampering across the grass as you approach.

The route soon swings west and reaches a junction (26). From here a dirt road leads to a gate and the park boundary, right. Your route, the Bay Leaf Trail, continues straight, then bends left and begins to descend. There are deep, tree-filled ravines on both sides of you now, as you follow a spur ridge southwest. Soon the route swings sharply right and drops into the right-hand ravine on a moderate grade. Approaching the bottom of the ravine, you enter a shady realm of bay, black oak, and California buckeye, remarkably different from the open ridgetop you traversed earlier.

Now the route bends almost 180-degrees left, crossing two creeks that flow under the road through culverts. The freeway noise which accompanied the start of this hike has been replaced perhaps by a serenade of running water, coming from a creek in a gully to your left. After an open section, where bright sunlight encourages plants such as California sagebrush, coyote brush, and bush monkeyflower to take hold on a rocky hillside, you reach a junction, right, with the single-track Sinbad Creek Trail (25). The nearby trees are draped with lace lichen, which resembles the Spanish moss found in the South. (A trail post here shows the Sinbad Creek Trail also continuing downhill.)

Your route follows the road downhill and soon reaches Sinbad Creek, at the bottom of Kilkare Canyon, just before the 6-mile point. Step across the creek on rocks, and at a T-junction with a dirt road, turn left (24). Walking downstream along the creek and following a level course, you pass large western sycamore trees and groves of bay and coast live oak, interspersed with shrubs such as hillside gooseberry and coyote brush. After about 0.7 mile of pleasant streamside walking, you reach another T-junction (23), where you turn left, recross the creek, and begin climbing steeply—this is the hardest part of the entire trip—on the Sinbad Creek Trail, a dirt road.

As the road winds uphill, you may notice some rock layers that appear to have been tilted from horizontal to vertical, an indication of the powerful forces that formed these hills. Two parallel fault systems border Pleasanton Ridge, and violent upheavals during the past two to three million years have twisted and rearranged the marine sediments that underlie this area. Passing a large water tank, the route emerges from dense forest into oak savanna, then swings east and crosses a notch in the ridgeline.

Ahead you can see the frog pond you passed earlier, and the large coast live oak growing at its edge. On your right is a water fountain. Passing a dirt road, left, you soon come to a T-junction with the Ridgeline Trail (22). Turn right and follow the Ridgeline Trail, bearing left at a fork about 250 feet past the end of the pond. You are now retracing your steps to the junction of the Ridgeline and Thermalito trails, at about the 8.5-mile point. When you reach that junction, which is in Augustin Bernal Park, you turn right on the Thermalito Trail, a dirt road, passing a drinking faucet and watering trough, and begin a moderate climb in the shade of valley oaks and coast live oaks. Soon you come to a gate (20) that marks the boundary between the city and regional parks. Now the route descends over rocky ground, steeply in places, following a southwest course. After passing a picturesque pond, left, which may have schools of small fish, the road rises steeply through a serene forest and then comes into the open.

The Thermalito Trail runs parallel to the Ridgeline Trail, making many ups and downs along the way. Watch for red-tailed hawks slowly circling overhead and acorn woodpeckers flashing through the trees. Mission Peak is once again in view to the south, across Interstate 680. Passing a connector, left, to the Ridgeline Trail

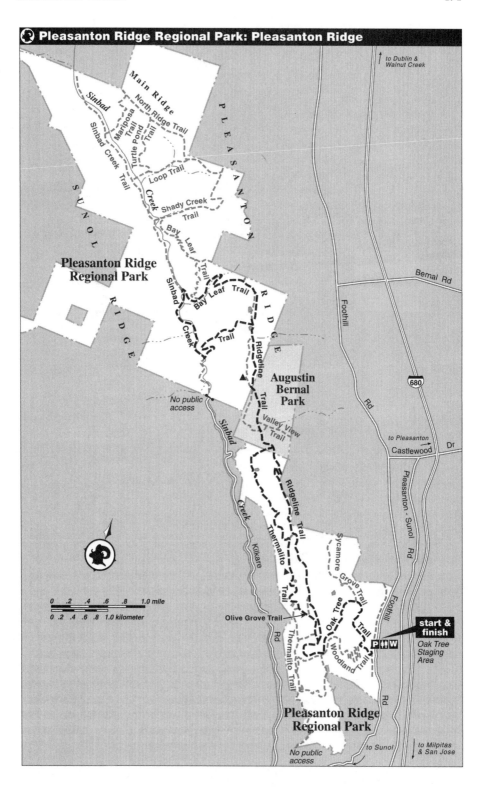

Pleasanton Ridge Regional Park: Pleasanton Ridge

(17), you continue on a rolling course, alternating between pockets of forest and open areas. Just shy of the 10-mile point, you reach a T-junction (15), where another connector to the Ridgeline Trail heads left, and your route, the Thermalito Trail, bears right.

Out in the open now, the road descends past a stock pond and a ground-squirrel colony to a small ravine, which may hold water during wet weather. Crossing to the other side of the ravine, the route climbs slightly, bringing you to another stock pond, right, and a junction. Leaving the Thermalito Trail where it turns right (13), you continue straight on a connector to the Olive Grove Trail. Walking east about 100 yards, you come to a junction with the Olive Grove Trail (12), which heads both left and straight. Continue straight, passing the olive grove on your left as you make a moderate descent on a rutted road. At the next junction (11), where the Olive Grove Trail swings right, continue straight on a connector to the Ridgeline Trail, which you soon reach. At the junction with the Ridgeline Trail (10), bear right and retrace your route on the Ridgeline and Oak Tree trails to the parking area.

◆ Mission Peak Regional Preserve ◆

MISSION PEAK

Length: 6.3 miles

Time: 3 to 5 hours

Rating: Difficult

Regulations: EBRPD; no bicycles on the single-track part of the Peak Trail.
Facilities: Water, toilet, horse staging.
Directions: From Interstate 880 in Fremont, take the Mission Blvd./Warren Ave. exit and go northeast on Mission Blvd. 1.8 miles to Stanford Ave. Turn right and go 0.6 mile to a parking area at the end of Stanford Ave. The trailhead is on the east side of parking area.

From Interstate 680 in Fremont, take the Mission Blvd./Warm Springs District exit and follow signs for Mission Blvd. eastbound. Once on Mission Blvd., follow it for 0.6 mile to Stanford Ave. Turn right and go 0.6 mile to a parking area at the end of Stanford Ave. The trailhead is on the east side of parking area.

(Note: On weekends the parking area can fill up. Don't be tempted to park in unofficial spots along the edge of the road—the Fremont police write tickets here frequently. You can find parking on Stanford Ave., a few blocks away from the parking area.)

A steady climb of more than 2000 feet in just over 3 miles, most of it on the Hidden Valley Trail, a well-graded dirt road, brings you to the top of Mission Peak, one of the East Bay's most dramatic summits, offering views of the entire Bay Area. If you plan your trip for a clear day in winter or spring, after a storm front has moved through, most of the Bay Area will be revealed, from Mt. Tamalpais to the

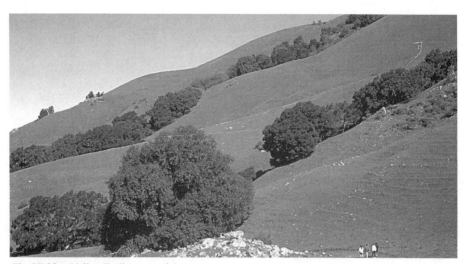

The Hidden Valley Trail is one of the routes up Mission Peak.

Santa Cruz Mountains. This is *not* a trip for hot weather—the out-and-back route offers little shade. Even on a warm day, however, take extra clothes and a wind shell—this is a mountain environment which can quickly turn hostile. Along the way to Mission Peak's summit, a number of paths—short cuts and cow trails—leave the main route: ignore these and stay on the wide dirt road. Please respect all signs regarding areas closed for restoration. (The letters MP, for Mission Peak, OT, for Ohlone Trail, and numbers in parentheses in the route description below refer to numbered junctions on the park map.)

From the parking area, the Hidden Valley Trail, a dirt road, heads uphill toward Mission Peak. Stay left at the first fork, an unsigned junction with the Peak Meadow Trail. On your right is a line of eucalyptus trees and just beyond them, Agua Caliente Creek, which drains Hidden Valley. Your route passes stands of coast live oak, western sycamore, California buckeye, and blue elderberry. (Use caution: vehicles transporting hang gliders and parasailers to their launch site may be on the road for the first few miles.)

The Ohlone Wilderness Regional Trail, a 28-mile trek through some of the East Bay's most scenic and remote territory, begins at the Stanford Ave. parking area and follows the Hidden Valley Trail up the west side of Mission Peak, though many people shun this steep climb and instead hike between Sunol and Del Valle regional parks, a trip described elsewhere in this book. The emblem for the Ohlone Wilderness Regional Trail, which you may see on trail posts here, is a white oak leaf in a red disk. You may also see numbers on some of the trail posts; these refer to numbered junctions on EBRPD's Ohlone Wilderness Regional Trail map, which is posted at the trailhead.

After about 0.3 mile, begin a gentle climb which soon becomes moderate. The terrain in the 2999-acre Mission Peak Regional Preserve is rolling; the hills are green in winter and spring, brown in summer and fall, with tree-filled canyons. Most of the route stays in the open, so as you climb, be sure to stop often and enjoy the view. Mission Peak (2517') sits atop a long ridge that trends northwest–south-

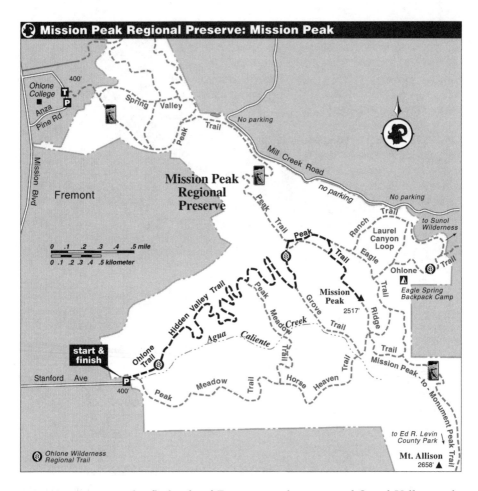

Mission Peak Regional Preserve: Mission Peak

east, towering over the flatlands of Fremont to the west and Sunol Valley to the east. Immediately southeast of Mission Peak is another ridge, running northeast–southwest, crowned by Mt. Allison (2658'). Farther still to the southeast is Monument Peak (2594'), on the border of Santa Clara County's Ed R. Levin Park. Combined, these three peaks make up a massif that from many places around the East Bay appears to rival Mt. Diablo in stature.

You route passes through a small wooded area—mainly coast live oak and California bay—near a stream, then bends south through a rocky area and continues to climb. Except from the air, no other vantage point offers such extensive views this close to San Francisco Bay. Turning back toward the peak, which exposes more of its rocky backbone the higher you get, you soon come to a short, steep section and then pass a junction (OT 2) with the unsigned Peak Meadow Trail, right. Now the road begins a series of switchbacks that will carry you to the summit. On most of the way you will have the parking area at the end of Stanford Ave. in view, so you can gauge your progress in both distance and elevation.

After 2 miles or so, the terrain around you becomes more rugged—a steep, grassy field strewn with boulders, and the dramatic rock cliffs of Mission Peak's summit. Lovers of wilderness often travel many hours for scenes such as this, yet you are only about an hour's walk from a trailhead in one of California's busiest urban areas.

Just below the cliffs you come to a T-junction (MP 26/OT 3), where you turn left. Nearby are rocks to sit on and enjoy thrilling views west to San Francisco Bay. The buildings to the southeast are used by EBRPD rangers, and looming above them is Mt. Allison, bristling with communication towers. Alfred A. Moore, an early California settler and attorney for the railroad, once owned several thousand acres on Mission Peak, including a ranch with exotic animals, which he used as a weekend retreat for family and friends. The Grove Trail, which goes right (southeast) from the T-junction, visits the A.A. Moore Memorial Grove.

Raptors and turkey vultures may look down from above as you struggle steeply upward. Respite arrives just as you crest the ridge in the form of a broad, flat area. Several dirt paths head right, but you continue straight, getting your first view today of Mt. Diablo and Pleasanton Ridge. At about the 2.5-mile point, you come to a barbed-wire fence with a gap. The Hidden Valley Trail ends at a four-way junction just beyond the fence (MP 25/OT 4). The Peak Trail goes straight and right; a dirt road heads left. There is a toilet nearby.

Here you turn right and follow the Peak Trail, a dirt road that parallels the fence and heads uphill. The Peak Trail, part of the Bay Area Ridge Trail, runs between Ohlone College in Fremont and the summit of Mission Peak. Just as your route veers left, away from the fence, you pass a wide trail continuing straight. (This alternate trail is steep but offers views of the Bay on its way to rejoin the Peak Trail near the summit of Mission Peak.)

If you opt to stay on the Peak Trail, continue to climb east, toward a flat spot on the skyline ridge, passing a connector to the Hidden Valley Trail, right. Here you have a chance to appreciate the tenacity of plants growing in this barren and often windy environment. Clumps of blue bush lupine cling to the rocky soil in the company of California buttercup, and a few bay trees grab footholds farther downhill. You may see a common bird of open places, the horned lark. Slightly larger than a sparrow, this brown and yellow bird is found on fields, ridges, and beaches across North America.

Soon you reach a fork (OT 5): right is the continuation of the Peak Trail; left is the Eagle Trail, the continuation of the Ohlone Wilderness Regional/Bay Area Ridge Trail. Turn right and begin a gentle climb that soon turns steep. If the winter or spring day you've chosen is especially clear, you may be thrilled, when you crest the ridge, to see a line of snow-capped peaks in the distance—the Sierra Nevada—rising behind Livermore and Altamont Pass. Ahead, to the east, the land drops away to the Alameda Creek drainage, then rises up on the other side to form the highlands of the Sunol/Ohlone Wilderness. At the end of the road, there are two garbage cans and a wooden hitching post for horses. (The alternate trail you passed earlier ends here.)

From road's end, several dirt paths head southeast, steeply uphill to the summit. As you climb, the waters of San Antonio Reservoir come into view to your left, but San Francisco Bay is hidden by a ridge, right. The dirt path quickly gives way to dirt and rock, and you top several false summits, staying just left and below the ridgecrest, until San Francisco Bay is back in view. Before reaching the true summit, you come to a metal post, anchored in rock, with holes drilled through it and each hole fitted with a pipe, 19 in all. These pipes are keyed to numbered plaques attached to the post. This clever, if low-tech, observation device allows you to identify more than two dozen Bay Area landmarks in a 360-degree circle around Mission Peak. Besides the ones already mentioned, some of the most notable include Mt. Hamilton's Lick Observatory (4209'); Rose Peak (3817') in the Ohlone Wilderness; Flag Hill, behind the visitor center in Sunol Wilderness; Moffett Field in Mountain View; Mt. Tamalpais; San Francisco; and Coyote Hills Regional Park.

A few steps bring you at last to the top of Mission Peak, a climb of about 2250 feet in a little more than 3 miles, for an average grade of about 7%. Congratulations, and welcome to one of the premier vantage points in the East Bay! When you have finished enjoying this exhilarating and hard-won summit, retrace your route to the parking area. (You can also vary the descent by retracing to the Peak Meadow Trail, then descending this lesser-used and shadier route south, then west, to the parking area.)

◆ Sunol Wilderness ◆

LITTLE YOSEMITE

Length: 3 miles

Time: 2 to 3 hours

Rating: Moderate

Regulations: EBRPD; fees for parking and dogs when entrance kiosk is attended.

Facilities: Visitor center, picnic tables, water, toilets, phone.

Directions: From Interstate 680 northbound, northeast of Fremont, take the Calaveras Road exit and bear right onto Calaveras Road. Go 4.2 miles to Geary Road, turn left, and go 1.8 miles to the entrance kiosk. At 0.1 mile past the kiosk, there is a parking area, left, beside the visitor center, a green barn. Continue about 100 yards to the next parking area, also left. (If this parking area is full, there is another on the right, or you can use the one beside the visitor center.) The trailhead is at the north corner of parking area.

From Interstate 680 southbound, south of Pleasanton, take the Calaveras Road exit, and at the stop sign at the bottom of the ramp turn left onto Paloma Road (signed PALOMA WAY). Go under Interstate 680, stay in the left lane, and at the next stop sign continue straight, now on Calaveras Road. Then follow directions above.

This loop is a fine introduction to Sunol Wilderness, one of the gems of the regional park system, and at nearly 7000 acres one of its largest holdings. A scenic trek along the Canyon View Trail, through oak savanna and grassland, brings you to Little Yosemite, a rocky gorge carved by Alameda Creek. Easily accessed on foot,

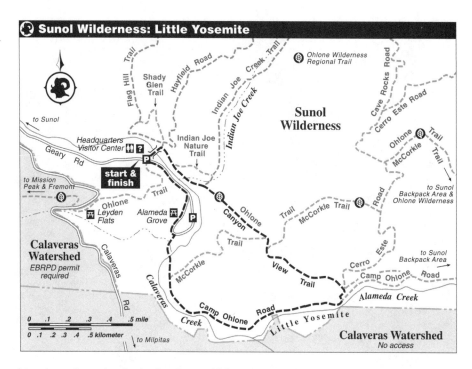

bicycle, or horseback via the Camp Ohlone Road, Little Yosemite is a popular destination for families with children. The return part of the loop, Camp Ohlone Road, takes you beside the tree-lined creek, especially lovely in fall.

(The letters SO, for Sunol/Ohlone, OT, for Ohlone Trail, and numbers in parentheses in the route description below refer to numbered junctions on the park map. These markings can be found on trail posts along the trail.)

From the trailhead, turn right and cross a wood bridge over Alameda Creek. Many of Sunol's trails use this bridge, including the Ohlone Wilderness Regional Trail, a 28-mile route from Mission Peak Regional Preserve to Del Valle Regional Park, parts of which are described elsewhere in this book. After crossing Alameda Creek and turning right, you are on the Canyon View Trail, a wide dirt path lined with white alder, bigleaf maple, western sycamore, and willow, with the creek on your right. (The first part of the Canyon View Trail is also part of the Indian Joe Nature Trail, a self-guiding route with numbered trail posts that correspond to text in a booklet available at the visitor center.)

Other trees and shrubs in this area include California bay, California buckeye, coast live oak, California sagebrush, bush monkeyflower, and poison oak. About 100 feet past the bridge, Hayfield Road climbs left, and some 30 feet beyond, a road leads to the creek, right. Continuing straight on the Canyon View Trail, you soon pass the Indian Joe Nature Trail, left, and then cross Indian Joe Creek. Follow the Canyon View Trail over rolling terrain to a fork with the Indian Joe Creek Trail (OT 14).

Where the Indian Joe Creek Trail veers left, continue straight on the Canyon View Trail, a single track, and climb on a moderate, then steep grade through an area shaded by coast live oak, blue oak, and bay. The view, right, takes in the

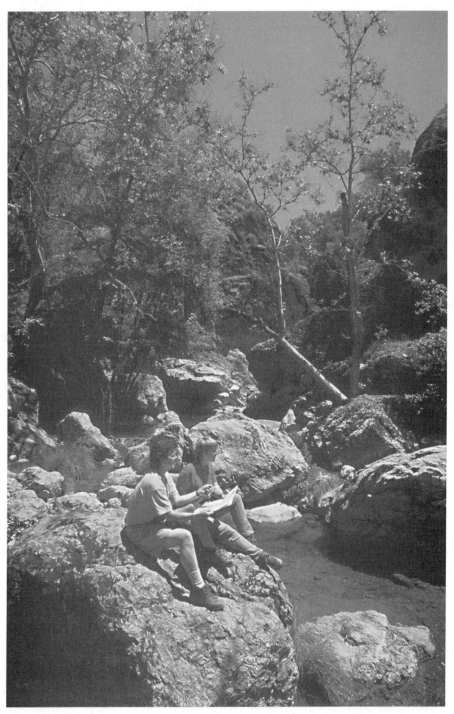

Little Yosemite is a rocky gorge on Alameda Creek, perfect for picnicking and nature study.

Alameda Creek valley and the highlands of Mission Peak Regional Preserve, crowned by three summits—from north to south, Mission Peak (2517'), Mt. Allison (2658'), and Monument Peak (2594'). After passing through a cattle gate, you come into the open atop a narrow ridge. As the grade eases and you pass through a savanna of blue and valley oak, you may be serenaded by a chorus of bird song. Groves of oaks are like islands in a sea of grass, providing shelter and food for a wide variety of birds, including jays, woodpeckers, yellow-billed magpies, western meadowlarks, brown creepers, and kinglets.

Serpentine and sandstone rock boulders and outcrops, seen here on the ridgetop, are evidence of Sunol's rocky foundation. From this vantage point, the exposed cliffs of Flag Hill, northwest, appear to tower over the visitor center and parking area. At a four-way junction (OT 15), cross the McCorkle Trail, a dirt road, and continue on the Canyon View Trail, climbing moderately across a steep, grassy hillside. If the deciduous oaks are leafless, you may notice clumps of mistletoe, a parasitic plant, growing in their branches. The sticky seeds of mistletoe, a photosynthesizing plant that has lost its ability to produce roots, are contained in berries eaten by birds. As the bird cleans its beak by wiping it against a tree branch, it "plants" the mistletoe seeds.

The route now traverses along the edge of a steep, south-facing hillside that leads down to Alameda Creek, about 200 feet below. Looking east, you can see the rugged hills that form the heart of the Ohlone Wilderness. After descending to a gully, possibly muddy, and crossing a small wood-plank bridge, you traverse an open expanse of grass dotted with rock outcrops which are tinged orange by lichen. The trail, rocky and eroded in places, rounds the end of a ridge, where a steep drop, right, reveals Camp Ohlone Road, your return route. The canyon below, containing Alameda Creek, is called Little Yosemite, and you may hear the sound of running water as the creek tumbles through its rocky gorge.

Pass through a rocky area shaded by valley oaks, then descend on a gentle grade, passing an open field with a fenced-off marshy area, left. Birds may be active here, including western scrub-jays and dark-eyed juncos. Crossing a culvert that drains water from the marshy area, you reach, in about 100 feet, a four-way junction with Cerro Este Road (SO 42). Turn right and follow the dirt-and-gravel road 0.2 mile downhill, via S-bends, to a junction with Camp Ohlone Road. (There's a toilet on the right.)

One of the scenic jewels of the regional park system, Little Yosemite features in miniature some of the wonders of its Sierra Nevada namesake, including water rushing through a boulder-strewn gorge, sheer cliffs, forested hillsides, and towering rock formations. A variety of trees and shrubs thrive here, including coast live oak, bay, California sagebrush, toyon, and bush monkeyflower. Stands of western sycamore add color in the fall.

After exploring to your heart's content, begin a gentle descent southwest on well-graded Camp Ohlone Road, soon reaching a fenced area, left, and several faint paths heading left toward the creek. Continuing on the road, you make a gentle climb past stands of willow, blue elderberry, and buckeye. Here you may see the bright red flowers of California fuchsia, a late bloomer, on a south-facing hillside. Now descending through an open area, you can see Flag Hill ahead, and when the route forks, stay right, soon passing the McCorkle Trail and a corral, right (SO 41).

A wooden bridge takes you across Alameda Creek, whose banks here are lined with white alder, willow, and sycamore.

Once across the creek, you are on a paved road (SO 40). About 50 feet past the bridge, a dirt path merges from the left. Continue straight, and after another 200 feet or so, you come to a large parking area. Proceed on the paved road, passing the Leyden Flats picnic area, left, until you reach the trailhead parking area.

MAGUIRE PEAKS

Length: 5.9 miles

Time: 3 to 4 hours

Rating: Moderate

Regulations: EBRPD; to park on Welch Creek Road, you must have either a parking permit, available at the Sunol visitor center on Geary Road, or a Regional Parks Foundation membership card: leave it on your dashboard. No bicycles or horses on the Upper Peaks Trail. (Horses and bicycles should start at the visitor center and use Hayfield and High Valley roads to reach Welch Creek Road, then follow the Maguire Peaks Trail to the Maguire Peaks Loop.)

Facilities: None along Welch Creek Road. Water, toilets, phone, maps, and information are available at the Sunol visitor center.

Directions: from Interstate 680 northbound, northeast of Fremont: take the Calaveras Road exit and bear right onto Calaveras Road. Go south 3.9 miles to Welch Creek Road. Turn left and go to the 1.6 mile marker—paying close attention, as there are numerous turnouts along the way—where two turnouts have space for about 6 to 8 cars total. The trailhead is on the north side of small parking area.

From Interstate 680 southbound, south of Pleasanton: Take the Calaveras Road exit, and at the stop sign at the bottom of the ramp turn left onto Paloma Road (signed PALOMA WAY). Go under Interstate 680, stay in the left lane, and at the next stop sign continue straight, now on Calaveras Road. Then follow the directions above.

To reach the Sunol visitor center: Proceed past Welch Creek Road another 0.3 mile, turn left on Geary Road and go 1.8 miles to the entrance kiosk. Then continue 0.1 mile to the visitor-center parking area, left.

This circuit of Maguire Peaks, via the Upper Maguire Peaks and Maguire Peaks trails and the Maguire Peaks Loop, explores a hidden corner of Sunol Wilderness, divided by Welch Creek Road from the main part of the park. The scenery is beautiful and serene, and the vistas from several vantage points are superb. To top it off (literally), you can make an ascent of Maguire Peaks west summit (1688'), a mountain climb in miniature. Parts of this semi-loop route may be extremely muddy during and after wet weather.

(The letters SO, for Sunol/Ohlone, and numbers in parentheses in the route description below refer to numbered junctions on the park map. These markings can be found on trail posts along the trail.)

From the uphill parking area, walk north down a small embankment and cross Welch Creek on rocks, finding a trail post and the Upper Maguire Peaks Trail, a single track heading north. This is a lovely wooded area of California bay, California buckeye, coast live oak, bigleaf maple, and western sycamore—remote and secluded. About 50 feet past the trail post you step across a little tributary of Welch Creek, and then follow the trail as it curves right and wanders upstream on a level grade. At a fork in the trail, you bear left, away from the tributary, and begin to climb across a steep hillside loaded with poison oak, California sagebrush, and bush monkeyflower, on a generally northwest course.

Having gained elevation, you enter a forest of blue oak, then reach a clearing where you have a beautiful view north to Maguire Peaks, two rocky summits behind a foreground of rolling, grassy hills studded with oaks. The view here also extends west toward San Francisco Bay, although it is often obscured by fog. This 6858-acre wilderness park is one of the best places in the East Bay to see yellow-billed magpies, large black-and-white birds with a long tail, usually found in flocks. Another sociable bird, the band-tailed pigeon, is also here, and the noise of their wings as they take off through the trees is startling. Now you follow an indistinct path across grassland, marked by metal trail posts, to a T-junction (SO 07) with the Maguire Peaks Trail, a dirt road signed MAGUIRE PEAKS ROAD.

This is the site of an old homestead, as evidenced by nearby eucalyptus and fruit trees, which are accompanied by pines and a large valley oak. You turn right and

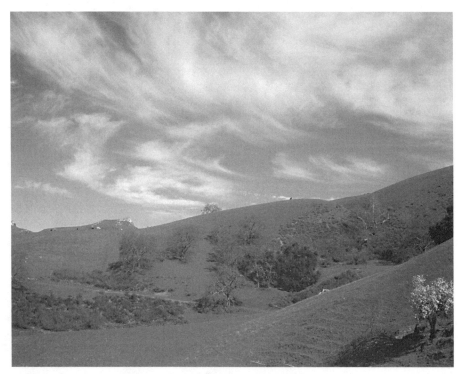

Cold, clear winter days are great for visiting the Maguire Peaks.

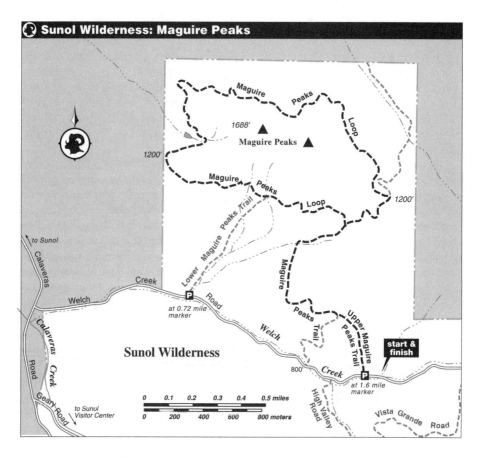

Sunol Wilderness: Maguire Peaks

then, after about 200 feet, curve sharply left and begin a moderate climb. Heading west, the route soon affords views of Mission Peak (2517') and antenna-topped Mt. Allison (2658'). The route here is mostly in the open, with a steep drop-off left. As you turn a corner and head north, you again have a view of Maguire Peaks, both just under 1700 feet high. Now you begin to descend via moderately graded S-bends into a forest of bay, blue oak, and coast live oak, where the silence is broken only by the twittering of birds.

Reaching the bottom of a shady canyon, the route crosses a tributary of Welch Creek flowing through a culvert, and then begins to climb, soon coming to an unsigned junction where you continue straight. Leaving the dense forest behind and entering oak savanna, you arrive at a junction with the Maguire Peaks Loop (SO 08). Here you continue straight, still on an ascending dirt road, and after about another 0.3 mile reach a junction (SO 09), marked by a metal trail post with an arrow pointing left, and sign for the Maguire Peaks Loop. Turn left, with Mt. Diablo just visible over hills to the north, and continue climbing. The route, a dirt road, bends north, skirts the end of a ridge topped by the easternmost of the two Maguire Peaks, left, and reaches level ground in a blue oak savanna. Ahead you can see San Antonio Reservoir, a large body of water about 1.5 miles north of the Sunol Wilderness boundary.

Circling around the north side of Maguire Peaks, you pass a hillside of blue bush lupine and reach an open area where the view extends northwest to Pleasanton and Sunol ridges. Now you have a better view of the Maguire Peaks themselves—the taller is the west peak, (1688'), directly ahead, its grassy summit guarded by a rock rampart. The route climbs on a moderate grade, aiming for a flat spot in a ridge extending northwest from the west peak. Along the way you may see two related shrubs (genus *Rhamnus*), coffeeberry and spiny redberry. Coffeeberry, appearing here as a small tree, has dark green elliptical leaves and purple berries. Spiny redberry has small, toothed leaves resembling those of holly or coast live oak, and red berries.

Spring wildflowers decorate the open hillsides here, but when the route enters a grove of coast live oak, ferns and moss take over, giving the shaded area a rain-forest feel. Two birds that seek dense cover, spotted towhee and wrentit, may be seen, or more likely heard, here. Now back in the open, the route crosses a rocky ridge, where a flat area with outstanding views of San Francisco Bay, Mt. Diablo, and Mission Peak makes a good rest stop.

To climb the westernmost and highest of the two Maguire Peaks, continue on the Maguire Peaks Loop, which now turns left and follows the ridgetop toward the peaks. Just before the route turns right and begins to descend, find an unsigned path, to the left of a bench, going straight and uphill, climbing southeast up a steep hillside of grass and lupine. After you gain the main ridge to the summit, staying well to the right of a severe drop-off, the grade eases. Soon you cross a rocky area, then tackle the final pitch up a grassy slope to the summit. A path leads across the summit, past low-growing coast live oak and blue elderberry, to a 360-degree view-point. From here you can see the east summit of Maguire Peaks, the high ground on the other side of Welch Creek Road (which you can explore on the "Vista Grande" hike, below), and the waters of Calaveras Reservoir.

Backtracking to the Maguire Peaks Loop, you then follow a winding course downhill through a grassy valley, where a kestrel may be hovering overhead, soon reaching level ground. Heading generally west, the route comes to the end of a long ridge, then bends around it to the south, crossing a culvert that drains a marshy area with a stock pond, right. Eventually the route finds a southeast course, and just shy of the 4-mile point, reaches a junction (SO 12) with the Lower Maguire Peaks Trail. (This alternate route leads to a parking area at mile marker 0.72 on Welch Creek Road, SO 12.)

From here the route climbs slightly, passing a number of creeks that flow down from Maguire Peaks, left, and run under the road through culverts. Now in oak woodland, you may hear the sharp cry of a northern flicker or the soothing call of a mourning dove. At about the 4.5-mile point, you come to the junction (SO 08) of the Maguire Peaks Loop and the Maguire Peaks Trail (signed MAGUIRE PEAKS ROAD). From here, turn right and retrace your route to the parking area, making sure to turn left on the Upper Maguire Peaks Trail at the old homestead (SO 07).

VISTA GRANDE

Length: 6.1 miles

Time: 3 to 5 hours

Rating: Difficult

Regulations: EBRPD; fees for parking and dogs when entrance kiosk is attended; no bicycles or horses.

Facilities: Visitor center, picnic tables, water, toilets, phone.

Directions: From Interstate 680 northbound, northeast of Fremont, take the Calaveras Road exit and bear right onto Calaveras Road. Go 4.2 miles to Geary Road, turn left, and go 1.8 miles to the entrance kiosk. At 0.1 mile past the kiosk, there is a parking area, left, beside the visitor center, a green barn. Continue about 100 yards to the next parking area, also left. (If this parking area is full, there is another on the right, or you can use the one beside the visitor center.) The trailhead is at the north corner of parking area.

From Interstate 680 southbound, south of Pleasanton, take the Calaveras Road exit, and at the stop sign at the bottom of the ramp turn left onto Paloma Road (signed PALOMA WAY). Go under Interstate 680, stay in the left lane, and at the next stop sign continue straight, now on Calaveras Road. Then follow directions above.

High vantage points and great views reward hikers who tackle this loop, which uses the Canyon View, Indian Joe Creek, Eagle View, and Flag Hill trails, along with parts of Eagle View, Flag Hill, and Vista Grande roads. Climbing from tree-lined Alameda Creek through oak woodland to the high ground of Vista Grande Road and then Flag Hill, you experience a wide variety of terrain and plant life. Best on a clear, windless day, the route crosses some very steep hillsides, where caution is advised.

(The letters SO, for Sunol/Ohlone, and numbers in parentheses in the route description below refer to numbered junctions on the park map. These markings can be found on trail posts along the trail.)

From the trailhead, turn right and cross a wood bridge over Alameda Creek. Many of Sunol's trails use this bridge, including the Ohlone Wilderness Regional Trail, a 28-mile route from Mission Peak Regional Preserve to Del Valle Regional Park, parts of which are described elsewhere in this book. After crossing Alameda Creek and turning right, you are on the Canyon View Trail, a wide dirt path lined with white alder, bigleaf maple, western sycamore, and willow, with the creek on your right. (The first part of the Canyon View Trail is also part of the Indian Joe Nature Trail, a self-guiding route with numbered trail posts that correspond to text in a booklet available at the visitor center.)

Other trees and shrubs in this area include California bay, California buckeye, coast live oak, California sagebrush, bush monkeyflower, and poison oak. About 100 feet past the bridge, Hayfield Road climbs left, and some 30 feet beyond, a road leads to the creek, right. Continuing straight on the Canyon View Trail, you soon pass the Indian Joe Nature Trail, left, and then cross Indian Joe Creek.

California sagebrush, toyon, snowberry, and bush monkeyflower flourish in this sun-warmed area. As you climb higher, more of Sunol's rolling, oak-dotted hills

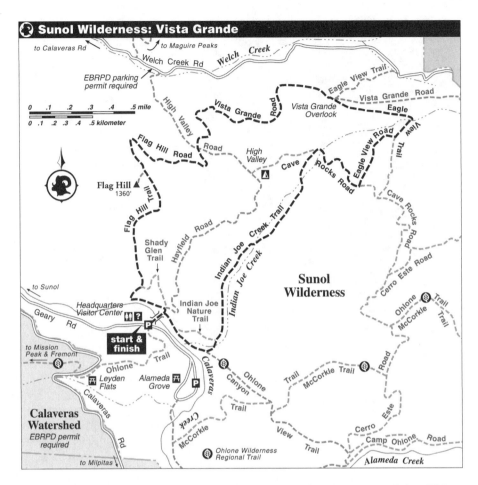

Sunol Wilderness: Vista Grande

come into view. At a fork, the Canyon View Trail, a segment of the Ohlone Wilderness Trail, veers right, but you take the left-hand fork, the Indian Joe Creek Trail. This single track descends from the ridge toward Indian Joe Creek, left, and wanders for a while in the shade of large coast live oaks. The route follows the creek northeast, passing a junction where the self-guiding Indian Joe Nature Trail turns left and crosses the creek. Continuing straight, you pass through a cattle gate, cross the creek's shallow water on rocks, then walk upstream in a narrow canyon filled with California sagebrush, bush monkeyflower, toyon, and coffeeberry. In the fall, sycamore and bigleaf maple add gold and orange to this wonderful area, helping it live up to its "wilderness" name.

A short, steep section, which soon levels, brings you to an open hillside, then two more creek crossings. As the canyon that holds Indian Joe Creek steepens, you cross again, and now on its right bank begin a moderate climb, turning temporarily away from the creek. Once on top of a ridge, you have a great view south toward the Alameda Creek canyon and the start of this loop. Valley oaks here are loaded with mistletoe, and you begin to see rock outcrops, colored green and orange by lichen.

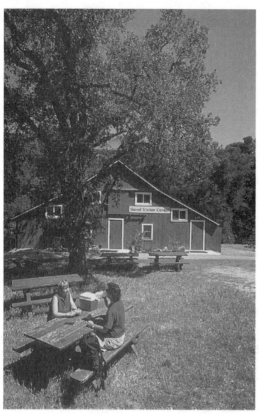

Trip to Vista Grande begins near the Sunol Visitor Center, a beautifully restored barn.

At about the 1.5-mile point (SO 23), an unnamed trail, left, connects to Hayfield Road, and a narrow path, also unnamed, heads right. Your route continues straight to Indian Joe Cave Rocks, a fantastic jumble of cliffs and boulders towering next to Indian Joe Creek. This is a popular bouldering location, and you may spot climbers testing their skills on these nearly vertical rock faces. Small informal trails trace the perimeter of this pile of boulders. One climbs the hill to the top of the pile, offering exceptional views over the rocks and back down the valley carved by Indian Joe Creek. Use caution: rattlesnakes frequent this area.

The trail here may be covered with leaf litter, prompting you perhaps to ponder the variety of leaf sizes. Plants use their leaves as collectors of sunlight, hence bigger leaves collect more light. This is helpful for plants that grow in shady areas. But leaves also are a source of moisture loss, with large leaves losing more moisture than small ones. So a plant must balance these two factors, and come up with the perfectly sized leaf to match its habitat. For example, valley oak and western sycamore are both large trees, ranging from 40 to 80 or 100 feet tall. Valley oaks typically grow in open areas, whereas sycamores inhabit shady canyons. As you might expect, the valley oak's leaf, at 2 to 4 inches long, is dwarfed by the sycamore's 6- to 9-inch leaf.

From here, switchbacks take you to the top of another ridge, this one more exposed to wind, but with grander views. The Indian Joe Creek Trail ends at the next junction, (SO 24), where you turn right on Cave Rocks Road, a dirt road, and make a moderate climb through an open area heavily used by cows. The view southwest from this wind-swept vantage point takes in the high ground of Mission Peak Regional Preserve, dominated by three summits—from left to right, Monument Peak (2594'), Mt. Allison (2658'), and Mission Peak (2517').

When you reach a trail post and a junction (SO 25), turn left on Eagle View Road. Just above the trail is a bench with a grad view of Mission Peak. Continue your moderate, sometimes steep climb on a rutted dirt road, with views now west toward San Francisco Bay. Soon Eagle View Road ends at a T-junction with the

Eagle View Trail, (SO 27). A warning sign here urges caution: the dropoff toward the creek is precipitous. Turn left and descend on a single-track trail into a wooded ravine, with the upper reaches of Indian Joe Creek at the bottom. The trail hugs a steep wall of the ravine as it loses elevation, makes a short climb via wooden steps, and then drops and crosses the creek on rocks.

About 100 feet past the crossing, the route turns sharply left and begins a moderate climb out of the ravine, then levels to cross a very steep hillside loaded with California sagebrush, blue bush lupine, and toyon. California fuchsia, a lover of rocky soil, may be blooming here as late as Thanksgiving. As the route begins to gain elevation again, two bodies of water—Calaveras Reservoir, south, and San Francisco Bay, west—come into view. This is one of the prettiest spots in the East Bay, but please be careful: the dropoff to your left is hazardous.

Finally you reach Vista Grande Overlook, a level area and important junction (SO 28), giving you a place to relax and take in the stunning 360-degree views, which include Pleasanton and Mt. Diablo (north); Apperson Ridge (northeast), site of an environmental battle in the late 1960s and early 1970s over a proposed rock quarry; and Maguire Peaks (northwest), two craggy summits described elsewhere in this book. Here a stone marker with attached wooden signs has directions and mileages to various points in the wilderness, but you have to walk around to the marker's north side to see them. From this point, the Eagle View Trail, now a dirt road, continues northeast across Vista Grande Road, which runs east–west.

Turn west on the dirt-and-gravel Vista Grande Road and walk downhill, past large valley oaks, on a moderate grade. The route turns south, reaches a narrow saddle (a bench is on a rise to the left), and then climbs to another terrific viewpoint, from where most of the Sunol Wilderness is visible. A moderate, then steep descent via S-bends, past stands of black oak, coast live oak, almond, and peppertree, brings you to an old homestead in High Valley. This bucolic area, with its large barn, windmill, water tower, and grazing cows, is used by EBRPD as an outdoor campsite. Other trees here include eucalyptus, cottonwood, fig, and walnut.

Just shy of the 4-mile point, you come to a four-way junction with High Valley Road (SO 4), and another stone marker, right, noting routes and mileages. From here, High Valley Road heads right to Welch Creek Road and left to the campsite. To find your route, Flag Hill Road, cross High Valley Road just right of a massive eucalyptus. Then bear left on a dirt road heading southeast and uphill through a cattle gate. This road, muddy in wet weather, makes an end run around a low, grassy ridge, turning first south, then southwest. As you gain back some of the elevation lost in the descent on Vista Grande Road, you begin to glimpse some of the now-familiar landmarks, such as Mission Peak and Maguire Peaks.

Now atop a ridge, in the realm of grasses and oaks, you travel south to a junction (SO 3), left, and a third stone marker. To visit Flag Hill, named for an American flag displayed here by a picnicking family on July 4th, 1903, continue straight. From where the road ends in a few hundred feet at a turn-around, follow a dirt path to the edge of a steep, rocky promontory—use caution! The sweeping view from here takes in Calaveras Reservoir, Alameda Creek canyon, Camp Ohlone Road, Mission Peak Regional Preserve, and Maguire Peaks. After relaxing for a while on the summit of Flag Hill, return to the stone marker and begin a moderate descent southeast on the Flag Hill Trail, a single track, with the visitor center and parking area in sight.

The trail now crosses steep open hillsides and descends through mixed woodland. After passing an eroded area (please stay on the trail), you pass through a cattle gate and fence guarding a beautiful grove of trees near Alameda Creek, which can be a torrent in winter or a trickle in summer. The trail continues to wind downhill, past an area of star thistle and beard grass, to a barbed-wire fence with a gate. Soon the Shady Glen Trail heads right (SO 2), but you continue straight and downhill to a T-junction near Alameda Creek. Turn left on a wide dirt path and follow it to the bridge, then turn right and retrace your route across the creek to the parking area.

◆ Ohlone Wilderness Regional Trail ◆

SUNOL TO DEL VALLE

Length: 19.4 miles

Time: Three days

Rating: Very difficult

Regulations: EBRPD; permit, camping reservations, and sign-in required; no bicycles; no pets in campsites overnight. The Ohlone Wilderness Regional Trail permit, good for one year, is a large map with route description, distances, trail elevations, and regulations. Trail permits are available for a small fee at the entrance kiosks at Sunol Wilderness and Del Valle Regional Park, the visitor center at Coyote Hills Regional Park in Fremont, and the EBRPD reservation office, 2950 Peralta Oaks Ct., Oakland. Permits for overnight parking are available at the entrance kiosks. Reservations for backpacking camps are required; phone EBRPD reservations, (510) 636-1684, 8:30 A.M. to 4 P.M., Monday through Friday.

If you are taking three days to complete the route, it is best to spend the second night at Stewart's Camp, on the road to Murietta Falls, but the camp has only one site and should be reserved far in advance. (Otherwise, you will end up spending the second night at Maggie's Half Acre, which makes for a very long and challenging third day.)

Facilities: Visitor center, picnic tables, water, toilet, phone, and horse staging at Sunol trailhead. Nonpotable water and unimproved campsites along the trail; plan on treating or filtering the water along the trail. Picnic tables, water, toilet, phone, and horse staging at Del Valle trailhead.

Directions: This is a car shuttle trip, starting at **Sunol Wilderness** and ending at **Del Valle Regional Park.** Drive first to Del Valle Regional Park, leave a car there, then proceed to Sunol Wilderness.

To reach **Del Valle Regional Park:** From Interstate 580 in Livermore, take the North Livermore Ave./Downtown Livermore exit, and follow North Livermore Ave. south through Livermore, where it becomes South Livermore Ave., and then, at a sharp left-hand bend on the outskirts of town, Tesla Road. At 3.7 miles from

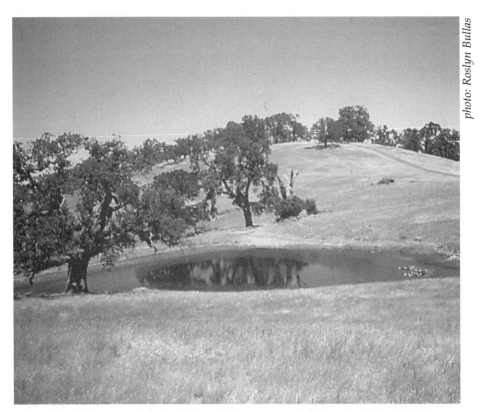

Numerous small cow ponds in the Ohlone Wilderness provide habitat for birds, amphibians, and fish.

Interstate 580, you reach a junction of Tesla and Mines roads. Turn right and go 3.6 miles to a junction with Del Valle Road; here Mines Road bears left. Stay straight on Del Valle Rd 3.2 miles to the entrance kiosk. Go another 1.2 miles past the kiosk, crossing a bridge and turning right at a T-junction, until you reach a large parking area at the end of the road, near the Lichen Bark picnic area.

To reach **Sunol Wilderness** via Highway 84: Return to central Livermore and follow 1st St. west 0.6 mile to Holmes St. Bear left onto Holmes St., go 2.1 miles and bear right onto E. Vallecitos Road. Follow E. Vallecitos and Vallecitos roads 6.6 miles to the Highway 84/Sunol/Dumbarton Bridge exit. Go under Interstate 680 and, at a stop sign, turn left onto Paloma Road (signed PALOMA WAY). Go back under Interstate 680, stay in the left lane, and from the next stop sign continue straight, now on Calaveras Road. Go 4.2 miles to Geary Road, turn left, and go 1.8 miles to the entrance kiosk. Go 0.1 mile past the kiosk and turn left into a parking area in front of the visitor center, a green barn. The trailhead is at the information panel and trail register on the south side of Geary Road, about 100 yards east of the visitor center.

To reach **Sunol Wilderness** from Interstate 680 northbound, northeast of Fremont: take the Calaveras Road exit and bear right onto Calaveras Road. Go 4.2 miles to Geary Road, turn left, and go 1.8 miles to the entrance kiosk. Go 0.1 mile

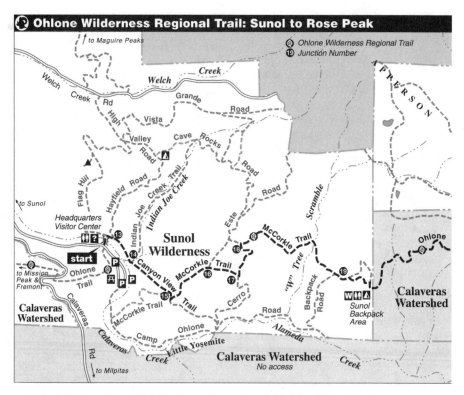

past the kiosk and turn left into a parking area in front of the visitor center, a green barn. (If this parking area is full, there are two more about 100 yards ahead, on both sides of Geary Road.) The trailhead is at the information panel and trail register on the south side of Geary Road, about 100 yards east of the visitor center.

From Interstate 680 southbound, south of Pleasanton: Take the Calaveras Road exit, and at the stop sign at the bottom of the ramp turn left onto Paloma Road (signed PALOMA WAY). Go under Interstate 680, stay in the left lane, and at the next stop sign continue straight, now on Calaveras Road. Then follow the directions above.

This backpacking point-to-point trip, the only one of its kind in the East Bay Regional Park system, puts you in the heart of the Ohlone Wilderness, a rugged, remote, and beautiful area. Along the way, you will also pass through Sunol Wilderness and Del Valle Regional Park, and spend two nights (or more if you like) camped in oak woodland, surrounded by wildflowers and birds, perhaps listening to the howl of a coyote or the hoot of an owl.

(**Boldface** numbers in the route description refer to numbers on the Ohlone Wilderness Regional Trail map. These numbers can be found on trail posts along the trail.)

After signing the trail register at the trailhead, walk north about 150 feet, across Geary Road and through a small parking area, to a wooden bridge over Alameda Creek. The entire Ohlone Wilderness Regional Trail is made up of many trails

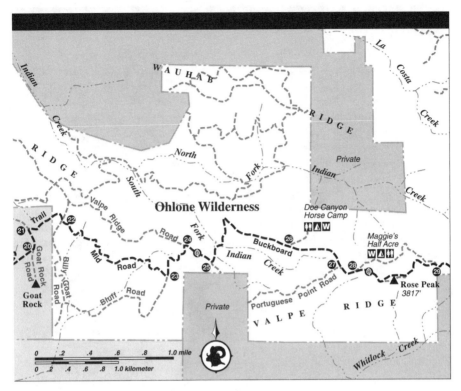

which, joined together, stretch 28 miles, from Stanford Ave. at the base of Mission Peak in Fremont, to the Lichen Bark picnic area on the shore of Lake Del Valle. For the next three days you will be following the Ohlone Wilderness emblem on trail posts: a white oak leaf in a red or brown disk.

After crossing Alameda Creek and turning right, you follow the Canyon View Trail, a wide dirt path lined with white alder, bigleaf maple, western sycamore, and willow, with the creek on your right. (The first part of the Canyon View Trail is also part of the Indian Joe Nature Trail, a self-guiding route with numbered trail posts that correspond to a pamphlet available at the visitor center.) You may also notice here some of the trees and shrubs that will keep you company for most of the way to Lake Del Valle, including California bay, California buckeye, coast live oak, California sagebrush, bush monkeyflower, and poison oak.

About 100 feet past the bridge, Hayfield Road, **13**, climbs left, and some 30 feet beyond, a road leads to the creek, right. Continuing straight on the Canyon View Trail, you soon pass the Indian Joe Nature Trail, left, and then cross Indian Joe Creek. Follow the Canyon View Trail over rolling terrain to a fork, **14,** with the Indian Joe Creek Trail.

Here you bear right on the Canyon View Trail and begin a steep climb through mixed oak woodland and grassland colored blue and yellow by Ithuriel's spear and Mariposa lily. Your chance of seeing a yellow-billed magpie, a large black-and-white member of the crow family, is better on this route than almost anywhere else in the East Bay, and it should be easy to spot other common birds, such as

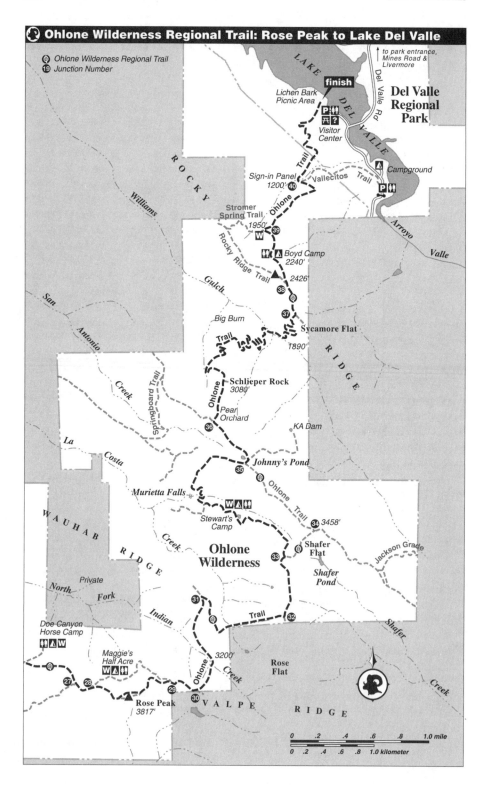

Ohlone Wilderness Regional Trail: Rose Peak to Lake Del Valle

Ohlone Wilderness Regional Trail
19 Junction Number

LAKE DEL VALLE

to park entrance,
Mines Road &
Livermore

finish

Lichen Bark
Picnic Area

Del Valle
Regional
Park

Del Valle Rd

Visitor
Center

Campground

Sign-in Panel
1200' 40

Vallecitos Trail

Ohlone Trail

Ohlone Trail

ROCKY

Williams

Stromer
Spring Trail
1950' 39

Rocky Ridge Trail

Boyd Camp
2240'

2426'
38

Arroyo

Valle

Gulch

37

Big Burn

Sycamore Flat
1890'

RIDGE

Trail

San

Antonio

Creek

Springboard Trail

Ohlone Trail

Schlieper Rock
3080'

Pear
Orchard

KA Dam

La

Costa

36

Johnny's Pond

35

Ohlone Trail

Murietta Falls

Stewart's
Camp

34 3458'

WAUHAB

RIDGE

Creek

Ohlone
Wilderness

33

Shafer
Flat

Shafer
Pond

Jackson Grade

North

Private

Fork

Indian

31

Trail

32

Shafer

Doe Canyon
Horse Camp

Maggie's
Half Acre

Ohlone

Creek

3200'

Rose
Flat

Creek

27   28

29

30 VALPE   RIDGE

Rose Peak
3817'

0   .2   .4   .6   .8   1.0 mile
0   .2   .4   .6   .8   1.0 kilometer

California towhee, American kestrel, turkey vulture, and western meadowlark. At a four-way junction, **15,** you leave the Canyon View Trail, which continues straight, and turn left on the McCorkle Trail. The route, now a dirt road, continues climbing steeply, then gradually levels to contour around a rocky ridge, and finally switchbacks upward toward a notch in the hills to the northeast.

At about the 1.3-mile point, you reach the notch and a junction with a connector to Cerro Este Road, **16.** The large bulk of Mission Peak (2517'), with its companion summits Mt. Allison (2658') and Monument Peak (2594'), appears to the west, while the waters of Calaveras Reservoir shimmer to the south. Bear right, staying on the McCorkle Trail, here a narrow track, and begin descending through an area of chaparral, a striking contrast to the oak woodland and rolling grassland of a few minutes ago. California quail and wrentits may be heard and sometimes seen here, as you climb on a steep, rocky course through a wooded area to a high ridge, where California poppies dot the grassy hillsides with orange.

At a T-junction, **17,** you come to the Cerro Este Road. Here your route, still part of the McCorkle Trail, turns left and continues uphill in the open to another T-junction, **18.** Now you turn right, staying on the McCorkle Trail, here a dirt road. A nearby cow pond provides habitat for a robin-sized bird called the killdeer, which you may hear giving its alarm call, "kill-dee, kill-dee." This shorebird, a member of the plover family, is at home in many areas besides the shore, and can be found throughout North America. In addition to cows and birds, other wildlife here includes amphibians: watch the ground closely for baby frogs in spring. Now heading east again and descending slightly, you pass large rock outcrops and a barbed-wire fence, where a narrow dirt path heads left and your route bends right.

After ambling a while on level ground, you descend via switchbacks to a small valley, where a wet area may provide a colorful display of spring wildflowers, including lupine, Ithuriel's spear, blow wives, owl's clover, and Mariposa lily. If the creek that drains this valley is running, you may have to cross it on rocks. At about 3.4 miles, you cross another creek and reach a junction, **19,** with Backpack Road. A gate ahead marks the entrance to the Sunol Backpack Area, and a signboard lists campsites—Eagles Eyrie, Hawks Nest, Sycamore Camp, Stars Rest, Sky Camp— reached by a steep uphill trail. Water and a toilet are available in the backpack area.

If you are spending the night here, Eagles Eyrie is an excellent campsite, but like all the others it requires advance reservation. To find it, climb about 0.3 mile from the backpack-area entrance and watch for a junction with a signed spur trail veering right. This trail leads to several campsites, including Eagles Eyrie, which is perched at about 1600 feet. The main trail continues straight and is rejoined by the spur trail, in about 0.3 mile, at a gate on the border of San Francisco Water Department land. Eagles Eyrie is a grassy area in the shade of a large blue oak, which is a magnet for birds such as woodpeckers, western bluebirds, nuthatches, and hummingbirds. Water is available from a faucet beside the trail, just below the campsite in a muddy area where you may find golden monkeyflower blooming in the spring. Expansive views west from a rock outcrop above the campsite—a great spot to watch the sunset—reveal much of the terrain back to the visitor center.

To rejoin the main route from Eagles Eyrie, walk northeast on an unsigned path across a grassy hillside, past a huge valley oak, joining a trail coming up from the water faucet and a lower campsite. A steep climb brings you to the San Francisco

Water Department gate. Once through the gate, now back on the main route, you continue climbing through open grassland, above 2000 feet for the first time on this route, heading generally northeast. Heavily forested Alameda Creek canyon is downhill and right; beautiful oaks grace the hillsides ahead.

Your route dips to cross several small creeks lined with bay and sycamore, then passes through an area of rock outcrops colored by orange lichen. From time to time, dirt paths take off from the main route; ignore them. In open grassland here you may find bluedicks and winecup clarkia, spring bloomers. This part of the route has a supreme feeling of isolation, with no signs of civilization other than jets on approach to Bay Area airports.

At about the 5-mile point you come to a trail post and an unsigned trail joining from the left; soon you reach a junction, **20,** with unsigned Goat Rock Road, right. Here your route turns left and climbs north toward the skyline ridge. In the distance to the south rise the Santa Cruz Mountains. At the next trail post, **21,** the route bends right, and in 100 yards reaches a fork, where you bear left. After climbing a slight rise, you descend to a four-way junction, **22,** with Billy Goat Road.

After crossing Billy Goat Road, you continue straight on Mid Road and contour southeast, reaching a gully with oak, blue elderberry, and California buckeye—the first shade in miles. Soon you reach a high point with views west, and then come to another gully with a culvert under the road. At about the 7-mile point, there is a T-junction, **23,** with Bluff Road, where your route turns left and climbs steeply. After cresting a small ridge near a cattle pond, you continue across grassy hillsides and through oak woodland to a junction, **24,** with Valpe Ridge Road, left. Here you walk through a cattle gate and turn right, passing another pond, and in about 0.3

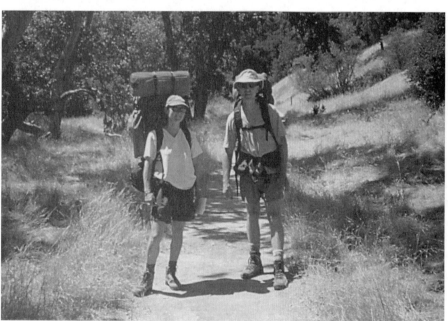

photo: Roslyn Bullas

Even experienced backpackers agree that the Ohlone Trail is a challenging, though rewarding, hiking trip.

mile make a sharp left, **25.** Now descend steeply on rocky ground into a small canyon which holds the south fork of Indian Creek.

In this oasis of shade and water, you may find an abundance of spring wild-flowers in bloom, including fiddleneck, a coiled stem with orange flowers, and Chinesehouses, pagoda-like tiers of purple flowers. A steep climb brings you out of the canyon and into a beautiful savanna—a haven for birds—where the grass, brown elsewhere by late spring, stays green in the shade of tall oaks. At a bend in the route, you get your first good look on this route of San Francisco Bay, and at the next bend, just above 3000 feet, you encounter a stunning vista that sweeps from Mt. Diablo to the Santa Clara Valley and Santa Cruz Mountains. If you like being up high, with unobstructed views, this is the place!

As the route, here called the Buckboard Trail, swings southeast, you have a pleasant walk along a ridgecrest, and soon reach a road, **26,** descending steeply left to Doe Canyon Horse Camp, where a water faucet and toilet await. (Water and a toilet are also available at Maggie's Half Acre campsite, about 0.8 miles ahead.) Now you continue east through oak savanna, home to acorn woodpeckers, toward Rose Peak (3817'), the high point on the Ohlone Wilderness Regional Trail. At a junction with Portuguese Point Road, **27,** you turn left, pass a small pond on your left, and soon reach a road, **28,** heading left to Maggie's Half Acre. (If you are doing this trip in four days instead of three, Maggie's Half Acre, with three sizable sites, makes a good second camp, about 6 miles from the Sunol backpack area. This is also where you'll spend the second night on a three-day trip, if you are unable to reserve the campsite at Stewart's Camp.)

Continuing east, the route steepens and passes over rocky terrain as you near the summit of Rose Peak, the highest point in Alameda County. About 0.2 mile past the last junction, an unsigned road, steep and rocky, heads left and climbs Rose Peak, while the main route skirts the peak's south side. Having come this far, be sure not to miss the 360-degree views from the summit, which is often above the Bay Area fog. After some effort, you arrive, seemingly, on top of the world. Using your map and compass, you can pick out many features of the Bay Area, including Altamont Pass, Mt. Diablo, Pleasanton Ridge, Coyote Hills, Mission Peak, the Santa Cruz Mountains, and Mt. Hamilton. Beyond the Central Valley lies the Sierra Nevada, visible on clear days. You have come nearly 10 miles from the Sunol visi-tor center; Rose Peak marks the halfway point to Lake Del Valle.

After you have relaxed for a while, continue east and descend steeply to the main road, which you can see below and right. Once back on the main road, you may notice as you continue your descent two trees not seen so far, black oak and gray pine, both found in hotter, drier areas of the East Bay. Canyon live oak is also here, along with blue oak, loaded with mistletoe, and valley oak, making this a good place to compare these species. Just past the 10-mile point, you pass the road, **29,** coming from Maggie's Half Acre, left.

At the next junction, **30,** a road goes straight to the wilderness boundary and Rose Flat, but you turn left and continue downhill, under large black oaks and gray pines—notice the huge pine cones—to the north fork of Indian Creek, losing the most elevation so far, more than 600 feet. The steep, rocky descent brings you to the bottom of a cool, shady canyon, where maple, alder, and bay line the creek, which may be flowing over the road. Climbing back into the open, you have views west to San Francisco Bay and Mission Peak.

As you begin to get a good view southwest across the canyon to Rose Peak, a road joins from the left, **31,** and your route bends sharply right and continues climbing. As you gain a ridgetop, you can look left into Box Canyon, headwaters of La Costa Creek. Descending beside a barbed-wire fence to the head of this canyon, you pass beautiful hillsides of colorful Chinesehouses that lie in the shade of gray pines. A small pond, left, may have many water lilies and lots of small fish. With La Costa Creek on your left, the route climbs gently past large rock outcrops through a little valley at the head of Box Canyon. A road to the wilderness boundary and Rose Flat joins your route at a T-junction, **32,** where you turn left and begin a gradual descent. From here, the Ohlone Wilderness Regional Trail, generally eastbound since the Sunol visitor center, begins a northward march to Lake Del Valle, about 7 miles away.

If you are staying at Stewart's Camp, angle left when you reach the next junction, **33,** leaving the Ohlone Wilderness Regional Trail. Otherwise, continue on the main route by heading right (northeast) to junction **34,** then turning left (northwest) to junction **35,** and pick up the route description below, just before the 15-mile point.

Descend to Stewart's Camp via a series of gentle switchbacks through an oak-and-pine forest, past stumps of old oaks riddled with woodpecker holes and fine displays of Chinesehouses. The camp is located just above a pond, where red-winged blackbirds nest in marsh vegetation and the surrounding hillsides are decorated with lupine. Water and a toilet are located near the only marked campsite, a rough area with hardly enough level ground for a small tent.

At just over 3000 feet, a night at Stewart's Camp can be a cold one, and don't be surprised by serenades from owls and coyotes. No need for an alarm clock here, as the chattering of birds at sunrise will get you started early. After passing the pond, you soon come to a junction with a road heading left to the wilderness boundary; your route continues straight and arrives at a small grove of trees. To visit seasonal Murietta Falls, turn left here, before crossing a tributary of La Costa Creek, and follow a narrow path that traverses and then winds behind large rock outcrops. Be careful here as you approach steep terrain. After a short distance the waterfall comes into view, tumbling perhaps 100 feet from a narrow channel in the rocks to a gully below.

The Murietta Falls area is a perfect spot to lounge in the sun, especially if the night has been cold. Once underway again on the main route, you cross the creek and immediately begin to climb north, out of a valley. Yellow Mariposa lilies and goldfinches add touches of color to the scene. At a T-junction, turn right and walk along the open crest of a ridge, toward Johnny's Pond and your reunion with the Ohlone Wilderness Regional Trail.

Just before reaching the 15-mile point of this route, you rejoin the Ohlone Wilderness Regional Trail at a junction, **35,** and turn left. Much of the land that became the Ohlone Wilderness was at one time owned by a rancher and cowboy named Harry Rowell. Rowell, a British merchant seaman who jumped ship in 1912 when he was 21 years old, settled in Alameda County and had a ranch on Dublin Canyon Road. Rowell died in 1969, but his legacy lives on in the form of the Rowell

Ranch Rodeo, which he started in 1920, and Rowell's Saddlery in Castro Valley, founded in 1942. Farther along the trail is Schlieper Rock, named for Fred Schlieper, a silversmith at Rowell's Saddlery in the 1940s; a bronze plaque embedded in the rock mentions that Schlieper's ashes are buried here. Johnny's Pond, left, was named for John Fernandes, who worked in Rowell's slaughterhouse and was his occasional sparring partner.

After descending slightly, the route climbs to a great vantage point, with views of Mt. Diablo, Morgan Territory Regional Preserve, Livermore, Altamont Pass, and the Central Valley. Shade is at a premium here, offered by a few groves of oak, oases for birds. California quail, western tanager, and lark sparrow may be found nearby. Even in death, oaks attract birds, providing nesting habitat and food storage for species as varied as woodpeckers and swallows.

At a fork in the route, **36,** bear right past an old pear orchard and begin descending steeply on loose ground. At about the 3000-foot level, the route becomes a narrow trail and begins to drop across a steep, brushy hillside on switchbacks built by the California Conservation Corps. Poison oak is rampant here. As you enjoy this well-graded descent, you may be treated to a fine display of spring wildflowers, such as Chinesehouses, Ithuriel's spear, bluedicks, and globe lilies.

Alternately open and wooded, the trail makes a long, switchbacking traverse across a north-facing hillside, where you may find canyon live oak and black oak; here the trees may be alive with dark-eyed juncos. In season, the sound of rushing water rises from Williams Gulch, a deep canyon ahead. When you reach its shady bottom, after putting your knees and hiking boots to the test, you will have dropped nearly 2000 feet from the route's high point, the summit of Rose Peak. Now is the time to relax and enjoy cool, peaceful surroundings. Two seasonal creeks—one from the southwest, the other from the southeast—join in Williams Gulch, and the resulting stream flows northwest, eventually reaching San Antonio Creek. Your route crosses the creeks on rocks, then emerges as a steep dirt road on an open hillside.

Maples and sycamores growing here indicate a high water table, but as you turn left at a T-junction, **37,** and gain Rocky Ridge, the dryland species—gray pine, black oak, blue oak—again become dominant. California buckeye, with its spring profusion of white, candle-like blooms, is also here. You have just completed the most remote section, from Rose Peak to Williams Gulch, of the Ohlone Wilderness Regional Trail. (When I reached this point, I had not seen any other people for 24 hours, a level of seclusion I have encountered only once before, on the John Muir Trail.)

At a fork, **38,** bear right and descend toward Boyd Camp; there is a toilet here, but water is available only at Stromer Spring, just west of the next junction, **39,** about 0.3 mile farther. (This is the last water until you reach Lake Del Valle.) After getting water, return to the main road, turn northeast and walk steeply downhill through an area of bush monkeyflower, toyon, and coyote brush to the Ohlone Wilderness Regional Trail sign-in board, **40,** and a junction with the Vallecitos Trail, right. To reach the parking area at the Lichen Bark picnic area, continue straight and continue to descend through an area of chaparral, mostly chamise, and wildflowers. Several switchbacks finally bring you to your goal—Lake Del Valle and the parking area.

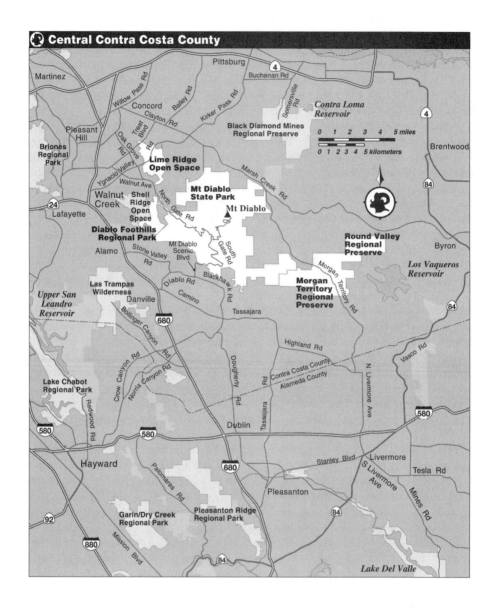

Central Contra Costa County

Martinez

Pittsburg

Buchanan Rd

Willow Pass Rd

Bailey Rd

Concord

Clayton Rd

Kirker Pass Rd

Somersville Rd

Contra Loma
Reservoir

Black Diamond Mines
Regional Preserve

0 1 2 3 4 5 miles

0 1 2 3 4 5 kilometers

Brentwood

Pleasant
Hill

Treat Blvd

Oak Grove Rd

Briones
Regional
Park

Lime Ridge
Open Space

Marsh Creek Rd

Ygnacio Valley

Walnut Ave

Walnut
Creek

Shell
Ridge
Open
Space

Mt Diablo
State Park

North Gate Rd

Mt Diablo

24

Lafayette

Diablo Foothills
Regional Park

Stone Valley Rd

Mt Diablo
Scenic
Blvd

South Gate Rd

Round Valley
Regional
Preserve

Byron

Los Vaqueros
Reservoir

Alamo

Diablo Rd

Blackhawk Rd

Morgan
Territory
Regional
Preserve

Morgan Territory Rd

Upper San
Leandro
Reservoir

Las Trampas
Wilderness

Danville

Camino

Tassajara

680

Bollinger Canyon Rd

Highland Rd

Vasco Rd

Lake Chabot
Regional Park

Crow Canyon Rd

Norris Canyon Rd

Dougherty Rd

Contra Costa County
Alameda County

N Livermore Ave

580

Redwood Rd

580

580

Dublin

Tassajara Rd

580

Hayward

Palomares Rd

680

Stanley Blvd

Livermore

Tesla Rd

92

Pleasanton

S Livermore Ave

Mines Rd

84

880

Garin/Dry Creek
Regional Park

Pleasanton Ridge
Regional Park

84

Mission Blvd

84

Lake Del Valle

♦ Central Contra Costa County ♦

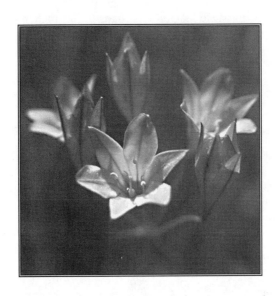

LIME RIDGE OPEN SPACE

Length: 3.3 miles

Time: 2 to 3 hours

Rating: Moderate

Regulations: City of Walnut Creek; no dogs; bikes are not allowed on the Lime Ridge Trail, and must instead stay on dirt roads to complete the route.

Facilities: None.

Directions: From Interstate 680 in Walnut Creek, or Highway 24 eastbound (just before the merge with Interstate 680), take the Ygnacio Valley Road exit and go northeast 3.5 miles to Oak Grove Road. Turn right and go 0.4 mile to Valley Vista Road. Turn left and go 0.8 mile to a parking area, right. The trailhead is at the end of parking area.

This athletic loop, a perfect cool-weather outing, uses the Ohlone, Manzanita, Lime Ridge, and Paraiso trails to explore the rugged, chaparral-clad hills northwest of Mt. Diablo on the border of Concord and Walnut Creek.

You go through a gate and walk uphill to an information board and the Ohlone Trail. Bearing left, you climb moderately on a dirt road to a junction, where the Paraiso Trail, which you will use later, joins from the right. Turning left, you soon go through a gate into the Walnut Creek Open Space Lime Ridge Preserve, which

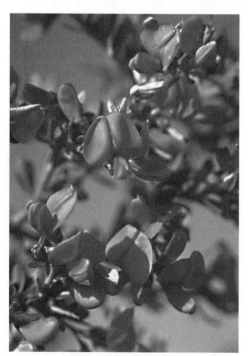

Magenta flowers of chaparral pea appear in the late spring.

is closed to dogs. Coast live oaks, blue oaks, and California buckeyes line the route, which also passes hillsides of chaparral, mostly chamise, toyon, California sagebrush, yerba santa, manzanita, and black sage.

Descending through a narrow ravine, you come to a T-junction, where you turn right on the Manzanita Trail. Climbing steeply, you follow a rocky dirt road that soon provides great views in exchange for the effort. After passing the Buckeye Trail, left, you reach a saddle where a number of trails meet. Turning right, you follow the Lime Ridge Trail, a dirt road, through a corridor of chaparral. At an unsigned fork, bear left and descend a set of steps, then follow a single-track trail to the base of a power-line tower.

With the tower on your right, follow the trail alongside, and then atop, Lime Ridge. A rolling course

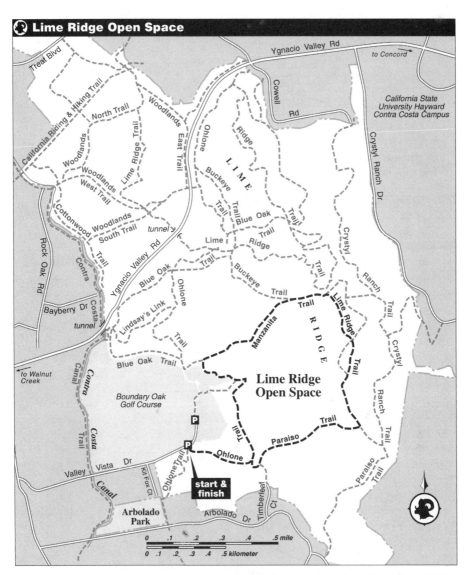

Lime Ridge Open Space

soon brings you to a junction with a dirt road, where you angle right. After 100 feet or so, you rejoin the Lime Ridge Trail by veering left. The trail soon merges with the dirt road you just left, and now you have an open, ridgetop climb. Topping a rise, you descend to a saddle and a junction with the Paraiso Trail, where you turn right.

Descending a dirt road on a gentle grade, you pass stands of chaparral pea, which produce beautiful magenta flowers in late spring and early summer. After meeting the Timberleaf Court Trail, left, your road curves right and closes the loop by joining the Ohlone Trail. Here you turn left and retrace your route to the parking area.

DIABLO FOOTHILLS REGIONAL PARK

Length: 6.1 miles

Time: 3 to 4 hours

Rating: Difficult

Regulations: EBRPD, City of Walnut Creek.
Facilities: None.
Directions: From Interstate 680 in Walnut Creek, or Highway 24 eastbound (just before the merge with Interstate 680), take the Ygnacio Valley Road exit and go northeast 2.3 miles to Walnut Ave. Turn right, go 1.6 miles to Oak Grove Road, and turn right. At 0.1 mile, Oak Grove Road changes to Castle Rock Road, and you continue straight. At 1.7 miles you come to the trailhead parking area. The trailhead is at the north end of the parking area, on the west side of road.

If you enjoy a challenging route, take this roller-coaster ride through the foothills just west of Mt. Diablo State Park. Using the Castle Rock, Shell Ridge Loop, Briones-to-Mt. Diablo Regional, Twin Ponds, Hanging Valley, and Stage Road trails, you'll make two connected loops through the park, with a short jaunt into neighboring Shell Ridge Open Space, enjoying oak savannas, wildflower-dotted hillsides, and a variety of birds.

You climb on a single-track trail, past a gate that prevents access by bikes and horses during wet weather. Meeting the Castle Rock Trail, a dirt road, you turn sharply right, then stay left at a fork. The road climbs on a gentle and then moderate grade. Wildflowers on display include California poppies, paintbrush, Ithuriel's spears, asters, bellardia, Mariposa lilies, and clarkias. At the next junction you also stay left, passing through a blue oak savanna. Gaining a ridgetop, you wind uphill through chaparral—chamise, black sage, toyon, California sagebrush—with a view, left, of impressive sandstone cliffs.

Climbing very steeply over rough ground, you meet the Shell Ridge Loop Trail at a T-junction. Turning left, you roller-coaster along an exposed ridgetop to a junction, where you stay right. Now descending on a moderate and then steep grade past a trail, left, you drop into a wooded valley and a junction with a connector to the Briones-to-Mt. Diablo Regional Trail. Turn right and walk through a canyon, passing the Buckeye Ravine Trail, left. When you meet the Briones-to-Mt. Diablo Regional Trail, a dirt road, turn right and go through a gate into Shell Ridge Open Space.

Where a dirt road veers right at about 2 miles, you continue straight past the Borges Ranch Trail, which leads to the Borges Ranch. The ranch is the former home of Walnut Creek pioneers Frank and Mary Borges, and is used today as a base of activities for Shell Ridge Open Space. The ranch has livestock and displays of ranching life, and also serves as a ranger station and residence. (For information about educational programs and group use, call (925) 942-0225 or visit www.ci.walnut-creek.ca.us/openspace/osborges.htm.)

Oak-topped hill frames view of Mt. Diablo's west side.

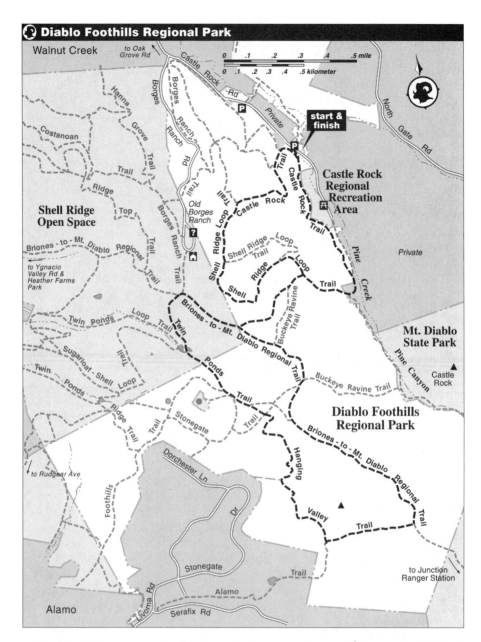

Diablo Foothills Regional Park

Bearing left, you come to a fork, where you again stay left, now on the Twin Ponds Trail, a dirt road that goes between two ponds. Beyond the ponds is a junction, where you continue straight and soon return to the regional park. Climbing moderately past a water tank and a paved road, you veer right at a fork and come to a four-way junction with the Stonegate Trail, signed in places as the Stone Gate Trail. (To shorten the route, turn left on the Stonegate Trail, go about 0.2 mile to a junction with the Briones-to-Mt. Diablo Regional Trail, and follow the description below.)

Go straight on the Hanging Valley Trail, following a rolling course until the trail climbs steeply over a rise. The view of a housing development from here reinforces the importance of protecting open space. Stay on the Hanging Valley Trail as it turns left at a junction with the Alamo Trail. Climbing on a moderate grade, with Mt. Diablo dominating the skyline, you reach a T-junction with the Briones-to-Mt. Diablo Regional Trail, a dirt road. Here turn left and continue climbing.

Spring brings birds in abundance to the Mt. Diablo area, and among the ones you may find nearby are Westerns scrub-jays, barn swallows, northern orioles, western bluebirds, northern mockingbirds, red-winged blackbirds, and flycatchers. Raptors, including a pair of peregrine falcons, have nested in the park.

Beyond a saddle, the road descends past a pond at about 4 miles, and then curves right and meets the Stonegate Trail, left. You veer right, then left at a junction with the Buckeye Ravine Trail. Still on the Briones-to-Mt. Diablo Trail, you come over a rise and then descend past a second Buckeye Ravine Trail to the junction that closes this loop. Here you turn right and retrace your route to the Shell Ridge Loop Trail. Turn right at the T-junction and follow a level course through a steep-walled canyon.

Soon the Shell Ridge Trail ends, and you turn left on the Stage Road Trail, a dusty dirt road. After about 0.1 mile, you branch left on the Castle Rock Trail, which skirts Castle Rock Regional Recreation Area. When you reach the short trail to the parking area, turn right and retrace your route.

◆ Mt. Diablo State Park ◆

According to a California Department of Parks and Recreation brochure, the history of Mt. Diablo as a state park goes back to 1921, when "a parcel of land on the mountain was designated a state park, and much of the rest of the mountain was declared a game refuge." In 1931, more land was acquired, and the park was formally dedicated and opened to the public. But tourists had been enjoying the mountain since the 1870s, especially the view from its 3849-foot summit, said to be surpassed in size only by that from the top of Africa's 19,340-foot Mt. Kilimanjaro. Toll roads, opened in 1874, brought visitors via stage from Walnut Creek and Danville to a 16-room hotel, Mountain House, located about three miles from the summit. The hotel, a site of frequent weddings, hosted guests from across the United States and as far away as Europe. The hotel and the summit observation platform were destroyed by fires in the 1890s, and the toll roads, closed to public access, did not reopen until 1915.

Prior to its days as the site of a swank resort, Mt. Diablo served as the reference point for surveys of most of California and portions of Nevada and Oregon. In 1851, Leander Ransome designated the summit as the crossing of an east–west Mt. Diablo baseline and a north–south Mt. Diablo meridian, reference points still used today in official surveys. In fact, the Mt. Diablo baseline passes between the Steam Trains and Vollmer Peak in Tilden Regional Park. According to Erwin G. Gudde, in *California Place Names*, the name "Mt. Diablo" may have come from a "fanciful" account of an 1806 battle told to the California state legislature in 1850 by Mariano G. Vallejo, formerly the Mexican governor of Alta California. When Spanish soldiers from the Presidio in San Francisco were fighting Indians in a battle near the mountain, they were scared off by a frightening personage they took to be the Devil, or *el Diablo*, but who perhaps may have been a medicine man in full regalia.

Although it looks like a volcano from afar, most of Mt. Diablo's rock is actually sedimentary, part of an ancient ocean floor that has been tilted and distorted within the last one or two million years by an uplifting core of hard Franciscan rock. Fossil hunters and rock hounds will enjoy areas such as Rock City, where rock formations are exposed and easily studied. Mt. Diablo is a botanist's delight: much of the upper mountain is

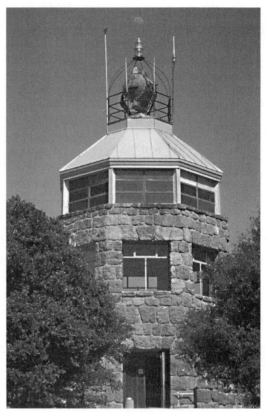

The tower atop Mt. Diablo's 3849-foot summit houses a museum and visitor center.

swathed in chaparral, while lower on its flanks grow pine, oak, and a host of other native trees, shrubs, and wildflowers. Birding is a popular pastime on the mountain, especially in Mitchell Canyon, and the Mt. Diablo bird list has more than 200 species.

Many groups, including the Sierra Club, the National Audubon Society, and the California Native Plant Society, schedule hikes and other programs on Mt. Diablo. A listing of these can be found in *Mount Diablo Review*, published twice yearly by Mount Diablo Interpretive Association (MDIA) and Save Mount Diablo in cooperation with Mt. Diablo State Park. The publication is sent free to MDIA members and is also available at the park's entrance kiosks. (See Appendix 3 for websites of these groups and organizations.)

There is a small entrance fee, payable at the North Gate and South Gate entrance kiosks, and a small parking fee at Mitchell Canyon. There are more than 50 picnic sites, each with table and barbecue, along the park's paved roads; there are also three group picnic sites for 25 to 100 people each. Group picnic site reservations and general park information can be obtained by calling Mt. Diablo State Park headquarters.

Mt. Diablo State Park: (925) 837-2525; open 8 A.M. to sunset.

Summit museum, visitor center, and store: for days and hours of operation, call (925) 837-6119.

Mitchell Canyon Interpretive Center: at the south end of Mitchell Canyon Road; open weekends and some holidays, 8 A.M. to 4 P.M., spring/summer; 8 A.M. to 3 P.M., fall/winter.

Camping: (800) 444-7275 or www.reserveamerica.com.

BACK CANYON

Length: 4.3 miles

Time: 2 to 3 hours

Rating: Moderate

Regulations: Mt. Diablo State Park; no bicycles, no dogs, no smoking.
Facilities: None.

Directions: From Interstate 680 in Walnut Creek, or Highway 24 eastbound (just before the merge with Interstate 680), take the Ygnacio Valley Road exit and go northeast 7.6 miles to Clayton Road. Turn right and go 2.9 miles (Clayton Road becomes Marsh Creek Road) to Regency Dr. Turn right and go 0.6 mile to a dead-end; park along the side of the street. The trailhead is on the north side of Regency Dr., about 200 feet from its end.

This loop, combining parts of the Donner Creek, Back Creek, and Meridian Point trails, and Back Creek, Meridian Ridge, and Donner Canyon roads, offers a wonderful sample of the joys the north side of Mt. Diablo has to offer. Cool, shady canyons, exposed rocky ridges, chaparral-covered hillsides, and oak woodlands compete for your attention with a terrific assortment of trees, shrubs, wildflowers, and birds. In spring, consider extending your trip to visit a set of hidden waterfalls by following the Middle and Falls trails as described in "Falls Trail," elsewhere in this book. The Back Canyon Trail and the lower part of Donner Canyon Road may be very muddy in wet weather.

On the north side of Regency Dr., about 200 feet before it dead-ends, find a gravel road, blocked by a gate, heading west. Follow this downhill, reaching in a few hundred feet a junction with the paved Donner Creek Trail (City of Clayton), just upstream from the confluence of Donner and Back creeks. Turn left and walk several hundred feet to the Mt. Diablo State Park boundary at Regency Gate. Immediately after entering the park, you pass a fire break leading right and uphill. In front of you are two dirt roads heading straight, parallel to each other, the left-hand one beside Donner Creek. Take the right-hand one, and after following it for about 100 yards you come to a fork marked by a trail post. Here your route, Back Creek Road, heads right and uphill, and Donner Canyon Road, which you will use later on the return, goes left.

As the route climbs in the open and you crest a small ridge, take a moment to admire the rugged north side of Mt. Diablo, at 3849 feet the East Bay's tallest mountain. To its left stands North Peak (3557'), admirable in its own right. Below

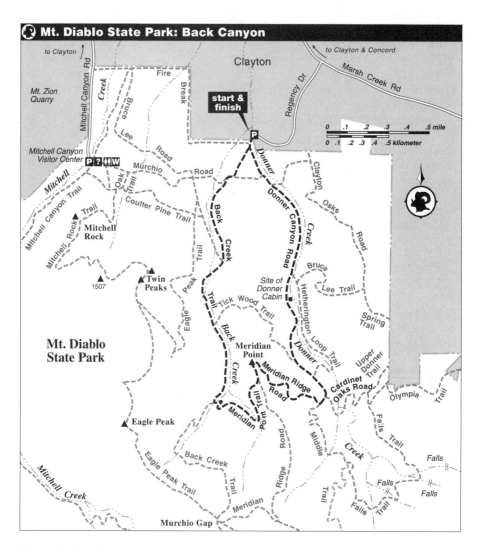

North Peak is Donner Canyon, whose upper reaches provide the source of the waterfalls you may wish to explore as an extension to this loop. Facing south, you have in front of you Meridian Ridge, which divides Donner and Back canyons. To your right, Eagle Peak (2369') and Twin Peaks (1507' and 1733') anchor a high ridge forming the border between Back and Mitchell canyons.

This route offers you ample opportunity to learn to identify some common East Bay trees. Two of our three common deciduous oaks, blue and valley, reside here. Blue oak has light gray bark divided into long strips, and blue-green leaves. Valley oak has checkered, dark gray bark and deeply lobed dark-green leaves. Valley oaks prefer moist soils found in canyon bottoms, and blue oak inhabits rolling foothills at higher elevations. Also here, especially along Donner Creek, is California buckeye, a deciduous tree with long, pointed leaves, arranged mostly in groups of five, like fingers on a hand. In late spring and early summer, buckeyes sprout long, upturned candles of white flowers.

Surrounded by open grassland, you come to a four-way junction. From here the Murchio Road heads right (west) to Mitchell Canyon and left (east) to Donner Canyon. Stay on Back Creek Road, which angles slightly left and contours around a ridge before dropping into Back Canyon. As you walk toward the ridge topped by Eagle Peak and Twin Peaks, Back Creek is to your right. Soon Back Creek Road turns right to cross Back Creek, but your route, the Back Creek Trail, a level dirt road, continues straight. Now enjoying an easy stroll, you have a chance to learn to recognize two more native trees.

The East Bay has three evergreen, or "live," oaks: coast, canyon, and interior. They are very similar, but the coast live oak, growing here beside the road, has spiny leaves that are glossy dark green and curled under at the edges. If you have a hand lens or a magnifying glass, you will see tiny tufts of hair attached to the veins on the underside of the leaf; the other two live oaks are hairless. California bay, related to the Mediterranean bay whose leaves are used in cooking, has long, dark green leaves that are pointed and shiny. If in doubt, rub a leaf and smell the distinctive odor on your fingers. Bay trees produce small clusters of yellow flowers in late winter. Shape, size, and habitat of bay trees varies greatly, from compact, round shrubs on wind-swept ridges to large trees with curved, drooping branches found in cool, dark canyons.

When the road reaches a gate, the Back Creek Trail becomes a single track that climbs gently over rocky terrain, alternating between open and wooded areas and making several crossings of Back Creek. At about the 1-mile point, you pass the Tick Wood Trail, left. Soon you will see a small canyon branching left from Back Canyon. The next segment of your route, the Meridian Point Trail, climbs this canyon. About 100 yards past where you can see the canyons branching, turn left on the Meridian Point Trail, a single track, and descend toward the creek. Cross Back Creek on rocks and begin to switchback up a steep embankment. The route climbs steeply on the east side of Back Creek and then enters the small canyon you saw earlier. Your efforts are rewarded by fine views north out Back Canyon to the residential developments of Clayton, and, beyond a set of rolling hills, the west delta. Paintbrush is plentiful along here, and soon you reach an area where manzanita and other chaparral plants cloak the rocky hillsides.

When the route reaches the head of the side canyon, you cross a small creek bed and turn sharply left to climb the canyon's exposed southwest-facing wall. Here the route is out in the open, hanging onto the edge of the hillside. More great views are in store, including one of Mt. Diablo's main summit ridge. A short while later, at about the 2-mile point, you reach a junction with Meridian Ridge Road. Here you turn left and descend steeply to Meridian Point, where the route bends sharply right. As you make the turn you can see North Peak rising in front of you, with Donner Canyon Road, the final leg of your loop, downhill and left.

You may be able to spot the difference here between two native pines, gray and Coulter. Gray pine, a tree well-adapted to dry conditions, has long gray-green needles in clusters of three, and big, spiny cones that fall to the ground when ripe. A close relative, the Coulter pine, has darker green, bushier needles, stout branches turning up at the ends, and even larger cones. Gray pines often have multiple trunks, but Coulter pines seldom do. Also found here, along with manzanita, are some of the other chaparral plants, including buckbrush, chamise, black sage, and yerba santa.

After descending steeply for about 0.5 mile from Meridian Point, you reach a junction with the Middle Trail heading right and uphill. (If you want to visit Mt. Diablo's hidden waterfalls, active during and after wet weather, turn right and follow the "Falls Trail" route description beginning on page 233. This loop will add about 2.3 miles to your hike.) The gray and twisted limbs of dead manzanita you see here are the result of a 1977 fire that swept across Mt. Diablo. Fire plays a beneficial role in the chaparral plant community, and you will see many young, healthy manzanitas here as well. Just downhill from the Middle Trail junction is the end of Meridian Ridge Road and a junction with Donner Canyon and Cardinet Oaks roads.

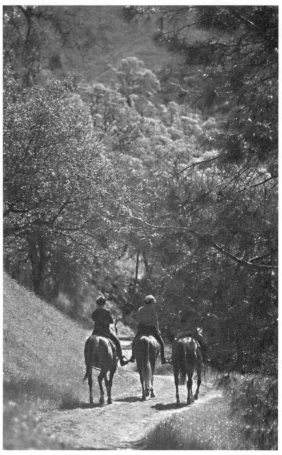

Equestrians on Back Creek Road enjoy early spring on Mt. Diablo.

At the junction, turn left and walk steeply downhill on Donner Canyon Road through an area of manzanita, chaparral, and blue oak, with Donner Creek on your right. A number of trails will join Donner Canyon Road on the way back to Regency Gate: ignore them. At about the 3-mile point you pass the Hetherington Loop Trail, right, and as the grade changes from steep to moderate, you enter a wonderful area containing most of Mt. Diablo's common trees and shrubs. Soon you pass the Tick Wood Trail, left; then, as the route steepens and you descend through oak woodland, you pass the other end of the Hetherington Loop Trail, right. Also right is a short trail leading to an old homesite called the Donner Cabin; all that remains is a brick fireplace foundation and other stone work.

Large valley oaks, along with California juniper, gray pine, and walnut, enhance this section of the route, a level walk along the west side of Donner Creek. Beautiful blue oaks dot the grassy hillside, left. At about the 4-mile point, you come to a trail to Clayton Oaks Road, right, heading across the creek. Continue straight, and in about 100 yards you reach Murchio Road, which goes left. Again continue straight, and in another 100 yards you reach a fork in the route: from here both paths lead to Regency Gate. From the gate, retrace your route to Regency Dr.

FALLS TRAIL

Length: 5.9 miles round-trip

Time: 3 to 4 hours

Rating: Moderate

Regulations: Mt. Diablo State Park; no bicycles, no dogs, no smoking.
Facilities: None.
Directions: From Interstate 680 in Walnut Creek, or Highway 24 eastbound (just before the merge with Interstate 680), take the Ygnacio Valley Road exit and go northeast 7.6 miles to Clayton Road. Turn right and go 2.9 miles (Clayton Road becomes Marsh Creek Road) to Regency Dr. Turn right and go 0.6 mile to a dead-end; park along the side of the street. The trailhead is on the north side of Regency Dr., about 200 feet from its end.

Best in early spring when the creeks are full, this scenic and strenuous semi-loop, using the Donner Creek, Middle, and Falls trails, and Donner Canyon, Meridian Ridge, and Cardinet Oaks roads, gives you views of hidden waterfalls cascading down from Mt. Diablo's North Peak. The Middle Trail takes you through an area that burned in 1977, providing a chance to see the regenerative effects of fire on manzanita and other chaparral vegetation. The lower part of Donner Canyon Road may be muddy during and after wet weather, but that's when the falls are running. (The Middle and Falls trails/Cardinet Oak Road segment of this route can be done as a 2.3-mile extension to the "Back Canyon" route.)

On the north side of Regency Dr., about 200 feet before it dead-ends, find a gravel road, blocked by a gate, heading west. Follow this downhill, reaching in a few hundred feet a junction with the paved Donner Creek Trail (City of Clayton). Turn left and walk several hundred feet to the Mt. Diablo State Park boundary at Regency Gate. Immediately after entering the park, you pass a fire break leading right and uphill. In front of you are two dirt roads heading straight, parallel to each other. Take the left-hand one, Donner Canyon Road, which hugs the west side of Donner Creek and heads into Donner Canyon. Soon you pass Murchio Road, right, and, in another 100 yards or so, a trail heading left across the creek to Clayton Oaks Road.

Nearby you may notice a large California ground-squirrel colony with dozens of holes on a southwest-facing hillside across the creek. Now you enjoy a straight and level walk past stands of valley oak, California juniper, gray pine, California buckeye, and walnut, soon passing Donner Cabin, site of an old homestead, left. Uphill and right, blue oaks and an occasional eucalyptus grace the hillsides. Be alert here for a hummingbird's fast buzz or the western meadowlark's liquid warble.

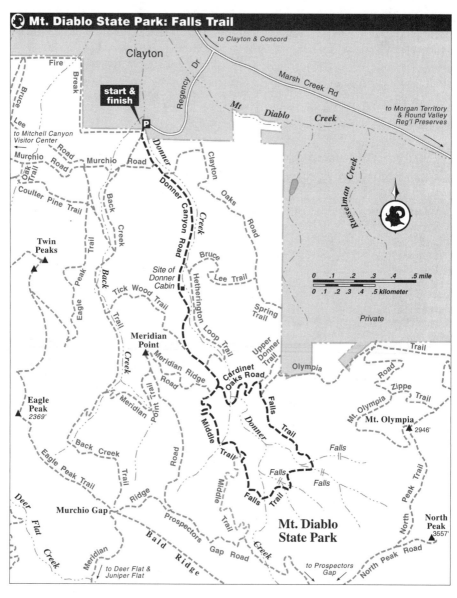

Mt. Diablo State Park: Falls Trail

As the route begins a steep climb through oak savanna, you pass the Hetherington Loop Trail, left, and the Tick Wood Trail, right. The grade eases somewhat, giving you a chance to notice more of the trees and shrubs common to this part of Mt. Diablo State Park, including coast live oak, gray pine, manzanita, coffeeberry, toyon, buckbrush, California sagebrush, chamise, and yerba santa. At about the 1-mile point the road steepens again, and you pass the uphill end of the Hetherington Loop Trail, left. Soon you come to a junction with Meridian Ridge and Cardinet Oaks roads.

Here you turn right and begin walking uphill on Meridian Ridge Road. After about 100 yards, you come to a trail post and a junction with a single-track trail heading left and uphill. This is the Middle Trail, which, as it climbs toward Prospectors Gap Road, brings you to the Falls Trail. You turn left onto it and begin a gentle climb through chaparral and stands of manzanita—tall, twisted remnants of a 1977 fire and shrubby new growth. The trail, an intimate path very different from the dirt roads that crisscross much of the mountain, alternates between open and wooded areas.

The route next climbs a series of switchbacks and then levels, giving you fine views southeast to Mt. Diablo's rugged North Peak (3557') and east to Mt. Olympia (2948'). You may hear the sound of running water coming from a tributary of Donner Creek, downhill and left. As the route comes into the open, it swings south toward Mt. Diablo's summit (3849') and crosses a hillside resembling a botanical garden, with manzanita, toyon, California sagebrush, black sage, chamise, buck-brush, and yerba santa.

Now back in the shade, the route meanders on a level grade, then makes a short climb. After crossing a small creek, the route becomes rocky, eroded, and possibly wet in places. As you gain elevation, you begin to have views north to Clayton, the west delta, and the hills of Napa and Solano counties. Continuing to climb on gentle and moderate grades, the trail slices across an open hillside which drops steeply left. Soon you are back in shady, cool thickets of shrubs and small trees.

At about the 2.3-mile point, you reach a junction. Here the Middle Trail turns right and climbs, but your route, the Falls Trail, a narrow track overgrown in places, heads straight. Continuing on the Falls Trail, you soon reach an open and very steep hillside above Donner Creek, hidden by trees below. Across Donner Canyon, left, rises the steep, rugged face of North Peak, one of the mountain's most impressive vistas. Please be careful as you gaze skyward: a misstep on these dizzying heights could be fatal. Look here for spiny redberry, a shrub with small, holly-like leaves. The route soon drops via switchbacks to the shady banks of Donner Creek, lined with California bay, and then begins a gentle climb on the creek's right-hand bank.

A short distance upstream, Donner Creek bends left around a rocky rib, but your route follows a tributary to the right. (This tributary is not shown on the Mt. Diablo State Park trail map.) A bit farther upstream, you cross the tributary, veer left, and begin climbing the opposite bank, now heading downstream. As you work your way up the rocky rib, you come to a fork in the trail. Angle left—the right-hand fork rejoins your route in a few hundred feet. Juniper trees thrive here, and may be loaded with gray berries that when crushed smell like gin. Once around the rocky rib, the trail leads upstream through a deep, shady ravine on the right side of Donner Creek. In early spring, look here for milkmaids, a wildflower with four white petals tinged near the base with yellow.

Soon you cross Donner Creek and continue to climb, sometimes steeply, across an open hillside. Mountain mahogany, a tree-like shrub with silver-gray bark and small, serrated leaves, grows here, along with large clumps of California sage-brush. After considerable effort, you are rewarded by a beautiful vista stretching north from Donner Canyon all the way to the hills of Napa and Solano counties. And after reaching a flat area, you see the first seasonal waterfall just ahead, a cascade of water tumbling over a large rock cliff. The trail climbs, descends to another seasonal creek, and then climbs again, until you are perched on a cliff above the waterfall. A rough path leads left to the edge of the cliff: use extreme caution!

The view from here includes all of Donner Canyon, Mt. Olympia, Mitchell Canyon Road, and quarry-scarred Mt. Zion (1635'). This is one of the great vistas on Mt. Diablo, but there is more to come. As the route swings east, passing through chaparral, more waterfalls pop into view, spilling across eroded, rocky cliffs. Now directly under North Peak, you step across a seasonal creek and then pass a stream flowing out of Wild Oat Canyon.

Now the trail bends west and then northwest, descending beneath impressive rock cliffs. Ahead a ridge sweeps down from Mt. Olympia to Donner Canyon; your route crosses it and another just beyond. Layers of rock, exposed in places here along the trail, are bent and tilted almost to the vertical, a vivid display of the forces that uplifted Mt. Diablo millions of years ago. Stop from time to time and look downhill to your left: more falls may be visible in the upper reaches of Donner Canyon. In early spring the hillsides here are lush green; within a few months they will turn brown and remain so until the rains arrive in autumn. Lupine in bloom may add dabs of blue to the scene.

The view along the final stretch of the Falls Trail is superb. To the west, Eagle Peak (2369') caps the ridge separating Mitchell and Back canyons. Across Donner Canyon is Meridian Ridge, leading uphill to Bald Ridge and the summit, which is due south. A level walk soon brings you to Cardinet Oaks Road, which you descend via S-bends to Donner Creek. If the creek is overflowing the road, step across on rocks and proceed uphill on a moderate grade, passing another creek flowing under the road through a culvert. At about the 4-mile point, you reach the junction of Cardinet Oaks, Meridian Ridge, and Donner Canyon roads. Retrace your route from here, descending through Donner Canyon to Regency Dr.

GRAND LOOP

Length: 6.5 miles

Time: 3 to 5 hours

Rating: Very difficult

Regulations: Mt. Diablo State Park; entrance fee; no bicycles, no dogs, no smoking.

Facilities: Picnic tables, water, toilet at trailhead; visitor center (may be closed), restrooms, phone, and water at summit.

Directions: From Interstate 680 in Danville, take the Diablo Road/Danville exit and follow Diablo Road 3 miles east to Mt. Diablo Scenic Blvd. Turn left onto Mt. Diablo Scenic Blvd.—which soon becomes South Gate Road—and go 3.7 miles to the South Gate entrance station. Continue on South Gate Road another 3.2 miles to Park Headquarters and a junction with North Gate and Summit roads. Turn right onto Summit Road and go 2.3 miles to Diablo Valley Overlook, a large parking area at a sharp bend in the road, at the entrance to the Juniper Campground. The trailhead is at the north end of Diablo Valley Overlook.

A complete circle around Mt. Diablo, the East Bay's tallest peak, plus a trip to the summit, makes this one of the region's premier trips, and a great way to learn more about the trees, shrubs, and wildflowers that struggle for survival on the rugged mountain's upper reaches. This strenuous route uses Deer Flat, Meridian Ridge, and Prospectors Gap roads, and the North Peak, Summit, and Juniper trails.

At the north end of the parking area and just to the right of the entrance to the campground, there is a picnic site with water. From there, follow either of two paved roads downhill into the Juniper Campground. On your left is a grassy area on a steep slope, a favorite jumping off point for hang gliders. From the point where the roads join, continue walking northwest on a gated dirt road, signed DEER FLAT ROAD/MITCHELL CANYON FIRE ROAD but called Deer Flat Road on the Mt. Diablo State Park trail map. Many of the trees and shrubs growing here are adapted to hot, dry conditions, including gray pine, California juniper, manzanita, and chamise. Other trees which manage somehow to survive here are coast live oak and California bay, normally associated with cooler, wetter terrain. Looking west across Pine Canyon, you have expansive views of the Interstate 680 corridor and the hills of Oakland and Berkeley, with Mt. Tamalpais in distant Marin county visible on a clear day. To the north, the vista extends past Walnut Creek and Concord to Suisun Bay and the west delta.

Soon you pass Burma Road, left; continue straight and then bear right as the road descends via well-graded S-bends, giving you a look at Mt. Diablo's 3849-foot summit, today's goal. The northward view takes in the rock quarry on Mt. Zion, and extends beyond to the west delta, home of the "mothball fleet," a collection of decommissioned naval vessels. The variety of trees and shrubs increases dramatically as you near Deer Flat, adding to your list such species as canyon live oak, blue oak, hoptree, toyon, coffeeberry, and yerba santa. Despite all this plant life, the route is open with no shade. When the road levels in a little valley, you have reached Deer Flat, one of the prettiest spots on Mt. Diablo, especially in fall when bigleaf maple, California wild grape, and poison oak add touches of color to the scene.

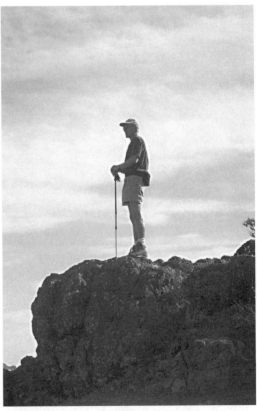

The Grand Loop features stunning scenery and superb vantage points.

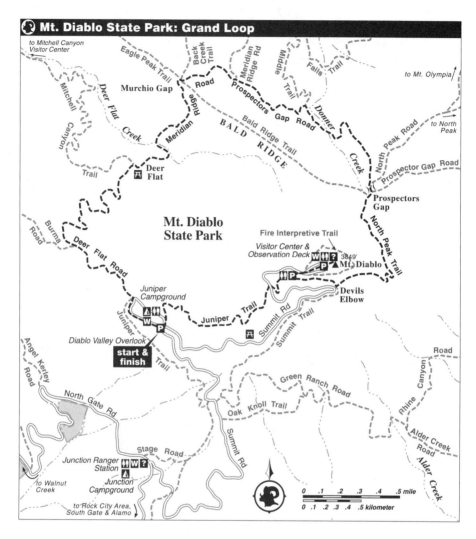

Mt. Diablo State Park: Grand Loop

Soon you come to a junction marking the end of Deer Flat Road. Here, Mitchell Canyon Road goes left, but your route, Meridian Ridge Road, turns right and heads for Murchio Gap. Descending on a gentle grade from Deer Flat, the route next turns north and skirts Bald Ridge as it begins to climb. A relentless, steep climb in the open helps you win back elevation lost in the descent from Juniper Campground. This is the domain of manzanita, with some species growing as tall as trees and others hugging the ground. Also here are chaparral pea, a thorny, three-leaved shrub that produces magenta flowers in late spring, and toyon, a tree-like shrub with oval leaves that are stiff and serrated.

At about the 2.2-mile point, you reach Murchio Gap, an important junction with many trails. Clockwise from the left as you face north, they are: Eagle Peak Trail, Back Creek Trail, Meridian Ridge Road, and Bald Ridge Trail. Murchio Gap is home to leather oak, a low-growing shrub with curly, gray-green leaves, confined in the East Bay mostly to Mt. Diablo. As you follow Meridian Ridge Road east, you have a fine view, left, of Clayton, the west delta, and the hills of Napa and Solano counties. Also left is a dark ridge leading northwest to Eagle Peak (2369'); and ahead of you, from left to right, are North Peak (3557'), Prospectors Gap—a notch on the skyline—and Mt. Diablo's summit.

After a gentle descent, you come to a junction; here Meridian Ridge Road turns left, but your route, Prospectors Gap Road goes straight. As you follow Prospectors Gap Road southeast, it holds a level course—savor this, as a long climbs is ahead. Where the Middle Trail comes in from the left, near Big Spring, you descend slightly to within earshot of Donner Creek. Here you may see canyon live oak, and on the ground big cones from gray pines. Now comes a steep climb, fortunately in the shade of bay and coast live oak, but soon the shade ends and the road, now rocky in places, makes a switchback, easing the grade somewhat as you struggle toward Prospectors Gap.

On your left is the steep, rocky face of North Peak. On your right, the top of Mt. Diablo, with its domed summit museum, comes into view. This long, steep climb is a great conditioning hike, but not for the weak-kneed or faint-of-heart. A final pitch brings you, with relief, to Prospectors Gap, at about the 3.5-mile point. From here, Prospectors Gap Road drops steeply in front of you; North Peak Road heads left to North Peak; and your route, the North Peak Trail, goes uphill and right. (The North Peak Trail is one of the few single tracks on Mt. Diablo open to bicycles.) Views here south and east extend to Curry Canyon, the Black Hills, Morgan Territory, and the Central Valley.

The North Peak Trail, rutted and rocky in places, climbs across an open hillside and soon passes an unsigned trail, right. Gray pine, interior live oak, canyon live oak, and blue oak dominate here; their shade is welcome on a hot day. A rocky ridge, dropping steeply from Devils Pulpit, just east of the summit, forms the near skyline to the south. As you near this ridge, the terrain becomes rockier, with a severe drop-off, left, and a steep uphill slope, right. As you come into the open and switchback across the ridge, you are rewarded with a stunning 180-degree view, which takes in the west delta, the Central Valley, Livermore, Pleasanton, the Sunol/Ohlone Wilderness, and Mission Peak.

As the route turns west and you begin walking toward Devils Elbow, a sharp bend in Summit Road, you can see the summit museum and communication towers on Mt. Diablo's summit. Low-growing bay and juniper join pine and oak on a windswept hillside. California fuchsia, a late bloomer, may add a touch of vivid red to the scene. A short climb on loose rock and dirt brings you to Summit Road at Devils Elbow. As you reach the pavement, make a sharp right and begin climbing the Summit Trail, which rises through chaparral to the summit's lower parking area, at about the 5-mile point.

To reach the mountain's 3849-foot summit from the lower parking area, turn right and follow signs for the continuation of the Summit Trail, which runs between the paved roads that link the parking area with the summit. Take this trail uphill for about 0.2 mile. The summit museum, which has an observation deck on top, was built by the Civilian Conservation Corps from 1938 to 1940, but remained mostly unused until 1993, when the Mount Diablo Interpretive Association opened its visitor center there. The center has information about the mountain's geology, flora, and fauna, as well as a small bookstore; for days and hours of operation, call (925) 837-6119. Also available are restrooms, telephone, and water. Climb to the rooftop observation deck for spectacular 360-degree views, enhanced by free binoculars; it is said that the only vantage place with more land in view on a clear day is the summit of Africa's Mt. Kilimanjaro. On clear days, look eastward to glimpse snow-capped Sierra peaks.

After resting and enjoying the scenery, retrace your steps to the lower parking area, then continue walking west across pavement until you find a trail post marking the Juniper Trail, a single track heading downhill from the edge of the parking area. From here, make a steep, rugged descent past several fenced-in communication towers on loose dirt, rocks, and railroad ties. Soon you reach Summit Road; cross carefully, turn right, and walk uphill a short distance to a trail post, left, marking the continuation of the Juniper Trail.

Now the route loses elevation via a series of switchbacks and passes through an area of pine, oak, bay, and chaparral. You head west and continue to descend along the crest of a broad ridge, with a sea of chaparral on both sides of the trail. As the route flattens out at a saddle, you come to a junction. Here an unsigned trail heads northwest to a high point on Moses Rock Ridge; and a trail post with an arrow pointing left directs you to the continuation of the Juniper Trail, which descends through groves of bay and juniper to the parking area.

JUNIPER AND SUMMIT TRAILS

Length: 4.2 miles

Time: 2 to 3 hours

Rating: Moderate

Regulations: Mt. Diablo State Park; entrance fee; no dogs, no smoking, no bicycles.

Facilities: Picnic tables, water, toilet at trailhead; visitor center (may be closed), restrooms, phone, and water at summit.

Directions: From Interstate 680 in Danville, take the Diablo Road/Danville exit and follow Diablo Road 3 miles east to Mt. Diablo Scenic Blvd. Turn left onto Mt. Diablo Scenic Blvd.—which soon becomes South Gate Road—and go 3.7 miles to the South Gate entrance station. Continue on South Gate Road another 3.2 miles to Park Headquarters and a junction with North Gate and Summit roads. Turn right onto Summit Road and go 2.3 miles to Diablo Valley Overlook, a large parking area at a sharp bend in the road, at the entrance to the Juniper Campground. The trailhead is at the north end of Diablo Valley Overlook.

This loop trip to the summit of Mt. Diablo uses the Juniper and Summit trails, and provides unrivaled views on a clear day, when most of the Bay Area, the Central Valley, and the Sierra Nevada appear before you. The mountain's upper reaches contain fine examples of chaparral plants, along with other trees and shrubs adapted to this harsh environment.

After you've had your fill of the fine views from the overlook—and they just get better as you ascend—walk east past the campground entrance and find a trail post with a sign for the Juniper Trail pointing uphill. The distance given on this sign, 1 mile to the lower summit parking area, somehow has lengthened by the time you get there, where a sign indicates 1.24 miles back to the campground. You will also see a sign for the Juniper Trail to Deer Flat Road, left, which is your return route.

The trail, a gravelly single track, passes the Laurel Nook picnic area, home to a large grove of California bay, and then heads steeply uphill via a series of switchbacks in the shade of bay and gray pine. As you climb, be sure to pause often and admire the view, which extends west across the Interstate 680 corridor and the towns of Walnut Creek, Alamo, Danville, and San Ramon. An explosion of growth

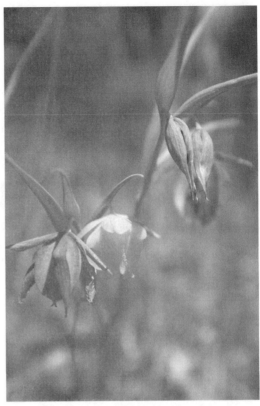

Mt. Diablo hikers may catch a glimpse of the rare Mt. Diablo globe lily.

in these areas has brought housing developments right up to the state park boundary, and offers strong testimony for the value of preserving open space.

As you climb to the crest of Moses Rock Ridge, you may notice the California juniper trees that give the trail its name. This evergreen, which produces small gray berries that smell like gin when crushed, is able to withstand the hot, dry conditions found here for much of the year. Once atop the ridge, you pass an unsigned trail heading left and uphill along the ridgecrest. Your route now swings right and crosses a rocky area that is home to a variety of wildflowers, making it a colorful place to visit in spring. In places the trail climbs steeply and relentlessly, but each step brings new views: north toward Suisun Bay, the west delta, and the towns of Concord, Pittsburgh, and Clayton; south and southeast across Curry Canyon and the Black Hills.

After about 0.5 mile of steady climbing, the trail levels, and you can see the communication towers on Mt. Diablo's summit directly ahead. In this area you may hear a California quail giving its loud and distinctive "chi-ca-go" call. The route returns briefly to a wooded area of bay and coast live oak, switchbacking uphill in the shade, before breaking into the open to climb a steep, rocky section beneath the first of several communication towers. The trail skirts to the north side of this

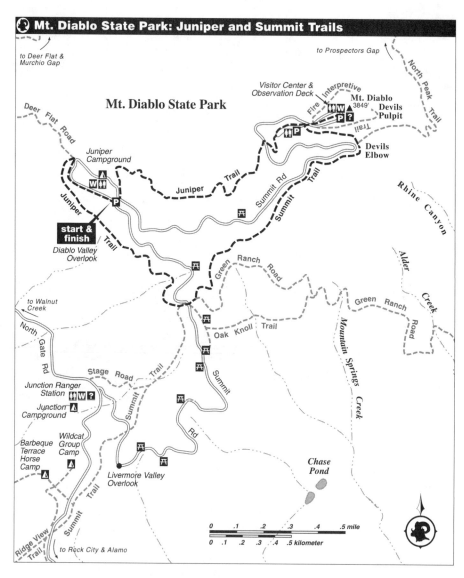

Mt. Diablo State Park: Juniper and Summit Trails

to Deer Flat &
Murchio Gap

to Prospectors Gap

North Peak Trail

Visitor Center &
Observation Deck

Mt. Diablo State Park

Mt. Diablo
3849'

Devils
Pulpit

Fire Interpretive

Deer Flat Road

Trail

Devils
Elbow

Juniper
Campground

Rhine Canyon

Juniper   Trail

Juniper

Summit Rd

Summit Trail

start &
finish

Juniper Trail

Alder Creek

Diablo Valley
Overlook

Green Ranch Road

to Walnut
Creek

Green Ranch Road

North Gate Rd

Oak Knoll Trail

Mountain Springs Creek

Stage Road

Summit Trail

Summit

Junction Ranger
Station

Junction
Campground

Rd

Barbeque
Terrace
Horse
Camp

Wildcat
Group
Camp

**Chase
Pond**

Livermore Valley
Overlook

Ridge View Trail

Summit Trail

to Rock City & Alamo

0   .1   .2   .3   .4   .5 mile
0   .1   .2   .3   .4   .5 kilometer

tower and then levels. About 100 feet farther, the trail begins climbing through a narrow corridor of chaparral to Summit Road.

At about the 1-mile point, after an almost continuous climb from the trailhead, you reach Summit Road. Cross carefully, turn right, and walk about 50 feet to find the trail, left, to the lower summit parking area. Now you climb on switchbacks and walk beside a barbed-wire fence surrounding another communication tower. California poppies and lupine dot the exposed rocky hillside with color in spring and summer. Soon, out of breath perhaps, you reach the lower summit parking area. As you continue through the parking lot uphill, you meet the Summit Trail. One branch of this trail, left, goes about 0.2 mile uphill, between the paved roads that link the parking area with the summit. The other branch, right, which you will use later, drops to South Gate Road and Devils Elbow.

The summit stands 3849 feet above sea level and is the highest point in the East Bay. You've climbed roughly 850 feet in about 1.5 miles, so take a moment to enjoy your achievement. The summit museum, which has an observation deck on top, was built by the Civilian Conservation Corps from 1938 to 1940, but remained mostly unused until 1993, when the Mount Diablo Interpretive Association opened its visitor center there. The center has information about the mountain's geology, flora, and fauna, as well as a small bookstore; for days and hours of operation, call (925) 837-6119. Also available are restrooms, telephone, and water. Climb to the rooftop observation deck for spectacular 360-degree views, enhanced by free binoculars; it is said that the only vantage place with more land in view on a clear day is the summit of Africa's Mt. Kilimanjaro.

On clear days, look eastward to glimpse snow-capped Sierra peaks. To the northeast is North Peak (3557'), home to more communication towers, and reachable only by foot, horseback or bicycle. Beyond it is the confluence of the Sacramento and San Joaquin rivers—the delta. To the west are San Francisco Bay, the Golden Gate, and the Pacific Ocean, landmarks unfortunately often lost in fog or haze. Scattered around the mountain are the suburban communities of Concord, Walnut Creek, Clayton, Alamo, Danville, San Ramon, and Pleasanton.

According to an informational placard placed near the summit, Mt. Diablo was a sacred place for Native Americans and a landmark for Spanish explorers and California settlers in the 18th and 19th centuries. In 1851 a survey led by Colonel Leander Ransome designated the summit as the crossing of an east–west Mt. Diablo baseline and a north–south Mt. Diablo meridian, so that the summit served as a reference point for future surveys of California and parts of Oregon and Nevada. In 1982, the National Park Service designated Mt. Diablo a National Natural Landmark.

The Fire Interpretive Trail, the trailhead for which is on the northeast side of the lower summit parking area, is a 0.7-mile loop encircling the summit. This self-guiding nature trail, which is disabled-accessible as far as Ransome Point Overlook, was built following a 1977 fire, using contributions from more than 1100 individuals, groups, and businesses. The trail, whose purpose is to show visitors the role fire plays in the chaparral ecosystem, is dedicated to Mary Leolin Bowerman, a pioneer Mount Diablo botanist.

Now that you've had your fill, for the time being, of Mt. Diablo's heights, retrace your route on the Summit Trail to the lower summit parking area, turn left, and find the continuation of the Summit Trail, which heads southeast to South Gate Road and Devils Elbow. As you look out over the southern expanse of Mount Diablo State Park, you can see the suburban communities and housing developments pressing up against the mountain's foothills. Your route now winds through an area of gray pines, chaparral, and wonderful wildflowers as it descends to meet Summit Road at Devils Elbow.

At about the 2-mile point, you reach Devils Elbow, a sharp bend where Summit Road turns west almost 180 degrees to make its final climb to the summit. On your left is a junction with the North Peak Trail to Prospectors Gap, part of the route described in "Grand Loop." Here you keep walking straight on the road and find the continuation of the Summit Trail as it continues to descend, now heading southwest. The descent is steep and rocky over the first few yards, then less so. Summit Road is above and to your right.

At a junction with a dirt road, you turn right on the Summit Trail and follow it uphill to Summit Road. Once you reach the pavement, leave it after a few steps, where the Summit Trail immediately descends to the left. Watch your footing here on loose gravel. The route passes through an area full of yerba santa, woody shrubs with white trumpet flowers. Now traversing southwest across a shrubby hillside, the trail next passes under an open scree slope before descending gradually into a grove of gray pine and bay. In places vegetation crowds the trail, but there are also openings that afford sweeping vistas to the south. Soon you are hiking in open grassland, with a large water-storage tank downhill to the left.

At about the 3-mile point, you reach Old Pioneer Horse Camp, with toilets, cooking grills, and a bathtub for watering horses. Walk straight ahead, past Green Ranch Road, left, keeping the bathtub on your left and the big pink water-storage tank on your right. Climb a small dirt embankment and follow the Summit Trail. Continue to descend on a rocky trail through a large area of chaparral, mostly chamise, in places too high to see over.

Out of the chaparral at last, you reach a paved service road and, passing another sign for Green Ranch Road, go straight to a gate at Summit Road. (A sign here reads SUMMIT TO THE RIGHT; ROCK CITY TO THE LEFT.) Carefully cross Summit Road and begin descending the Summit Trail, now a substantial dirt road that eventually leads to Park Headquarters at the junction of North and South Gate roads. As the road turns left and descends (about 150 feet downhill from Summit Road) look for the Juniper Trail, signed TO LOWER SUMMIT PARKING LOT, climbing to your right.

The trail immediately begins to switchback up the side of a small gully, in a corridor of chamise and other chaparral plants. A couple of switchbacks bring you to an open, rocky area and a sign for the Juniper Trail, straight. When you reach this point, walk uphill and right, toward Summit Road. Before reaching the road, look left and get on a small trail going west down the side of an embankment. This is the continuation of the Juniper Trail, which contours north and then northwest across a southwest-facing hillside. On a clear day this vantage point gives you fine views of the Bay Area, including Mount Tamalpais, the Golden Gate Bridge, and the hills of Oakland and Berkeley.

The open, grassy expanse of Mt. Diablo's southwest flank is dotted with groves of blue oak, gray pine, and juniper. On the way back to Juniper Campground, the route dips into several small canyons which may have running water—cool shady areas with stands of bay and coast live oak. When the route breaks into the open again, you climb a narrow track cut into the steep, grassy hillside. Here you may see raptors soaring on thermals rising from Pine Canyon, left. This is a wonderful part of the hike, giving you the feeling of being high on the slopes of a grand mountain—which you are! The route, which has taken you to the top of the East Bay's tallest peak, nears its end as you reach the open area just below Juniper Campground. From here, you turn right and walk uphill on the paved campground road to the parking area.

MITCHELL AND DONNER CANYONS

Length: 8.6 miles

Time: 5 to 7 hours

Rating: Difficult

Regulations: Mt. Diablo State Park; parking fee; no dogs, no smoking.

Facilities: Visitor center, water, phone, toilets, horse staging. The Mitchell Canyon Interpretive Center, at the south end of Mitchell Canyon Road, has displays, interpretive materials, maps, and a docent on duty. The center is open weekends and some holidays, 8 A.M. to 4 P.M., spring/summer; 8 A.M. to 3 P.M., fall/winter.

Directions: From Interstate 680 in Walnut Creek, or Highway 24 eastbound (just before the merge with Interstate 680), take the Ygnacio Valley Road exit, right, and go northeast 6.9 miles to Pine Hollow Road. Turn right and go 1.7 miles to Mitchell Canyon Road. Turn right and go 1.3 miles to the Mt. Diablo State Park entrance. Pay a parking fee at the automated ticket machine, then continue 0.1 mile to a large parking area. The trailhead is on the south side of the parking area.

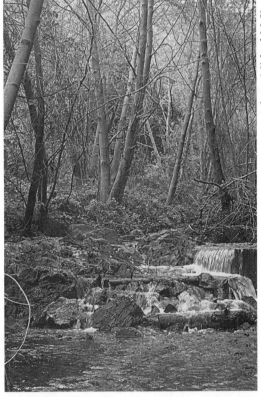

photo: Michael McKay

Climbing 1800 feet to Murchio Gap, a high point on Mt. Diablo's north side, this rigorous loop uses Mitchell Canyon, Meridian Ridge, and Donner Canyon roads to let you sample the wonders of our premier East Bay park: great views, spring wildflowers, migrating songbirds, and an abundance of native trees and shrubs. The first part of Mitchell Canyon Road is a self-guiding nature trail, with a descriptive leaflet available at the trailhead.

Mitchell Canyon is a great birding area, and if you are here in spring, check the parking area for western bluebirds and other songbirds in the trees before starting your hike. Wildflower enthusiasts will want to pick up a copy of the full-color "Mt. Diablo Wildflowers" brochure published in 2005 by the Mount Diablo Interpretive Association. As you stand in the parking area and look south, the hills in front

Deer Flat Creek is a clear, fast-running stream in the winter and spring.

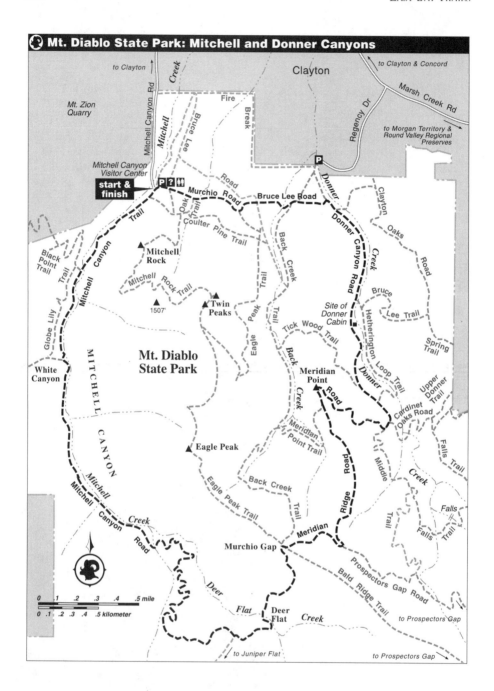

Mt. Diablo State Park: Mitchell and Donner Canyons

of you are the Twin Peaks (1733', 1507'), with Eagle Peak (2369') in the background. Mt. Diablo's summit (3849') is hidden from view, but an hour or two of hiking, some of it steeply uphill, will reveal the mountain's upper reaches.

Leaving the south side of the parking area, follow Mitchell Canyon Road, which is shared by hikers, bicyclists, and equestrians. Continue past a gate and walk uphill on a gentle grade. About 150 feet beyond the gate, you pass a connector to the Mitchell Rock Trail, left. Continuing straight on Mitchell Canyon Road, you pass the park ranger's residence, right, and behind it, heavily quarried Mt. Zion (1635'). Fall brings a spectacle of New England–like color to Mitchell Canyon, thanks to black walnut, bigleaf maple, California wild grape, and poison oak. The woodlands here also contain coast live oak, valley oak, blue oak, gray pine, blue elderberry, and California buckeye.

Look for a large coast live oak on your right; this is the Bicentennial Tree, dedicated in 1987 by the Daughters of the American Revolution. Some of the shrubs here include California sagebrush, bush monkeyflower, coffeeberry, spiny redberry, and narrow-leaf bush sunflower. As you begin a moderate climb, Mitchell Creek is on your right, and soon you pass a marshy area, remnant of an artificial pond, filled with poison hemlock.

Just past the 0.5-mile point, you come to a junction with the Black Point Trail, a dirt road heading right. Continue straight, walking along Mitchell Canyon, with the creek, bordered by willows, now on the left. California bay, toyon, yerba santa, and wild rose also thrive here. As the canyon walls begin to close in, notice the chaparral growing high on the rocky hillsides. This plant community, composed of hardy, heat-tolerant shrubs such as manzanita, buckbrush, chamise, and black sage, depends on fire to regenerate itself by recycling nutrients into the soil and cracking the plants' hard seed coats.

Among the profusion of spring wildflowers common in lower Mitchell Canyon are California buttercup, blow wives, blue-eyed grass, bluedicks, Ithuriel's spear, larkspur, California poppy, Chinesehouses, lupine, paintbrush, and various clarkias. Two exquisite flowers to look for are the multi-hued Mariposa lily and the lantern-shaped Mt. Diablo globe lily, a specialty in this state park. In the fall, California fuchsia is one of the last flowers to remain in bloom here.

At about the 1-mile point, Red Road starts a climb into White Canyon, right, but your route, Mitchell Canyon Road, holds a level course into the ever-narrowing canyon. Here the creek is on your left, close to the road. On your right is a steep, east-facing hillside of chaparral. Ground cover beside the trail includes blackberry and periwinkle, a nonnative plant with dark green leaves and five-petaled, lavender flowers. Two additions to your tree list here are white alder and Fremont cottonwood, species associated with water. If you hear a flock of noisy birds flitting in the trees, they could be bushtits. These tiny gray birds resemble chickadees but are slightly smaller, with a long tail. You may see golden-crowned sparrows on the ground, scraping in the leaf litter for food. And do not be surprised, in the fall, to come upon a tarantula walking slowly along the side of the road. These large, sluggish spiders are generally not poisonous to humans, although they can bite. Unfortunately, they can easily be crushed by a hiking boot, a bicycle tire, or a horse's hoof.

Prospectors Gap, a saddle between Mt. Diablo's summit, right, and North Peak (3557'), left, soon comes into view. At about the 2-mile point the route begins to climb, first in shade, then via steep switchbacks in the open. This is a great part of the route for scenery and birds. You have a great view of Mitchell Canyon and its chaparral-clad walls. Look up and you may see turkey vultures or red-tailed hawks gliding overhead; look down and you may spot a secretive hermit thrush.

As you gain elevation, Deer Flat Creek, a tributary of Mitchell Creek, is at the bottom of a canyon, left. Stay on the road, and ignore any single-track trails that branch from it. Across this canyon is a steep, rocky ridge running between Eagle Peak, an impressive summit in its own right, and Murchio Gap, a place you will visit later today. Ahead of you, unseen, is Deer Flat, gained only by more steep climbing. But the enticement of high ground and the reward of expanding vistas help you overcome the relentless grade. From time to time, take a break from the climb and listen here for the California quail's three-part call: it sounds like "chi-ca-go." As you approach Deer Flat, the grade levels, and you can see North Peak and its communication towers to the east, just behind Bald Ridge.

At approximately the 3.5-mile point, you reach Deer Flat, a scenic area of gray pine and live oak, with several welcoming picnic tables and a horse watering trough. After stopping to rest and admire the scenery, resume your walk and soon come to a junction. From here, Deer Flat Road climbs right, toward Juniper Camp, but you turn left on Meridian Ridge Road and begin a gentle descent through an area, colorful in fall, of manzanita, hoptree, spiny redberry, poison oak, narrow-leaf bush sunflower, and wild rose. Be on the lookout here for golden eardrops, a 2- to 6-foot-tall wildflower with fern-like leaves and yellow blossoms that is abundant after fires.

After crossing a small streambed, the route begins to climb. Stay straight on Meridian Ridge Road, signed for Donner Canyon. As the

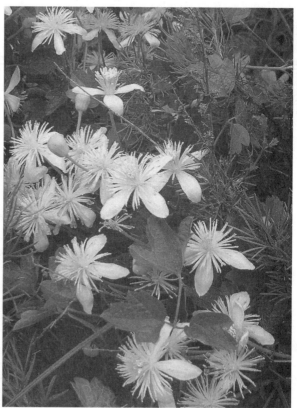

photo: Michael McKay

Clematis, a woody vine found at lower Mitchell Canyon, has impressive blooms in springtime.

route steepens, the air becomes fragrant with the smell of pine, and you begin to glimpse Eagle Peak ahead. Behind you is Mt. Diablo's summit, with its domed summit museum; to your right is the grassy expanse of Bald Ridge. Soon Murchio Gap, at 2320 feet the high point on this route, comes into view. As you near the gap, you pass through a lovely area where Manzanita, toyon, chamise, yerba santa, and chaparral pea thrive on a hot, dry hillside.

At Murchio Gap, at about the 4.3-mile point, you may notice a dense, low-growing shrub with gray-green leaves. This is leather oak, limited in the East Bay to Mt. Diablo and Mines Road. Murchio Gap is an important junction, so take a moment to admire the view and get your bearings. If you stand at the gap and face north, you are ringed by trails. Clockwise from the left these are: Eagle Peak Trail, Back Creek Trail, Meridian Ridge Road, and Bald Ridge Trail. The top-of-the-world feeling continues as you descend on the Meridian Ridge Road, right, with views north to Clayton, the west delta, and the hills of Napa and Solano counties. Also impressive is North Peak, with its furrowed, rocky ridges and canyons falling steeply from the skyline. We are lucky to have mountain scenery like this, reminiscent of the High Sierra, so close to home.

The descent steepens and covers some rough ground, rocky and rutted. Pay attention to your footing, but also be alert for unusual birds, such as Townsend's solitaire. This gray bird, slightly smaller than a robin, has a white eye-ring and white on the outside of its tail. Summer residents of the high mountains, solitaires migrate in the fall to lower elevations, where they are often seen feeding on juniper berries. After descending about 0.5 mile from Murchio Gap, you come to a junction with Prospectors Gap Road. Here the route to Mt. Diablo's summit goes straight, but you stay on Meridian Ridge Road by veering left. Now descend steeply along narrow Meridian Ridge to Meridian Point.

With Eagle Peak now to your left, the route heads north, alternating between steep and not-so-steep pitches on a ridge that is just wide enough for the road. This is an excellent place to study chaparral—it is everywhere you look. Four common chaparral plants seen here belong to the buckthorn (*Rhamnaceae*) family: jimbrush, buckbrush, coffeeberry, and spiny redberry. The first two are ceanothuses, or wild lilacs, and the second two belong to the genus *Rhamnus*. Jimbrush is a large shrub with small, dark green leaves having three main veins; it blooms in the spring with pale blue flowers. Buckbrush has small, paddle-shaped leaves, dark green on top, lighter green below; its spring blossoms are white. Coffeeberry has long, slender leaves, with veins that run almost to the leaf's edge, and dark berries. Spiny redberry resembles a miniature live oak, with stiff, rounded leaves that are spiny on the edges.

Just before reaching Meridian Point, you pass the Meridian Point Trail, left, coming from Back Creek. At Meridian Point, an unsigned viewpoint, your route veers sharply right and descends, steeply at times, toward Donner Canyon. Here you have a chance to compare two very similar pines, gray and Coulter: Coulter pines have longer cones, stouter limbs, and denser foliage. Before the junction with Donner Canyon and Cardinet Oaks roads, you pass the Middle Trail, right. (Return to this spot sometime in early spring and follow the "Falls Trail" route description to find Mt. Diablo's hidden waterfalls.)

248   EAST BAY TRAILS

Just past the 6-mile point, you reach a major intersection; here Cardinet Oaks Road heads right, but your route, Donner Canyon Road, turns left. Now you are on level ground, but soon the route begins to drop again. The variety of trees and shrubs here is stunning—almost everything you've seen so far, together in one area. On your way down Donner Canyon Road you will pass a number of trails: Hetherington , Tick Wood, and a trail to the Donner Cabin homestead site. Ignore them all and continue straight, descending steeply through blue-oak savanna until you are walking on level ground once again, with Donner Creek on your right. Steller's jays and dark-eyed juncos may follow your progress through their neighborhood with interest and an occasional comment.

About 0.5 mile past the trail to Donner Cabin, you pass a trail leading to Clayton Oaks Road, right. Here you continue straight, and almost immediately reach Murchio Road (unsigned), heading sharply left and uphill. Follow this road due west as it climbs west over a grassy hill, passing eucalyptus, black locust, and walnut trees on the way. The scenery is great—Mt. Diablo's summit, North Peak, Eagle Peak, and Twin Peaks are all in view.

Soon you reach a four-way junction with Back Creek Road. You go straight, still on Murchio Road, signed for the Mitchell Canyon staging area, dropping briefly to cross Back Creek. At the next junction, where Bruce Lee Road goes right, you stay on Murchio Road by going straight. With Twin Peaks uphill and left, your route maintains a level grade through oak savanna. Soon you pass a connector to the Eagle Peak Trail and the unsigned Oak Trail, a dirt road, both left. Where the Mitchell Rock Trail goes left at a T-junction, just past a water tower, you turn right and descend to the parking area.

SYCAMORE CREEK

Length: 5 miles

Time: 3 to 4 hours

Rating: Moderate

Regulations: Mt. Diablo State Park; entrance fee; no dogs, no smoking, no bicycles on the Devils Slide Trail.

Facilities: None.

Directions: From Interstate 680 in Danville, take the Diablo Road/Danville exit and follow Diablo Road 3 miles east to Mt. Diablo Scenic Blvd. Turn left onto Mt. Diablo Scenic Blvd.—which soon becomes South Gate Road—and go 3.7 miles to the South Gate entrance station. Continue on South Gate Road another 1.6 miles to Curry Point Overlook, right, located at a sharp left-hand bend in the road. The trailhead is at the east side of the parking area.

Most routes on Mt. Diablo involve a good deal of climbing, usually at the start. This semi-loop, which uses the Curry Canyon, Knobcone Point, Black Hawk Ridge, and Sycamore Creek roads, along with the Devils Slide Trail, is different. It starts at mid-mountain, just below 1800 feet, descends into the beautiful canyon that holds Sycamore Creek, explores the Blackhills addition to the park, and climbs

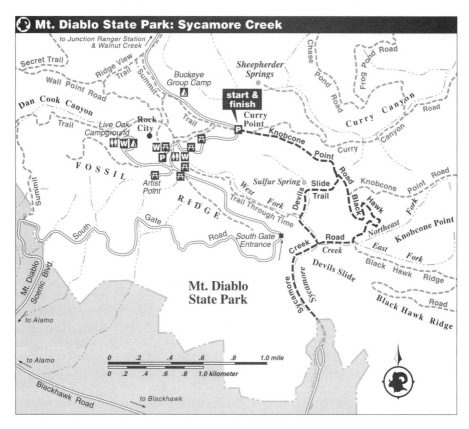

Mt. Diablo State Park: Sycamore Creek

about 1000 feet back up to the parking area. Two rare plants, Mt. Diablo manzanita and Mt. Diablo sunflower, are present, along with a fine array of other trees, shrubs, and wildflowers. This loop, best in spring and fall, may be extremely muddy in wet weather.

From the east side of the exposed and possibly windy parking area, follow a dirt-and-gravel road—signed here as Curry Canyon Road—on a level grade as it runs slightly south of east along the top of a broad ridge. Mt. Diablo's summit (3849') rises majestically to your left. This is open country, and in spring the grassy hillsides are speckled with wildflowers, including California buttercup, blue-eyed grass, wild pansy, and bluedicks. After about 150 yards you come to a junction. Here Curry Canyon Road heads downhill and left, but your route, Knobcone Point Road, a dirt road, continues straight and begins to climb slightly. A deep, forested canyon, right, holds Sulfur Spring and the headwaters of Sycamore Creek.

Here a few coast live oaks provide the only shade; otherwise this part of the route is in the open, providing great views east to the Central Valley and, on a clear day perhaps, beyond to the Sierra. The road, rocky in places, begins to descend gently, soon passing through a fence and then entering a wooded area of California bay, coast live oak, and gray pine. Poison oak is especially rampant here. The deep fold of Curry Canyon is left, and beyond it in the distance rises North Peak (3557'),

Mt. Diablo's twin summit. As the route begins to bend right, you pass the Devils Slide Trail, right, which you will use later on your return climb out of Sycamore Creek canyon.

Passing another fence, the road rises on an easy grade through a mixed forest, then breaks into the open at a T-junction. Here Knobcone Point Road turns left, but your route, Black Hawk Ridge Road, turns right. (You can make an interesting side-trip by turning left here and following Knobcone Point Road to Knobcone Point, named for a species of closed-cone pine found here and hardly anywhere else in the East Bay.) If you look left and uphill at this junction, you may notice a large sunflower-like blossom on a plant with gray, fuzzy leaves. This is mule's ear (genus *Wyethia*), a sunflower relative that grows low to the ground in large colonies.

Following Black Hawk Ridge Road, through oak and pine, you may notice heath warrior poking through the leaf litter and pine needles on the forest floor. This parasitic plant, related to paintbrush and owl's clover, is associated with madrone and manzanita, which are always nearby; it also attracts humming-birds. You may also notice huge fallen pine cones, belonging to gray pine, the dominant pine here. Soon you come to an area of chaparral, where the rare Mt. Diablo manzanita flourishes in company with more common shrubs such as chamise, toyon, bush monkeyflower, and silk tassel bush. You may also see here the Mt. Diablo sunflower, another plant confined to Mt. Diablo. This spring bloomer has green, lance shaped leaves and a bright yellow flower held aloft on a single slender stalk.

As the route descends via S-bends through rocky terrain, burned in the fall of 1996, you continue to see evidence of plant diversity, with wildflowers such as common star lily and shooting star, and clematis, a vine that overruns the toyon. In late spring, look for flowering shrubs such as buckbrush and narrow-leaf bush sun-flower to brighten this stretch of the route. Losing elevation on a moderate grade, you soon enter a wooded canyon where the sound of frogs may signal the nearby presence of water, and Steller's jays on patrol will probably give you a noisy wel-come. Slightly downstream from the confluence of the east and northeast forks of Sycamore Creek, just shy of the 2-mile point, you come to a junction marked by a trail post. Straight ahead is Black Hawk Ridge Road; to the right is your route, Sycamore Creek Road.

After turning right, you follow the east fork of Sycamore Creek downstream, walking on a dirt road along the creek's right-hand bank. Plants suited to a cool-er, wetter environment grow here, including western sycamore, bigleaf maple, white alder, California buckeye, snowberry, creambush, and wild rose. Crossing the creek twice—after the second crossing you pass the Devils Slide Trail, your return route, right—you continue walking downstream, now following the main branch of Sycamore Creek. Soon you pass a clearing where, in spring, blue bush lupine and California buttercup bloom on a steep, open hillside. The landscape becomes rockier as you continue to descend in the shade of bay and coast live oak.

Now the route emerges into the open, crosses the creek over a large culvert, and soon reaches a fence marking the boundary between the state park and the 252-acre Blackhills parcel, which was added to the park—thanks to a compromise negotiated with the parcel's owner by the group Save Mount Diablo—and official-ly dedicated in April 1997. Continue walking in the open, past clumps of California sagebrush and black sage, enjoying a vista that takes in rolling hills studded with oaks, and the Black Hills—high, rocky cliffs where endangered peregrine falcons were re-introduced from 1989 to 1993.

Large rock outcrops tower close to the road, which is carved out of a hillside that descends to Sycamore Creek, right. Here the creek and road are squeezed between the ends of Fossil and Black Hawk ridges, an area called Devils Slide. A short dis-tance downstream are piles of wood, remnants of several large water tanks that used to stand here, near a small dam.

About 100 yards past the dam, look for an overgrown trail, unsigned, going right at a sharp angle and downhill to the creek. Watch your footing to avoid tripping on a metal pipe that crosses your path, and descend carefully to the creek. Please avoid trampling any of the delicate streamside vegetation. The trail leads upstream to two pools, the second of which is filled by a lovely waterfall that tumbles over slick rock. After enjoying this secluded spot, retrace your steps to the junction of Sycamore Creek Road and the Devils Slide Trail, about the 3.5-mile point.

Turn left onto the Devils Slide Trail, a single track, and continue walking uphill in dense forest, following Sycamore Creek, which is on your right, upstream. About 100 yards past the junction, search the area between the trail and the creek for giant trillium, a large, three-leaved plant with a single maroon, pink, or white flower that appears in spring. Another unusual plant, California barberry, can be found here, along with the more common coffeeberry, creambush, and snowberry; you may also see a delicate white spring wildflower called woodland star. Soon you cross the creek on rocks and continue upstream with the creek now on your left. After a short distance, the route recrosses the creek and comes to a junction. Here the Trail Through Time goes straight, but you say on the Devils Slide Trail by veering right.

Now on a moderate grade, you climb to the next creek crossing, just below Sulfur Spring, where the smell of sulfur is noticeable. Turning right and stepping across the creek here, you follow the rocky and eroded trail uphill past a signpost. A faint path on your left goes upstream toward the spring. Another tributary of Sycamore Creek, not on the park map, is to your right. The route, mostly shaded, passes stands of bay, buckeye, coast live oak, and toyon. At about the 4-mile point you reach a fork with another faint path. Bearing right, you descend to the tribu-tary, then cross it and continue walking upstream on a slight uphill grade. The trail may be muddy at the crossing and overgrown farther on with creambush and poison oak.

Soon you merge with a trail, left, coming from the previous fork, then swing sharply left and climb across an open, grassy hillside, with the summit of Mt. Diablo just peeking over a ridge ahead. In spring this beautiful area is full of blue-eyed grass. Climbing a bit farther, you close the loop at Knobcone Point Road; turn left here and retrace your route to the parking area.

◆Morgan Territory Regional Preserve ◆

BOB WALKER RIDGE

Length: 5.9 miles

Time: 3 to 4 hours

Rating: Moderate

Regulations: EBRPD; no bicycles on the single-track part of the Coyote Trail.

Facilities: Picnic tables, water, toilet, horse staging; two toilets along the trail.

Directions: From Interstate 580 in Livermore, take the North Livermore exit and go north on North Livermore Ave., and then west on its continuation, Manning Road. At 4.4 miles from the interstate, just after a sharp bend to the west, you turn right onto Morgan Territory Rd., and go 6.3 miles to the Volvon staging area, right. (Use caution: after 0.7 mile, Morgan Territory Rd. becomes a one-lane road with turnouts.) The trailhead is at the northeast edge of parking area.

From Interstate 680 in Walnut Creek, or Hwy. 24 eastbound (just before the merge with I-680), take the Ygnacio Valley Rd. exit and go northeast 7.6 miles to Clayton Rd. Turn right and go 6 miles (Clayton Rd. becomes Marsh Creek Rd.) to Morgan Territory Rd. Turn right and go 9.4 miles to the Volvon staging area, left. (Caution is also advised along this road, which winds through the hills and is narrow in stretches.) The trailhead is at the northeast edge of parking area.

This is one of the most remote and scenic parks in the East Bay, perched at 2000 feet on the southeastern edge of Mt. Diablo State Park, within sight of Livermore, Altamont Pass, and the Central Valley. Seclusion and wilderness make hiking here a special experience. This loop, which uses the Coyote, Stone Corral, Volvon Loop, and Volvon trails, takes full advantage of these attributes, dropping into a deep canyon, then climbing lofty Bob Walker Ridge. This is a region of extremes: hot in summer, cold in winter, and potentially windy all year.

As soon as you leave the large gravel parking area, which may be windy, you have a choice of two trails, Coyote and Volvon. Left is the Coyote Trail, a single track for hikers only; the Volvon Trail, a dirt road straight ahead, is open to hikers, horses, and bicycles. These trail names are based on Native American history and tradition: Coyote is a mythic personality in Indian legends, and the Volvon were one of the East Bay groups that resisted the Spanish mission system. The preserve itself is named for Jeremiah Morgan, an early settler, gold miner, and rancher. Bob Walker Ridge and the Bob Walker Regional Trail honor a photographer and environmentalist whose efforts on behalf of EBRPD from 1984 until his death in 1993 led to additional land acquisitions in Morgan Territory and Pleasanton Ridge. The Bob Walker Regional Trail, combining parts of the Volvon, Volvon Loop, Eagle, and Highland Ridge trails, connects Morgan Territory with Mt. Diablo State Park.

Following the Coyote Trail, you descend through beautiful grassland, with oaks dotting the hillsides and Mt. Diablo visible to the northwest. At a stock pond with numerous water lilies, bear left, passing the Condor Trail, which continues straight

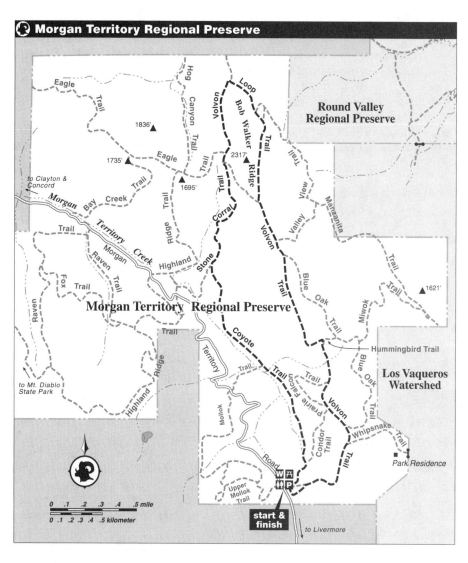

Morgan Territory Regional Preserve

through a gate. Your route climbs gently through stands of blue oak and coast live oak as it skirts the right side of the pond, which is shaded by a large valley oak. After passing the pond, the trail, which is indistinct in places, splits and continues along both sides of a narrow, rocky canyon. When water is flowing along this creek, stay on the right-hand trail; when no water is present, either side of the trail will do. As you descend, note that the canyon is lined with black oak, California bay, and manzanita, here growing as tall as a small tree. Poison oak is here too, so be careful. As beautiful views open up toward Mt. Diablo, resist the temptation to look and walk at the same time: the footing gets tricky here.

This is rugged terrain, colorful in fall, with a distinct wilderness feel. Above and right is a high, rocky ridge blanketed with chaparral. As the descent becomes steeper, the trail makes S-bends down the hillside. Toyon, coffeeberry, creambush, spiny redberry, and hoptree are some of the shrubs you may spot along the way. At about the 0.8-mile point, in the canyon bottom, you pass a junction with the Mollok Trail, left. A streambed lined with bigleaf maple and western sycamore is also left, and as you continue straight ahead, the canyon walls relax their grip and the terrain becomes more open and park-like.

Just past the 1-mile point, you come to a fork in the trail; the branches rejoin a short distance ahead at a gate. Passing through the gate, you emerge from forest into grassland and leave the canyon behind. The route, sometimes just a matted path in the grass, stays in the middle of a large valley, and soon reaches another fork. This time, follow the right-hand branch and walk uphill. The weedy plant with blue flowers growing beside the trail is called vinegar weed; rub the leaves and smell your fingers to find out why. Large oaks with clumps of mistletoe grace the hillsides. Ahead is junction with the Stone Corral Trail, a dirt road. Here you turn right and climb north on a gentle and then moderate grade through oak savanna; you will be on dirt roads until you return to the parking area. From his perch on an oak limb, a raucous Steller's jay may announce your arrival. You may also spot a northern flicker, a member of the woodpecker family, here. As you gain elevation via long switchbacks and gradually emerge from the trees, look up to check the sky for hawks.

At about the 2.3-mile point, you pass Volvon Loop Trail, right, leading up Bob Walker Ridge to join the Volvon Trail. Continue straight, past a disused cattle-loading pen on your right, and after a few hundred feet you reach a fork. Here the Eagle Trail branches left, and your route, the Volvon Loop Trail, goes right. As you continue climbing on a gentle grade, you are rewarded with fine views of Mt. Diablo's North Peak, and, in the distance, Clayton, Pittsburg, Antioch, and the west delta. When you reach the north end of Bob Walker Ridge, the route bends sharply right, presenting a vista that stretches east to the Central Valley and, on a clear day, the Sierra. Now heading southeast, the route stays just below the ridgecrest, right, and passes through lovely stands of blue oak and bay. From here you can see in the distance the windmills near Altamont Pass. At about the 3-mile point, you pass on your left the first of three connections to the Valley View Trail, the first two about 0.1 mile apart, the third about 0.8 mile farther along. Just ahead on the right is a good place for a picnic, with rocks to sit on.

Soon you reach a notch in the ridge, and a trail leading right and downhill to the Coyote Trail. Mt. Diablo looks impressive from here, dominating the northwest skyline. Continuing straight on the Volvon Trail, you pass the Valley View, left (a toilet is nearby), and Blue Oak trails, also left. In the bay trees here you may see flocks of dark-eyed juncos, a western scrub-jay, or perhaps a woodpecker. Tall manzanitas line the left side of the road. At about 4.5 miles, the Hummingbird Trail, a short connector to the Blue Oak Trail, goes straight, but you follow the Volvon Trail as it turns sharply right and passes through an area of chaparral, mostly chamise. Soon you pass two junctions, about 0.2 mile apart, with the Prairie Falcon Trail, right. Just beyond the second of these, a junction with the Condor Trail, also right. Beside the Condor Trail junction are a shaded picnic table and a toilet.

When you reach a junction with the Blue Oak Trail, follow the Volvon Trail as it veers right, and in about 150 feet you come to a T-junction with a dirt-and-gravel road. Turn right here and begin a gentle descent through open grassland, with Mt. Diablo visible on your right. At about the 5.5-mile point you arrive at a fork; stay to the right and follow the gently rolling road until you can see the parking area. As you approach it, another fork presents you with two options: a steep descent, right, or a more circuitous but moderate descent, left. Both arrive at the parking area.

ROUND VALLEY REGIONAL PRESERVE

Length: 4.8 miles

Time: 2 to 3 hours

Rating: Moderate

Regulations: EBRPD
Facilities: Picnic tables, water, toilets, emergency phone.
Directions: From Interstate 680 in Walnut Creek, or Highway 24 eastbound (just before the merge with Interstate 680), take the Ygnacio Valley Road exit and go northeast 7.6 miles to Clayton Road. Turn right and go 14.8 miles (Clayton Road becomes Marsh Creek Road) to the parking area, right. The trailhead is at the south end of the parking area.

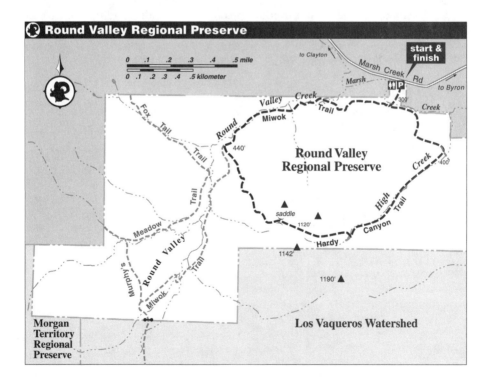

Loop through this preserve, which forms an important link in the East Bay's open space chain, using the Hardy Canyon and Miwok trails. The rolling, oak-shaded hills here are daubed with floral colors in spring, and the impressive expanse of Round Valley itself has few rivals in the Bay Area. This is a popular equestrian area, and the single-track Hardy Canyon Trail takes a beating.

Follow a path that curves left from the trailhead to a T-junction with a dirt road. Turn right and go across a bridge over Marsh Creek. The Miwok Trail, which you will use later, is right, but you turn left on the Hardy Canyon Trail and stroll beside Marsh Creek. Staying right at a fork, you follow a rutted track through an open field and curve away from the creek. Among the trees found in this preserve are California buckeye, valley oak, blue oak, coast live oak, Fremont cottonwood, hop-tree, Western sycamore, and California bay. The trail rises through a blue oak savanna and then enters the canyon holding High Creek.

Emerging into a wide valley at about 2 miles, you skirt a stock pond and cross the dam that forms it. The trail, just a narrow path through the grass, angles right and climbs to a saddle just north of Peak 1142. The stunning views here reward your efforts, and now you descend toward Round Valley, with Mt. Diablo rising in the distance. Switchbacks aid the descent, which crosses flower-filled slopes. Dropping on a moderate grade, you curve around a ridge and meet the Miwok Trail, a dirt road, at about 3.4 miles. (You can extend the route by circling Round Valley on the Miwok and Murphy Meadow trails.)

You veer right and follow Round Valley Creek through a broad canyon. At a fork with a closed road, you stay right and climb on a gentle grade. At the next fork, unsigned, you again stay right and soon wind moderately uphill. Crossing the end of a ridge, you descend and meet the trail coming from the previous fork. Continuing straight, you follow a rolling course to the junction that closes the loop. Here you turn left and retrace your route to the parking area.

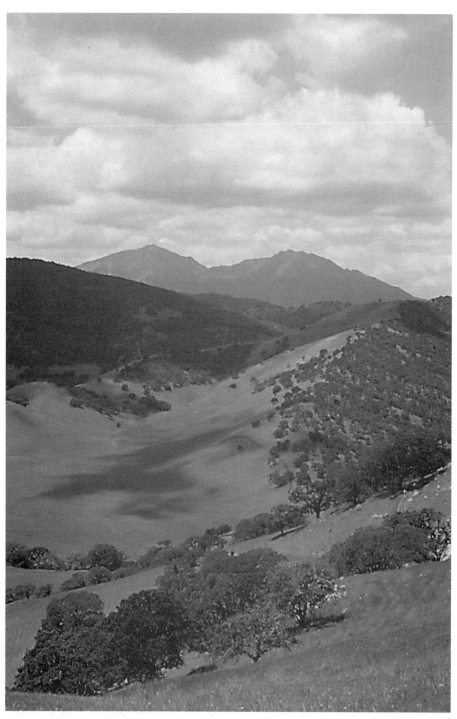

View west from saddle to Mt. Diablo.

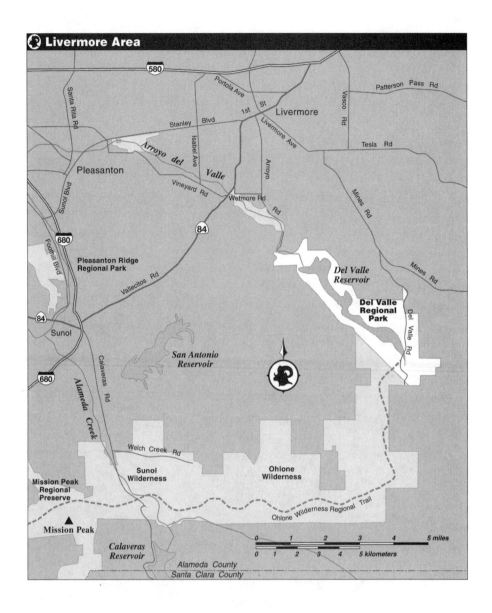

♦ Livermore Area ♦

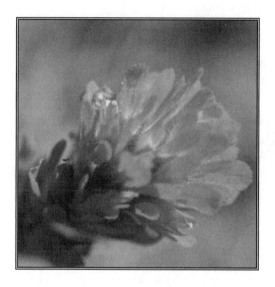

◆Del Valle Regional Park ◆

EAST SHORE TRAIL

Length: 8 miles

Time: 3 to 4 hours

Rating: Moderate

Regulations: EBRPD; fees for parking and dogs.
Facilities: Picnic tables, water, toilet.
Directions: From Interstate 580 in Livermore, take the North Livermore Ave./Downtown Livermore exit, and follow North Livermore Ave. south through Livermore, where it becomes South Livermore Ave., and then, at a sharp left-hand bend on the outskirts of town, Tesla Road. At 3.7 miles from Interstate 580, you reach a junction of Tesla and Mines roads. Turn right and go 3.6 miles to a junction with Del Valle Road; here Mines Road bears left. Stay straight on Del Valle Rd 3.2 miles to the entrance kiosk. Just past the kiosk, turn right and go 0.7 mile to a large parking area at the end of the paved road. The trailhead is at the northwest end of parking area.

Located on the flanks of the hot, dry Livermore Valley, Lake Del Valle is an artificial impoundment on Arroyo del Valle, and the lake's surrounding parklands contain many hiking trails, including connectors to the Ohlone Wilderness Regional Trail. The East Shore Trail is the longest of Del Valle's trails, running for more than 6 miles along the lake's indented shoreline. This out-and-back route explores the trail's first 4 miles, a fine combination of level shoreline, oak woodland, and hilly uplands.

From the northwest end of the parking area, beyond a boat ramp, toilets, information board, and gate, follow the East Shore Trail, a dirt road that leads on a level grade past stands of gray pine, oak, and white alder. The lake is on the left, and rock cliffs, home to California sagebrush and paintbrush, rise steeply from the road, on the right. Raucous western scrub-jays raise their alarm calls from the trees, tiny Bewick's wrens flit through the underbrush, and sleek cormorants fly low over the water.

Lake Del Valle is popular with boaters and fishermen, while hikers, equestrians, and bicyclists share trails along the shoreline or in the surrounding hills of this 4315-acre park. Because of its location—Del Valle is one of the easternmost of the East Bay regional parks—you are likely to find yellow-billed magpies and western bluebirds here, along with more common birds such as western meadowlarks, Brewer's blackbirds, American coots, and killdeer. At Hetch Hetchy Camp, a clearing with a water fountain, picnic table, and toilets, you pass the Hetch Hetchy Trail, right, and continue straight beside the lake, whose level fluctuates by about 25 feet during the year. Across the water, a high, forested ridge guards access to the Ohlone Wilderness, reached via a steep climb from the lake's southwest shore.

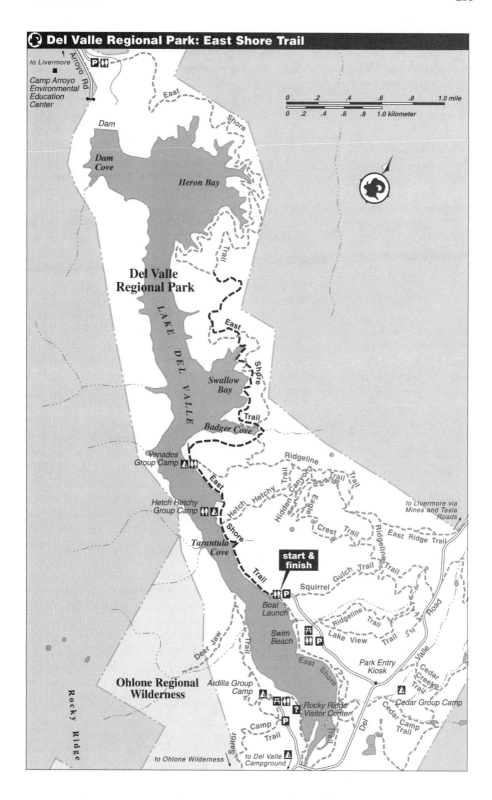

Del Valle Regional Park: East Shore Trail

to Livermore

Camp Arroyo
Environmental
Education
Center

Arroyo Rd

East

Shore

Dam

Dam
Cove

Heron Bay

0   .2   .4   .6   .8   1.0 mile
0   .2   .4   .6   .8   1.0 kilometer

**Del Valle
Regional Park**

Trail

LAKE DEL VALLE

East

Shore

Swallow
Bay

Trail

Badger Cove

Venados
Group Camp

East

Ridgeline

Hidden Canyon Trail

Trail

Trail

Hetch Hetchy
Group Camp

Hetch Hetchy Trail

Shore

Eagle

Crest   Trail

Ridgeline Trail

East Ridge Trail

to Livermore via
Mines and Tesla
Roads

Tarantula
Cove

**start &
finish**

Trail

Squirrel Gulch Trail

Boat
Launch

Ridgeline Trail

Swim
Beach

Lake View

Park Entry
Kiosk

Del Valle Road

**Ohlone Regional
Wilderness**

Deer Jaw

Trail

Ardilla Group
Camp

Rocky Ridge
Visitor Center

East   Shore

Cedar
Creek
Trail

Cedar Group Camp

Cedar Camp Trail

R o c k y   R i d g e

Sailor

Camp

Trail

to Ohlone Wilderness

to Del Valle
Campground

The road now rises moderately to cross a ridge jutting toward the lake, and soon reaches a junction with the Ridgeline Trail, right. Continuing straight, you pass Venados Group Camp, left, a level area atop another low ridge, then descend again almost to water level. Early spring wildflowers, such as California buttercup and shooting stars, bring bursts of color to the grassland here. Just past the camp site is a junction. Leaving the road, which descends and dead-ends at the lake, you turn right to stay on the East Shore Trail, now a single track. (In places, the East Shore Trail is signed as the Shadow Cliffs-to-Del Valle Trail.)

After passing through a gate in a barbed-wire fence, you enjoy a moderate climb through a beautiful, shady savanna of blue oak, coast live oak, and tree-sized spiny redberry. The hillside drops steeply left, and as you gain elevation you can look northwest to the far reaches of the lake.

The route rolls along, following Badger Cove—a narrow, northeast-pointing finger of the lake—to a T-junction, where you turn left to stay on the East Shore Trail and descend, now on a dirt road. Continue straight past the Venados Trail, left, and cross a creek flowing under the road through culverts. (Beyond here, a single-track trail, closed to bicycles, wanders back and forth across the road a number of times and can be used as an alternate route.)

Now you begin a steep climb in the open, soon reaching a promontory that divides Badger Cove and Swallow Bay. This lovely grassy area, shaded by oaks at about the 2-mile point, is a perfect spot for a picnic. As the road descends from the promontory, you see ahead a large cove called Swallow Bay. Here the road swings away from the water and begins to climb into rolling, oak-dotted hills. California ground squirrels scamper across the grass, perhaps communicating with each other in short, high-pitched whistles.

The route ascends moderately through a road-cut, then descends and bends right, following another narrow finger of the lake. After crossing a creek that flows through a culvert, you tackle a long, steep climb with no shade, on a rutted stretch of road. Your reward, upon reaching a high point, is a grand view of Lake Del Valle, silver water set amid wooded, dark-hued hills. After enjoying this well-earned vista, follow the road as it descends moderately, then levels in a quiet area of rolling hills and groves of oak. A narrow ravine, left, may hold running water, and the road climbs away from the lake to cross it. There is a stock pond here, and a creek that drains through a culvert under the road, which may be muddy and cut up by cows and horses.

The route bends left, and now a moderate climb to a ridgecrest puts you in view of the lake again, with the dam clearly visible in the distance. Here, at about the 4-mile point, you reach a junction with a single-track trail heading left and downhill to a promontory at the entrance to Heron Bay. If you wish to explore farther, you can stay straight on the road until it reaches a restricted area near the dam, or turn left and follow the single track through shady groves of California buckeye and oak toward the water's edge. Otherwise, retrace your route to the parking area via the East Shore Trail. (For an alternate return route, follow the description in "Ridgeline Loop," below, from the T-junction at the northeast end of Badger Cove.)

RIDGELINE LOOP

Length: 4.8 miles

Time: 2 to 3 hours

Rating: Moderate

Regulations: EBRPD; fees for parking and dogs. (Bicyclists wishing to ride this loop should follow the East Shore Trail to its junction with the Ridgeline Trail, turn right, and then follow the Ridgeline Trail as described below.)

Facilities: Picnic tables, water, toilet.

Directions: From Interstate 580 in Livermore, take the North Livermore Ave./Downtown Livermore exit, and follow North Livermore Ave. south through Livermore, where it becomes South Livermore Ave., and then, at a sharp left-hand bend on the outskirts of town, Tesla Road. At 3.7 miles from Interstate 580, you reach a junction of Tesla and Mines roads. Turn right and go 3.6 miles to a junction with Del Valle Road; here Mines Road bears left. Stay straight on Del Valle Rd 3.2 miles to the entrance kiosk. Just past the kiosk, turn right and go 0.7 mile to a large parking area at the end of the paved road. The trailhead is at the northwest end of parking area.

Although boating and fishing on artificial Lake Del Valle are the prime attractions of this regional park, there are also fine trails to explore in the surrounding hills. This loop follows the East Shore and Ridgeline trails, taking you from the water's edge through oak savanna to grassy ridgetops, where views extend north to the Livermore Valley, and south to the Ohlone Wilderness.

From the northwest end of the parking area, beyond a boat ramp, toilets, information board, and gate, follow the East Shore Trail, a dirt road beside the lake, which is left. From time to time on this route, narrow paths diverge from the road; unless indicated in the description, ignore them.

At Hetch Hetchy Camp, a clearing with a water fountain, picnic table, and toilets, you pass the Hetch Hetchy Trail, right, and continue straight beside the lake, whose level fluctuates by about 25 feet during the year. Across the water, a high, forested ridge guards access to the Ohlone Wilderness, reached via a steep climb from the lake's southwest shore.

The road now rises moderately to cross a ridge jutting toward the lake, and soon meets the Ridgeline Trail, right. Continuing straight, you pass Venados Group Camp, left, a level area atop another low ridge, then descend again almost to water level. Just past the camp site is a junction. Leaving the road, which descends and dead-ends at the lake, you turn right to stay on the East Shore Trail, now a single track. (In places, the East Shore Trail is signed as the Shadow Cliffs-to-Del Valle Trail.)

After passing through a gate in a barbed-wire fence, you enjoy a moderate climb through a beautiful, shady savanna. The route rolls along, following Badger Cove—a narrow finger of the lake—to a T-junction at the cove's northeast end. Here you turn right on an unsigned road and climb via well-graded S-bends through oak woodland. Forest birds such as nuthatches and titmice may be in evi-

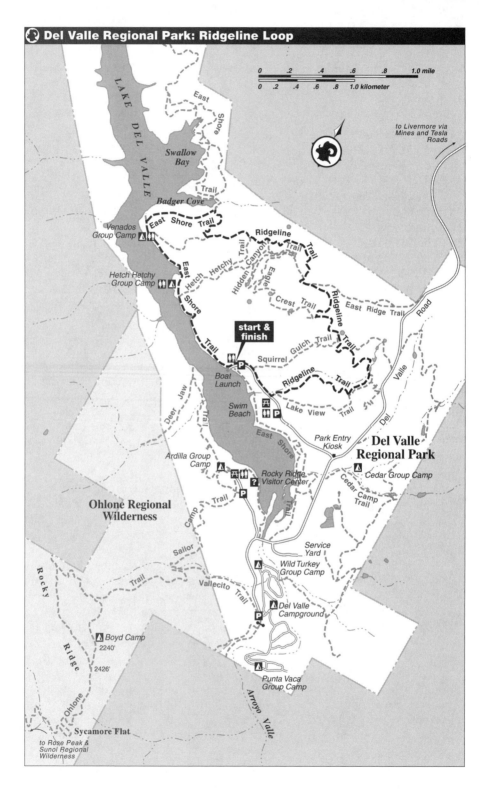

Del Valle Regional Park: Ridgeline Loop

Lake Del Valle

Swallow Bay

East Shore Trail

Badger Cove Trail

Venados Group Camp

East Shore Trail

Ridgeline Trail

Hetch Hetchy Group Camp

Hetch Hetchy Trail

Hidden Canyon Trail

Eagle Trail

Crest Trail

Ridgeline Trail

East Ridge Trail

start & finish

Squirrel Gulch Trail

Ridgeline Trail

Boat Launch

Ridgeline Trail

Swim Beach

Lake View Trail

Del Valle Road

East Shore Trail

Park Entry Kiosk

Del Valle Regional Park

Deer Jaw Trail

Ardilla Group Camp

Rocky Ridge Visitor Center

Cedar Group Camp

Cedar Camp Trail

Ohlone Regional Wilderness

Camp Trail

Service Yard

Wild Turkey Group Camp

Sailor Trail

Vallecito Trail

Del Valle Campground

Rocky Ridge

Boyd Camp 2240'

2426'

Punta Vaca Group Camp

Ohlone Trail

Arroyo Valle

Sycamore Flat

to Rose Peak & Sunol Regional Wilderness

to Livermore via Mines and Tesla Roads

0   .2   .4   .6   .8   1.0 mile
0   .2   .4   .6   .8   1.0 kilometer

dence, although you may hear many more birds than you actually see, especially if the trees have leafed out.

The moderate grade soon brings you to a cattle gate; beyond it you reach an open area atop a ridge and a T-junction with the Ridgeline Trail, here unsigned. Turning left, you follow the Ridgeline Trail, a dirt road, as it passes stands of California buckeye and spiny redberry, and then reaches a high vantage point with 360-degree views of the lake and its surrounding hills.

Just before going through the next cattle gate, you pass the Hetch Hetchy Trail, right, which connects with the East Shore Trail. Beyond the gate, at about the 2-mile point, the route passes an unsigned, gated road, left, and a connector to the Hidden Canyon Trail, right. Now you enjoy a peaceful ridgetop stroll, far removed from the lakeshore hubbub of picnickers and power boats; the lake itself is hidden from view here. At the next junction, the Eagle Crest Trail goes right, but you continue climbing to a low point on the ridge ahead, where a road leads to a viewpoint, right. Bear left and continue to climb, soon reaching a junction with the East Ridge Trail. Here you stay right, following the Ridgeline Trail on a mostly level course, punctuated by a moderate descent on loose dirt, with a steep ravine to your right.

Now on a narrow ridgecrest, you regain your view of the lake as you drop to a T-junction, where the Eagle Crest Trail heads right, and the Ridgeline Trail, your route, turns sharply left and continues descending on a gentle and then moderate grade. A short rise in the road puts you at a cattle gate; once through, you pass the Squirrel Gulch Trail, right, and continue straight, gaining back some lost elevation. The route hugs the ridgetop for a while, giving you a view east to the park entrance road, but soon begins a moderate and then steep descent to a marshy area where you may be greeted by a chorus of frogs. Here water flows under the road through a culvert and into a steep ravine, right. Now descending gently, you pass a road to the park boundary that joins sharply from the left. Continue straight through a moist, shady area where colorful plants such as blue witch and narrow-leaf bush sunflower thrive.

A short, steep pitch brings you to a four-way junction with the Lakeview Trail and another road to the park boundary. Stay on the Ridgeline Trail by turning right and continuing to descend gently through oak savanna toward the lake. Following a lovely ravine, right, you pass two entrances to the East Tank Loop, which circles a water tank. Still descending, you soon reach a gate and the paved East Shore Road. Here you turn right and walk a short distance to the parking area.

Appendix 1: Favorite Trails

Birding

Black Diamond Mines Regional Preserve:
    all trips
Coyote Hills Regional Park: Lizard Rock
Don Edwards San Francisco Bay National
    Wildlife Refuge: Tidelands Trail
Hayward Regional Shoreline: Cogswell Marsh
Martin Luther King, Jr. Regional Shoreline:
    Arrowhead Marsh
Mt. Diablo State Park: all trips
Point Pinole Regional Shoreline: Bay View Trail
Sunol Wilderness: all trips

Creekside Trips
(Fall Colors Possible)

Dry Creek Pioneer Regional Park: Tolman Peak
Garin Regional Park: Zeile Creek
Mt. Diablo State Park: Back Canyon, Falls Trail,
    Mitchell and Donner Canyons, Sycamore
    Creek
Ohlone Wilderness Regional Trail: Sunol
    to Del Valle
Pleasanton Ridge Regional Park:
    Pleasanton Ridge
Sunol Wilderness: Little Yosemite, Vista Grande
Tilden Regional Park: Lake Anza

Easy Trips, Good for Kids

Coyote Hills Regional Park: Lizard Rock
Don Edwards San Francisco Bay National
    Wildlife Refuge: Tidelands Trail
Hayward Regional Shoreline: Cogswell Marsh
Huckleberry Botanic Regional Preserve:
    Huckleberry Nature Path
Martin Luther King, Jr. Regional Shoreline:
    Arrowhead Marsh
Sibley Volcanic Regional Preserve: Round
    Top Loop
Sobrante Ridge Botanic Regional Preserve:
    Manzanita Grove
Tilden Regional Park: Lake Anza

Redwoods

Joaquin Miller Park: Redwood Forest
Redwood Regional Park: East Ridge,
    French Trail

Scenic Vistas

Black Diamond Mines Regional Preserve:
    all trips
Briones Regional Park: Briones Crest,
    Diablo View
Briones Reservoir: Reservoir Loop
Carquinez Strait Regional Shoreline:
    Franklin Ridge
Coyote Hills Regional Park: Red Hill
Del Valle Regional Park: all trips
Dry Creek Pioneer Regional Park: Tolman Peak
East Bay Skyline Trail: Wildcat Canyon to
    Lomas Cantadas, MacDonald Gate
    to Proctor Gate
Garin Regional Park: Garin Peak
Lafayette Reservoir: Rim Trail
Las Trampas Wilderness: all trips
Miller/Knox Regional Shoreline: Scenic Loop
Mission Peak Regional Preserve: Mission Peak
Morgan Territory Regional Preserve:
    Bob Walker Ridge
Mt. Diablo State Park: all trips
Ohlone Wilderness Regional Trail:
    Sunol to Del Valle
Pleasanton Ridge Regional Park:
    Pleasanton Ridge
Redwood Regional Park: East Ridge
Round Valley Regional Preserve
Sibley Volcanic Regional Preserve: Round
    Top Loop
Sunol Wilderness: all trips
Tilden Regional Park: Wildcat Peak
Wildcat Canyon Regional Park:
    San Pablo Ridge

Summer Trips

Joaquin Miller Park: Redwood Forest
Redwood Regional Park: French Trail
Tilden Regional Park: Lake Anza

Waterfalls

Mt. Diablo State Park: Falls Trail
Ohlone Wilderness Regional Trail

Wildflowers/Nature Study

Black Diamond Mines Regional Preserve:
    all trips
Briones Reservoir: Bear Creek Trail
Diablo Foothills Regional Park
Huckleberry Botanic Regional Preserve:
    Huckleberry Nature Path
Lime Ridge Open Space
Mt. Diablo State Park: all trips
Sobrante Ridge Regional Preserve:
    Manzanita Grove
Sunol Wilderness: all trips

Winter Trips

Don Edwards San Francisco Bay National
    Wildlife Refuge: Tidelands Trail
Hayward Regional Shoreline: Cogswell Marsh
Huckleberry Botanic Regional Preserve:
    Huckleberry Nature Path
Martin Luther King, Jr. Regional Shoreline:
    Arrowhead Marsh
Point Pinole Regional Shoreline: Bay View Trail

Trips that Don't Allow Dogs

Hayward Regional Shoreline: Cogswell Marsh
East Bay Skyline National Recreation Trail:
    Lomas Cantadas to Skyline Gate
Tilden Regional Park: Wildcat Peak
Huckleberry Botanic Regional Preserve:
    Huckleberry Nature Path
Upper San Leandro Reservoir: King
    Canyon Loop
Upper San Leandro Reservoir: Ramage Peak
Briones Reservoir: Bear Creek Trail
Briones Reservoir: Reservoir Loop
Lafayette Reservoir: Rim Trail
Lime Ridge Open Space
Mt. Diablo State Park: all trips

Appendix 2: Recommended Reading

Bay Area

Heid, Matt, *Camping and Backpacking in the San Francisco Bay Area.* Berkeley: Wilderness Press, 2003.

Lage, Jessica, *Trail Runner's Guide: San Francisco Bay Area.* Berkeley: Wilderness Press, 2003.

Margolin, Malcolm, *The East Bay Out.* Revised ed. Berkeley: Heyday Books, 1988.

Rusmore, Jean, *The Bay Area Ridge Trail.* 2nd ed. Berkeley: Wilderness Press, 2002.

Rusmore, Jean, et al., *Peninsula Trails.* 4th ed. Berkeley: Wilderness Press, 2005.

Rusmore, Jean, et al., *South Bay Trails.* 3rd ed. Berkeley: Wilderness Press, 2001.

Wayburn, Peggy, *Adventuring in the San Francisco Bay Area.* Revised ed. San Francisco: Sierra Club Books, 1995.

Weintraub, David, *North Bay Trails.* 2nd ed. Berkeley: Wilderness Press, 2004.

Weintraub, David, *Top Trails San Francisco Bay Area.* Berkeley: Wilderness Press, 2004.

Weintraub, David, *Afoot and Afield San Francisco Bay Area.* Berkeley: Wilderness Press, 2004.

Weintraub, David, *Peninsula Tales and Trails.* Portland: Graphic Arts Books, 2004.

History

Lavender, David, *California.* Lincoln: University of Nebraska Press, 1972.

Richards, Rand, *Historic San Francisco.* San Francisco: Heritage House Publishers, 1999.

Natural History

Alt, David, and Donald W. Hyndman, *Roadside Geology of Northern and Central California.* Missoula: Mountain Press Publishing Company, 2000.

Barbour, Michael, et al., *Coast Redwood.* Los Olivos: Cachuma Press, 2001.

Burt, William H., and Richard P. Grossenheider, *A Field Guide to the Mammals, North America, North of Mexico.* 3rd ed. Boston: Houghton Mifflin Company, 1980.

Clark, Jeanne L., *California Wildlife Viewing Guide.* Helena: Falcon Press, 1992.

Coffeen, Mary, *Central Coast Wildflowers.* San Luis Obispo: EZ Nature Books, 1996.

Faber, Phyllis M., *Common Wetland Plants of Coastal California.* 2nd ed. Mill Valley: Pickleweed Press, 1996.

Faber, Phyllis M., and Robert F. Holland, *Common Riparian Plants of California.* Mill Valley: Pickleweed Press, 1988.

Kozloff, Eugene N., and Linda H. Beidleman, *Plants of the San Francisco Bay Region.* Revised ed. Berkeley: University of California Press, 2003.

Lanner, Ronald M., *Conifers of California.* Los Olivos: Cachuma Press, 1999.

Little, Elbert L., *National Audubon Society Field Guide to North American Trees, Western Region.* New York: Alfred A. Knopf, 1994.

Lyons, Kathleen, and Mary Beth Cooney-Lazaneo, *Plants of the Coast Redwood Region.* Boulder Creek: Looking Press, 1988.

National Geographic Society, *Field Guide to the Birds of North America.* 3rd ed. Washington, D.C.: National Geographic Society, 1999.

Niehaus, Theodore F., and Charles L. Ripper, *A Field Guide to Pacific States Wildflowers.* Boston: Houghton Mifflin Company, 1976.

Pavlik, Bruce M., et al., *Oaks of California.* Los Olivos: Cachuma Press, 1991.

Peterson, Roger T., *A Field Guide to Western Birds.* 3rd ed. Boston: Houghton Mifflin Company, 1990.

Schoenherr, Allan A., *A Natural History of California*. Berkeley: University of California Press, 1992.

Sibley, David Allen, *The Sibley Guide to Birds*. New York: Alfred A. Knopf, Inc., 2000.

Stebbins, Robert C., *A Field Guide to Western Reptiles and Amphibians*. 2nd ed. Boston: Houghton Mifflin Company, 1985.

Stuart, John D., and John O. Sawyer, *Trees and Shrubs of California*. Berkeley: University of California Press, 2001.

Place Names

Durham, David L., *Place-Names of the San Francisco Bay Area*. Clovis: Word Dancer Press, 2000.

Gudde, Erwin G., *California Place Names*. 4th ed. Berkeley: University of California Press, 1998.

Marinacci, Barbara and Rudy Marinacci, *California's Spanish Place-Names*. 2nd ed. Houston: Gulf Publishing Company, 1997.

Appendix 3: Agencies and Information Sources

PARKS AND AGENCIES

California State Parks (CSP)
Mt. Diablo State Park
   General Information   (925) 837-2525
   Summit Museum, Visitor Center, Store   (925) 837-6119
   Camping   (800) 444-7275
   http://parks.ca.gov/default.asp?page_id=517
   www.reserveamerica.com

East Bay Municipal Utility District (EBMUD)   (510) 287-0459
http://www.ebmud.com/services/recreation/
east_bay/default.htm

East Bay Regional Park District (EBRPD)
Information   (510) 562-7275
Reservations
Oakland Area   (510) 636-1684
Hayward Area   (510) 538-6470
Contra Costa County   (925) 676-0192
Livermore Area   (925) 373-0144
www.ebparks.org

Oakland, City of, Office of Parks and Recreation   (510) 238-7275
Joaquin Miller Park   (510) 482-7856
http://www.oaklandnet.com/parks/facilities/
parks_joaquin_miller.asp

U.S. Fish and Wildlife Service (USFWS)   (510) 792-0222
Don Edwards San Francisco Bay National Wildlife Refuge
   http://desfbay.fws.gov

Walnut Creek Open Space & Trails Division (WCOSTD)   (925) 943-5860
Lime Ridge Open Space
www.ci.walnut-creek.ca.us/openspace

INTERNET RESOURCES

Organization	Website
AC Transit	www.actransit.org
Bay Area Hiker	www.bahiker.com
Bay Area Open Space Council	www.openspacecouncil.org
Bay Area Rapid Transit (BART)	www.bart.gov
Bay Area Ridge Trail Council	www.ridgetrail.org
Bay Nature magazine	www.baynature.com
California Native Plant Society	www.cnps.org
Greenbelt Alliance	www.greenbelt.org
Mount Diablo Interpretive Association	www.mdia.org
National Audubon Society	www.audubon.org
Golden Gate (San Francisco, East Bay)	www.goldengateaudubon.org
National Geographic Maps/TOPO!	http://maps.nationalgeographic.com/topo
Natural Resources DataBase	www.nrdb.org
San Francisco Bay Trail	www.baytrail.org
Save Mount Diablo	www.savemountdiablo.org
Sierra Club	www.sierraclub.org
San Francisco Bay Chapter	www.sanfranciscobay.sierraclub.org
Trail Center	www.trailcenter.org
University of California Natural Reserve System (UCNRS)	http://nrs.ucop.edu Weather
National Weather Service	www.nws.noaa.gov
Weather.com	www.weather.com
Whole Access (to increase recreational opportunities for people with disabilities)	www.wholeaccess.org
Wilderness Press	www.wildernesspress.com

Index

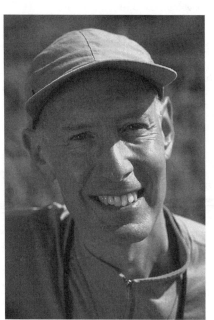

About the Author

David Weintraub is a writer, editor, and photographer based in South Carolina and Cape Cod. His other Wilderness Press titles are *North Bay Trails, Monterey Bay Trails, Top Trails: San Francisco Bay Area, Afoot & Afield: San Francisco Bay Area,* and *Adventure Kayaking: Cape Cod and Martha's Vineyard.* Visit David on the Web at www.wein-traubphoto.com.

Wilderness Press covers the San Francisco Bay Area

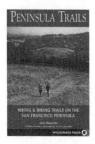

Peninsula Trails
Outdoor Adventures on the San Francisco Peninsula

The only guide that covers all the parks and open spaces from San Bruno Mountain to Saratoga Gap. Includes the vitally useful "Trails for all Seasons and Reasons," so you can choose just the right trail.

ISBN 0-89997-197-0

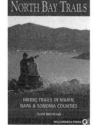

South Bay Trails
Outdoor Adventures in & around Santa Clara Valley

Explore Silicon Valley's 125,000 acres of public open space, from San Jose to the Santa Cruz Mountains. Over 100 routes and 568 miles of trails in the southern San Francisco Bay Area are described.

ISBN 0-89997-284-5

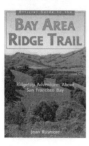

North Bay Trails
Hiking Trails in Marin, Napa & Sonoma Counties

Fifty-six routes in the coastal salt marshes, remote mountaintops, and shady redwood groves of the North Bay. Includes clear, easy-to-follow directions, photos, and maps.

ISBN 0-89997-378-7

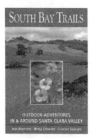

Bay Area Ridge Trail
Ridgetop Adventures Above San Francisco Bay

This official guide covers the 230 completed miles of the planned 425-mile recreation trail encircling the San Francisco Bay. Includes trailhead access, on-the-trail directions, side trips, facilities, and maps.

ISBN 0-89997-280-2

For ordering information, contact your local bookseller or Wilderness Press, www.wildernesspress.com.